Neurones communicate with each other and with other cells in the body by releasing chemicals known as neurotransmitters. These combine with specific receptors on the downstream cell to propagate the message. Neurotransmitter release in response to a nerve impulse is not fixed and constant, however, but is continually and subtly modified via the release-modulating action of substances in the immediate environment of the release sites. Effective modulators of neurotransmitter release include the neurotransmitter itself, or neurotransmitters released from adjacent nerves, hormones, a variety of chemical products of (non-neural) cells surrounding the release site and a variety of drugs, both medicinal and recreational or abused. Such subtle regulation has profound effect on the message transmitted. In this book, acknowledged authorities in the subject concisely and simply describe the basic phenomenon of neurotransmitter release and its modulation throughout the nervous system and the underlying biochemical mechanisms. A quantitative evaluation of the biological significance of release modulation and its possible clinical relevance is also given. The clear descriptions and many complementary illustrations provide an easy to read and valuable reference resource for both non-specialist readers and neuroscientists alike. Clinicians, research workers and students should all find its contents of interest and value.

# NEUROTRANSMITTER RELEASE AND ITS MODULATION

## Biochemical Mechanisms, Physiological Function and Clinical Relevance

# NEUROTRANSMITTER RELEASE AND ITS MODULATION

## Biochemical Mechanisms, Physiological Function and Clinical Relevance

Edited by

### David A. Powis
*Associate Professor of Human Physiology,*
*Faculty of Medicine, The University of Newcastle,*
*New South Wales, Australia*

### Stephen J. Bunn
*National Health and Medical Research RD Wright Fellow,*
*Faculty of Medicine, The University of Newcastle,*
*New South Wales, Australia*

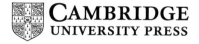
CAMBRIDGE
UNIVERSITY PRESS

Published by the Press Syndicate of the University of Cambridge
The Pitt Building, Trumpington Street, Cambridge CB2 1RP
40 West 20th Street, New York, NY 10011-4211, USA
10 Stamford Road, Oakleigh, Melbourne 3166, Australia

First published 1995

Printed in Great Britain at the University Press, Cambridge

*A Catalogue record for this book is available from the British Library*

*Library of Congress cataloguing in publication data*

Neurotransmitter release and its modulation : biochemical mechanisms,
physiological function and clinical relevance / edited by David A.
Powis, Stephen J. Bunn.
p.   cm.
Includes index.
ISBN 0 521 44068 8 (hc). – ISBN 0 521 44616 3 (pb)
1. Neurotransmitters.   2. Neurotransmitter receptors.
3. Neurochemistry.   4. Neuropsychiatry.   I. Powis, David A.
II. Bunn, Stephen J.
[DNLM:   1. Synaptic Transmission.   2. Neuroregulators.
3. Receptors, Neurotransmitter,   4. Signal Transduction.   WL 102.8
N4945 1995]
QP364.7.N4753   1995
612.8 – dc20
DNLM/DLC
For Library of Congress   94-24054 CIP

ISBN 0 521 44068 8 hardback
ISBN 0 521 44616 3 paperback

# Contents

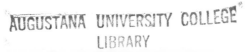

Contents                                                     ix

ixContents                                                     ix

# Contents

Contents

# Contributors

Michelle Barrington — Prince Henry's Institute of Medical Research, Clayton, Victoria, Australia

Maxwell R Bennett — Neurobiology Laboratory, Department of Physiology, The University of Sydney, New South Wales, Australia

David Bleakman — Lilly Research Centre, Erl Wood Manor, Windlesham, Surrey, England

Pierre Blier — Neurobiological Psychiatry Unit, Department of Psychiatry, McGill University, Montreal, Quebec, Canada

Michael R Boarder — Department of Cell Physiology and Pharmacology, The University of Leicester, Leicester, England

Kazimierz R Borkowski — Pharmaceuticals Division, Medical Affairs and Research and Development, Ciba-Geigy Canada, Mississauga, Ontario, Canada

James A Brock — Neuroscience Group, Faculty of Medicine, The University of Newcastle, New South Wales, Australia

Robert D Burgoyne — The Physiological Laboratory, University of Liverpool, Liverpool, England

Loris A Chahl — Neuroscience Group, Faculty of Medicine, The University of Newcastle, New South Wales, Australia

Timothy R Cheek — AFRC Laboratory of Molecular Signalling, Department of Zoology, University of Cambridge, Cambridge, England

| | |
|---|---|
| Bertil B Fredholm | Department of Physiology and Pharmacology, Karolinska Institutet, Stockholm, Sweden |
| Manfred Göthert | Institute of Pharmacology and Toxicology, University of Bonn, Bonn, Germany |
| Marian Joëls | Department of Experimental Zoology, The University of Amsterdam, The Netherlands |
| Zeinab Khalil | National Research Institute for Gerontology and Geriatric Medicine, North West Hospital, Parkville, Victoria, Australia |
| E Ronald de Kloet | Department of Pharmacology at the Center for Bio-Pharmaceutical Sciences, Leiden University, Leiden, The Netherlands |
| Henryk Majewski | Prince Henry's Institute of Medical Research, Clayton, Victoria, Australia |
| Philip D Marley | Department of Pharmacology, University of Melbourne, Parkville, Victoria, Australia |
| Richard J Miller | Department of Pharmacological and Physiological Sciences, University of Chicago, Illinois, USA |
| Claude de Montigny | Neurobiological Psychiatry Unit, Department of Psychiatry, McGill University, Montreal, Quebec, Canada |
| Graham M Nicholson | Department of Health Sciences, University of Technology, Sydney, New South Wales, Australia |
| Dennis A Przywara | Department of Pharmacology, Wayne State University School of Medicine, Detroit, Michigan, USA |
| Julianne J Reid | Department of Medical Laboratory Science, Royal Melbourne Institute of Technology, Melbourne, Victoria, Australia |
| Peter Sneddon | Department of Physiology and Pharmacology, University of Strathclyde, Glasgow, Scotland |

Lennart Stjärne          Department of Physiology and
                         Pharmacology, Karolinska Institutet,
                         Stockholm, Sweden

Arun R Wakade            Department of Pharmacology, Wayne
                         State University School of Medicine,
                         Detroit, Michigan, USA

Ben HC Westerink         University Centre for Pharmacy,
                         Department of Medicinal Chemistry,
                         State University of Groningen, The
                         Netherlands

Thomas C Westfall        Department of Pharmacological and
                         Physiological Science, Saint Louis
                         University School of Medicine, St
                         Louis, Missouri, USA

Max Willow               Department of Cell and Molecular
                         Biology, University of Technology,
                         Sydney, New South Wales, Australia

Susan A Wonnacott        School of Biology and Biochemistry,
                         University of Bath, Claverton Down,
                         Bath, England

and with an introduction by

Klaus Starke             Pharmakologisches Institut, Albert-
                         Ludwigs-Universität Freiburg,
                         Freiburg im Breisgau, Germany

# Preface

The idea for this book arose during the lead-up to the 13th International Congress of Neurochemistry, which was to be held in Sydney, Australia during July 1991. We were organising a colloquium for the congress on this aspect of neurotransmission, which, in 1991, had come of age by reaching the 21st anniversary of its first specific recognition in the scientific literature.

The notion that the amount of transmitter released by an effective action potential arriving at the nerve terminal is not constant but can be varied by the chemical environment in the vicinity of the secretory site, is now well accepted. There is a large specialist literature on the subject, but the phenomenon is not well covered in textbooks, and there are still conflicting views regarding its functional significance. We felt that it was timely to organise a review colloquium for this international forum of neurochemical scientists. However, mindful of the fact that the material presented and discussed at scientific meetings often has little lasting impact outside the immediate professional community, we thought that the topic, at this stage of its history, should be more amply reviewed and more permanently documented. The idea was discussed with Dr Richard Barling of Cambridge University Press who was then visiting Australia, and his enthusiasm at that point allowed the project to be developed. At that time, we envisaged that the nuclear chapters would be provided by the speakers from the colloquium at the conference and that their written contributions would be a global, but accessible, review of the areas in which they are acknowledged experts. These chapters would be complemented by others, which were to cover the areas that, because of time constraints, could not be addressed at the conference. The result, we hoped, would be a comprehensive account of the processes that occur at the nerve terminal which result in an alteration, up or down, of the amount of neurotransmitter released and which, thereby, modify the resultant effector response.

In the ensuing brief to our colleagues who agreed to contribute to the book, we asked them to deal with their topic so as to produce a balanced review of the current position and to include a discussion of the controversies as well as the accepted facts. We required them also to write for the interested outsider, not just the expert in the field. The result is printed here: a collection of essays by active researchers that present a broad account of the subject of neurotransmitter release modulation. Starting from a basic description of neurotransmitter release and the phenomenology of its modulation, the book then deals with the mechanisms by which modulation is brought about. Next there is discussion of its probable physiological significance and finally a collection of views of how the process of neurotransmitter release modulation may be exploited to therapeutic advantage. Each author has been encouraged to bring his or her particular style of presentation to their chapters and this has brought a breath of freshness to each point of the story as the subject unfolds. Readers will note that the authors' stylistic approach is also manifested in the depth to which their topics are discussed. We do not believe that the book suffers as a result of these individualistic traits.

We hope the result is appreciated and, more importantly, is helpful and informative to those who wish to learn more about this fascinating topic.

It is a pleasure to acknowledge the following people who have helped, in a variety of ways, with the preparation of the book. These we have listed alphabetically. We thank Robert Barber, Richard Barling (CUP), Ruth Barrett, Gillian Bennett (for the drawings in Chapter 3), James Brock, Jocelyn Foster (CUP), Bruce Gynther, Andy Hargreaves, Robert Henderson, Ena Mawer, Phillipa Powis, Alethea Taylor, Colin Taylor, Bruce Walmsley and Michael Williamson for their encouragement, help and patience. In addition we single out for special mention Professor Klaus Starke, who, we believe is still the central figure in this important area of physiology and is a leader of the scientific endeavour which is helping it to be understood. His seminal publications, now more than 20 years old, are still key references in the field; his own recent publications, and the mention of them in reviews of the field published by others, indicate the extent to which his work has provided the understanding we now enjoy. We have been privileged to enjoy his personal friendship for many years and, more recently, his encouragement and help with this project; we are doubly fortunate that he contributed the foreword to this book.

*David Powis*
*Stephen Bunn*
*Newcastle, New South Wales, July 1994*

# Abbreviations

| | |
|---|---|
| α,β-mATP | α,β-methylene ATP |
| α,β-mADP | α,β-methylene ADP |
| 11β-OHSD | 11β-hydroxysteroid dehydrogenase |
| 4-AP | 4-aminopyridine |
| 5-HT | 5-hydroxytryptamine (serotonin) |
| ACE | angiotensin converting enzyme |
| ACPD | (1$S$,3$R$)-aminocyclopentane dicarboxylic acid |
| ACTH | adrenocorticotrophic hormone |
| AHP | after hyperpolarisation |
| AMPA | α-amino-3-hydroxy-5-methyl-4-isoxozole |
| ANNAP$_3$ | arylazidoaminopropionyl-ATP |
| ANP | atrial natriuretic peptide |
| cAMP | cyclic adenosine monophosphate |
| CCK | cholecystokinin |
| cGMP | cyclic guanosine monophosphate |
| CGRP | calcitonin gene-related peptide |
| CICR | calcium-induced calcium release |
| CNS | central nervous system |
| CRH | corticotrophin-releasing hormone |
| DAG | diacylglycerol |
| dopa | dihydroxyphenylalanine |
| DPCPX | 1,3-dipropyl 1-8-cyclopentyl xanthine |
| DYN | dynorphin |
| EJC | excitatory junction current |
| EJP | excitatory junction potential |
| EPC | endplate current |
| EPP | endplate potential |
| EPSP | excitatory postsynaptic potential |
| fEPSP | fast excitatory postsynaptic potential |
| FMRF-amide | Phe-Met-Arg-Phe-amide |

| | |
|---|---|
| GABA | gamma-aminobutyric acid |
| GAL | galanin |
| GDPβS | guanosine 5′-$O$-(2-thiodiphosphate) |
| GH | growth hormone |
| GHRH | growth hormone-releasing hormone |
| GTPγS | guanosine 5′-$O$-(3-thiotriphosphate) |
| HPLC | high-pressure liquid chromatography |
| HVA | high-voltage activated |
| Ins(1,4,5)$P_3$ | inositol 1,4,5-trisphosphate |
| IPSP | inhibitory postsynaptic potential |
| LHRH | luteinising hormone-releasing hormone |
| LSD | lysergic acid diethylamide |
| LTP | long-term potentiation |
| LVA | low-voltage activated |
| MAO | monoamine oxidase |
| MAO-A | monoamine oxidase type-A |
| MDA | 3,4-methylenedioxyamphetamine |
| MDMA | 3,4-methylenedioxymethamphetamine |
| MEPP | miniature endplate potential |
| nAChR | nicotinic acetylcholine receptor |
| NANC | non-adrenergic, non-cholinergic |
| NIDDM | non-insulin-dependent diabetes mellitus |
| NMDA | $N$-methyl-D-aspartate |
| NPY | neuropeptide Y |
| NSAIDs | non-steroidal anti-inflammatory drugs |
| NSF | $N$-ethylmaleimide-sensitive fusion protein |
| NTS | nerve terminal spike |
| PAF | platelet activating factor |
| PG | prostaglandin |
| PNMT | phenylethanolamine $N$-methyltransferase |
| PSC | postsynaptic current |
| PSP | postsynaptic potential |
| ROC | receptor-operated channel |
| sEPSP | slow excitatory postsynaptic potential |
| SHR | spontaneously hypertensive rats |
| SNAP | soluble NSF attachment protein |
| SRIF | somatotrophin release-inhibiting factor |
| TEA | tetraethylammonium |
| VIP | vasoactive intestinal peptide |
| VSCC | voltage-sensitive calcium channels |
| WKY | Wistar Kyoto rats |

# Introduction

Klaus Starke

There are many reviews and several books on the modulation of neurotransmitter release[8,10]. David Powis' and Stephen Bunn's enterprise differs from previous ones: the aim was a readily accessible text for a wide readership rather than a detailed account for the specialist.

Why should a wide readership be interested in the subject?

Modulation of transmitter release is a general phenomenon. We have to realise – and have realised by now – that the average release of transmitter, per action potential per number of release sites, is neither constant nor changed only by built-in automatisms, such as depletion of transmitter pools. In fact it is subject to modulation by many chemical signals in the biophase around the terminal axons. These signals act at presynaptic receptors (for terminology see ref. 15). The average release of transmitter, per action potential per number of release sites, can be increased or decreased through presynaptic receptors. Certain presynaptic receptors, when activated, initiate release rather than modify release elicited by orthodromic action potentials; others modulate the biosynthesis of a transmitter, independently of changes in release. Much more common, however, are presynaptic receptors that either increase or decrease nerve impulse-evoked release. 'A real mosaic of receptors', as S. Z. Langer once wrote[9], may be present on terminal axons. Terminals are by no means only transmissive, they are also eminently receptive structures.

The science of presynaptic modulation has been, and is, vivid. A vivid science will solve riddles: so has the theory of presynaptic modulation. Best-known is the story of the increase in noradrenaline overflow from isolated organs caused by α-adrenoceptor antagonists, as originally observed by G. L. Brown and J. S. Gillespie[1]. First explained by blockade of postsynaptic α-adrenoceptors, which were thought to fix the transmitter in the tissue, then by inhibition of neuronal reuptake or extraneuronal uptake of noradrenaline, the increase eventually turned out to be the result of blockade of novel, presynaptic, release-inhibiting α-adrenoceptors (see refs. 10 and 13). The effect of nicotine on the heart is another example. In his contribution to the *Handbuch der experimentellen Pharmakologie*, W. E. Dixon showed in 1924 that nicotine, when injected into a rabbit isolated heart perfused according to Langendorff, caused bradycardia followed by tachycardia and an increase in the amplitude of contraction[5]. The bradycardia was explained by excitation of vagal ganglia, the positive chronotropic and inotropic effect by excitation of sympathetic ganglia[5]. Sympathetic ganglia, however, do not occur in the heart, so part two of the explanation was wrong. Nicotine acts on the terminal postganglionic sympathetic axons, and Dixon's study is, in fact, one of the first experiments demonstrating presynaptic receptors, in this case nicotine receptors that, when activated, trigger release of noradrenaline.

1

A vivid science will stimulate neighbouring fields: so has presynaptic modulation research. Presynaptic receptors were several times found to differ from hitherto known receptors and became prototypes of new classes such as $\alpha_2$-adrenoceptors, $GABA_B$ receptors, $H_3$ histamine receptors and, in a way, $5\text{-}HT_{1B}$ receptors. The pioneer role may continue: although the present subclassification of $\alpha_2$-adrenoceptors into $\alpha_{2A,B,C,D}$ is based on radioligand binding, non-homogeneity of the $\alpha_2$-type was first noticed in studies on presynaptic $\alpha_2$-autoreceptors[6]. For example, a species difference between rabbit and rat $\alpha_2$-autoreceptors, known for about 14 years, can now be explained by the existence of $\alpha_{2A}$-adrenoceptors in rabbit and (phylogenetically homologous but pharmacologically distinct) $\alpha_{2D}$-adrenoceptors in rat noradrenergic neurones[11,16].

A vivid science will create new tasks and may create new riddles: so does presynaptic modulation. Co-transmission, another theory that changed the face of neurotransmission[3], immediately raises the question of presynaptic effects of all of the co-transmitters. It seems likely now that postganglionic sympathetic axons possess receptors not only for noradrenaline ($\alpha_2$) but also for the co-transmitters neuropeptide Y and ATP ($P_2$ or possibly $P_3$). Furthermore, the $P_2$ purinoceptors are autoreceptors *sensu stricto* in that they are activated by an endogenous ligand, presumably ATP: $P_2$ purinoceptor antagonists, such as suramin and reactive blue-2, increase the release of noradrenaline in some tissues[17]. But studies on presynaptic modulation in co-transmission systems have also generated an apparent paradox: some presynaptic modulators seem to change the stimulation-evoked overflow of noradrenaline on the one hand, and of ATP on the other hand, to different degrees[7]. Is there, in fact, a differential modulation of neural noradrenaline versus ATP release, and if so, how is this brought about?

A review article in 1981 suggested that many presynaptic receptors may be 'without normal input, … vestiges of evolution that continue to exist because they do us no harm'[14]. While this may be so, it is clear now that presynaptic modulation serves essential functions for our body as a whole. Instances are discussed throughout this book. Another fascinating example is the role of $GABA_B$ autoreceptors in some brain circuits in which a glutamate neurone excites a postsynaptic cell C directly, but at the same time inhibits it indirectly through a GABA interneurone. When a single stimulus is applied to the glutamate neurone, the excitation of the postsynaptic cell C remains small because of simultaneous release of glutamate and gamma-aminobutyric acid (GABA). In a series of pulses at sufficient frequency, however, the release of GABA declines progressively as the result of activation of release-inhibiting presynaptic $GABA_B$ autoreceptors, and excitatory transmission to cell C is enhanced. This $GABA_B$ autoreceptor-mediated disinhibition underlies some forms of long-term potentiation, and it seems at least possible that it plays a role in learning on the one hand and epileptic discharges on the other[4].

Modulation of transmitter release has been studied most intensively for postganglionic sympathetic neurones. Modulation here doubtlessly is an essential feature. What we owe to the sympathetic nervous system can hardly be described better than in Thomas Mann's *Der Zauberberg*, *The Magic Mountain*, originally published in 1924, the year of Dixon's presynaptic nicotine experiment. The hero, Hans Castorp, has been staying in the *Internationales Sanatorium Berghof* in Davos, Switzerland for seven months (seven being a magic number in the novel), because of a doubtful diagnosis of tuberculosis, before approaching Clawdia Chauchat in the evening of Shrove Tuesday and declaring his love.

'*Er war totenbleich … Die Gefäßnervenleitung nach seinem Gesichte spielte mit dem Erfolg, daß die entglutete Haut dieses jungen Gesichtes blaßkalt einfiel, die Nase spitz erschien und die Partie unter den Augen ganz so bleifarben wie bei einer Leiche aussah. Aber Hans Castorps Herz ließ der Sympathikus in einer Gangart trommeln, daß von geregelter Atmung überhaupt nicht mehr die Rede sein konnte, und Schauer überliefen den jungen Menschen als Veranstaltung der Hautsalbendrüsen seines Körpers, die sich mitsamt ihren Haarbälgen aufrichteten.'*

'He was deadly pale ... The nerves controlling the blood-vessels that supplied his face functioned so well that the skin, robbed of all its blood, went quite cold, the nose looked peaked, and the hollows beneath the young eyes were lead-coloured as any corpse's. And the *Sympathicus* caused his heart, Hans Castorp's heart, to thump, in such a way that it was impossible to breathe except in gasps; and shivers ran over him, due to the functioning of the sebaceous glands, which, with the hair follicles, erected themselves.'[12]

What would Hans' experience have been without the intense vasoconstriction, tachycardia and contraction of the *Musculi arrectores pilorum*? We can be sure that presynaptic modulation of this or that kind took place in all three tissues the narrator mentions. The reader may think there is no evidence for modulation of transmitter release at the *arrectores pilorum* muscles, but then he is mistaken. In 1935, F. T. Brücke[2] showed that, in the cat tail, acetylcholine suppresses pilomotor responses to sympathetic nerve stimulation but not to adrenaline and concluded that 'acetylcholine acts at the sympathetic nerve endings; perhaps it inhibits the production of sympathin so that the pilomotor muscles cannot respond to the neural stimulus': perhaps the first recorded instance of muscarinic inhibition, 11 years after the first report on nicotinic excitation.

Modulation of transmitter release is ubiquitous, the subject of vivid research, solving and creating riddles and essential for a number of functions of our body.

## References

1. Brown GL and Gillespie JS (1957) The output of sympathetic transmitter from the spleen of the cat. *Journal of Physiology* **138:** 81–102
2. Brücke FT (1935) Über die Wirkung von Acetylcholin auf die Pilomotoren. *Klinische Wochenschrift* **14:** 7–9
3. Burnstock G (1986) The changing face of autonomic neurotransmission. *Acta Physiologica Scandinavica* **126:** 67–91
4. Davies CH and Collingridge GL (1993) The physiological regulation of synaptic inhibition by $GABA_B$ autoreceptors in rat hippocampus. *Journal of Physiology* **472:** 245–265
5. Dixon WE (1924) Nicotin, coniin, piperidin, lupetidin, cytisin, lobelin, spartein, gelsemin. In: Heffter A (ed), *Handbuch der experimentellen Pharmakologie*, vol II, pp 656–736, Springer, Berlin
6. Doxey JC and Everitt J (1977) Inhibitory effects of clonidine on responses to sympathetic nerve stimulation in the pithed rat. *British Journal of Pharmacology* **61:** 559–566
7. Driessen B, von Kügelgen I and Starke K (1994) $P_1$-purinoceptor-mediated modulation of neural noradrenaline and ATP release in guinea-pig vas deferens. *Naunyn-Schmiedeberg's Archives of Pharmacology* **350:** 42–48
8. Dunwiddie TV, Lovinger DM (eds) (1993) *Presynaptic Receptors in the Mammalian Brain.* Birkhäuser, Boston
9. Langer SZ (1981) Presynaptic regulation of the release of catecholamines. *Physiological Reviews* **32:** 337–362
10. Langer SZ, Starke K and Dubocovich ML (eds) (1979) *Presynaptic Receptors.* Pergamon, Oxford
11. Lattimer N and Rhodes KF (1985) A difference in the affinity of some selective $\alpha_2$-adrenoceptor antagonists when compared on isolated vasa deferentia of rat and rabbit. *Naunyn-Schmiedeberg's Archives of Pharmacology* **329:** 278–281
12. Mann T (1961) *The Magic Mountain*, 3rd edn. Translated by HT Lowe-Porter. Secker & Warburg, London
13. Starke K (1977) Regulation of noradrenaline release by presynaptic receptor systems. *Reviews of Physiology, Biochemistry and Pharmacology* **77:** 1–124
14. Starke K (1981) Presynaptic receptors. *Annual Review of Pharmacology and Toxicology* **21:** 7–30
15. Starke K and Langer SZ (1979) A note on terminology for presynaptic receptors. In: Langer SZ, Starke K, Dubocovich ML (eds) *Presynaptic Receptors*, pp 1–3, Pergamon, Oxford

16. Trendelenburg AU, Limberger N and Starke K (1993) Presynaptic $\alpha_2$-autoreceptors in brain cortex: $\alpha_{2D}$ in the rat and $\alpha_{2A}$ in the rabbit. *Naunyn-Schmiedeberg's Archives of Pharmacology* **348:** 35–45

17. von Kügelgen I, Kurz K and Starke K (1993) Axon terminal $P_2$-purinoceptors in feedback control of sympathetic transmitter release. *Neuroscience* **56:** 263–267

# 1 Neurotransmitter release

# 1 Mechanisms of exocytosis and the central role of calcium

Robert D. Burgoyne and Timothy R. Cheek

Before one can appreciate the notion of modulation of neurotransmitter release, it is necessary to have a basic understanding of the process of neurotransmitter release itself. While the mechanisms involved at the nerve terminal are not yet fully understood, there has been much progress made recently and a picture is gradually emerging. In this Chapter, Robert Burgoyne and Timothy Cheek describe the current concept of exocytotic neurotransmitter release at nerve terminals and and the crucial role of $Ca^{2+}$ influx in triggering that release. Because of their larger size and, consequently, the increased ease with which biochemical manipulations can be performed, much of our understanding of exocytotic neurotransmitter release has come from the study of chromaffin cells from the adrenal medulla – functional homologues of postganglionic sympathetic neurones – rather than from neurones themselves. The chapter focuses on the situation in the adrenal chromaffin cell but with appropriate cross-referencing to conventional nerve terminals.

## 1 The regulation of neurotransmitter release and $Ca^{2+}$

Neurotransmitters and hormones are released from their storage vesicles by exocytosis. This is the process by which secretory vesicles fuse with the plasma membrane; it is usually triggered by a rise in the concentration of cytosolic free calcium ($[Ca^{2+}]_i$). During the 1980s, substantial advances have been made in gaining understanding of calcium signals within cells, including detailed characterisation of plasma membrane $Ca^{2+}$ channels, through which $Ca^{2+}$ enters, intracellular $Ca^{2+}$ stores, which can be mobilised, and the role of plasma-membrane-derived inositol 1,4,5-trisphosphate ($Ins(1,4,5)P_3$) as a physiological trigger for internal $Ca^{2+}$ mobilisation. In the case of neurotransmitter release and the release of some hormones, it is apparent that $Ca^{2+}$ entry across the plasma

membrane is the usual effective trigger. A rise in $[Ca^{2+}]_i$ resulting from release from intracellular stores is usually poorly effective, if at all. This has resulted in attention being focused on the $Ca^{2+}$ channels and other $Ca^{2+}$ entry mechanisms that could be linked to exocytosis in various secretory cells.

The mechanisms by which local increases in $[Ca^{2+}]_i$ beneath the plasma membrane activate exocytosis and the nature of the components of the exocytotic machinery are now beginning to be resolved, but we still have only limited insight into these aspects at present. It seems likely that the intracellular $Ca^{2+}$ receptor mechanism and the exocytotic fusion machinery may involve several cytosolic and membrane-bound proteins acting in concert[16]. As well as the essential proteins of the machinery, a variety of other proteins are likely to be involved as modulatory components that allow the extent or rate of exocytosis to be increased or decreased.

This chapter deals with the relationship between $[Ca^{2+}]_i$ and exocytosis, the nature of the $Ca^{2+}$ channels and the proteins involved in the $Ca^{2+}$-signalling pathway leading to exocytosis. Considerable emphasis is given to studies on $[Ca^{2+}]_i$ and exocytosis in bovine adrenal chromaffin cells, where they have been extensively investigated, but reference is made to the specialisations found in neuronal synapses. Adrenal chromaffin cells are derived during embryogenesis from the same precursors as sympathetic neurones and have much in common with them. However, they have provided a more convenient model for the study of the molecular aspects of neurotransmitter release.

## 2   Exocytosis in adrenal medullary chromaffin cells

The physiological stimulus for catecholamine secretion from (bovine) adrenal chromaffin cells is acetylcholine acting through cholinergic nicotinic receptors. Nicotinic receptor activation of chromaffin cells results in the opening of receptor-associated channels allowing entry of $Na^+$ and $Ca^{2+}$, which leads to depolarisation and the subsequent opening of voltage-sensitive $Ca^{2+}$ channels in the plasma membrane (see also Chapter 10). The current view is that the major signal for exocytotic secretion is a rise in $[Ca^{2+}]_i$ resulting from $Ca^{2+}$ entry from the extracellular medium[19,26,28,35,60].

Pharmacological studies have shown that chromaffin cells possess L-type (dihydropyridine-sensitive) $Ca^{2+}$ channels[5,18], dihydropyridine-insensitive but ω-conotoxin-sensitive $Ca^{2+}$ channels (N-type) and other pharmacologically distinct $Ca^{2+}$ channels[6]. L-type channels are not the only channels involved in voltage-dependent $Ca^{2+}$ entry leading to secretion, because dihydropyridine antagonists do not completely block the rise in $[Ca^{2+}]_i$ or the secretion elicited by either nicotine or GABA[36]. Electrophysiological studies on single-channel kinetics have shown

that chromaffin cells express multiple distinct voltage-sensitive $Ca^{2+}$ channels whose role in exocytosis has yet to be determined[6] (see also Chapter 10).

### 2.1   The intracellular $Ca^{2+}$ signal in chromaffin cells

Many laboratories have used $Ca^{2+}$-sensitive fluorescent indicator dyes inside intact cells to follow the stimulus-induced changes in $[Ca^{2+}]_i$ in chromaffin cell populations or single cells. From these studies, resting $[Ca^{2+}]_i$ in the chromaffin cell appears to be within the range 10–100 nM, and, after stimulation with nicotinic agonists, this rises to 300–1000 nM.

#### 2.1.1   Spatial aspects of $Ca^{2+}$ entry

Spatial aspects of the $Ca^{2+}$ signal in single bovine chromaffin cells have been investigated using video imaging of the fluorescent $Ca^{2+}$ indicator fura-2 in intact cells[14,26,28,29,33,49] and fura-2 in whole cell patch-clamp recording[44]. Following stimulation with nicotine or during electrical depolarisation, the rise in $[Ca^{2+}]_i$ caused by $Ca^{2+}$ influx is initially restricted to the subplasmalemmal region of the cell[27,44,49]. An increase in $[Ca^{2+}]_i$ then spreads into the interior of the cell, either by diffusion or as a result of $Ca^{2+}$-induced $Ca^{2+}$ release from intracellular stores (see below), to give a more uniform elevation of $[Ca^{2+}]_i$ throughout the cytoplasm. Subsequently, a further increase in $[Ca^{2+}]_i$ may occur, which is sometimes localised to one area of the cell[49]. This latter response may also be the result of the release of $Ca^{2+}$ from internal stores.

The early ($< 1$ s) subplasmalemmal rise in $[Ca^{2+}]_i$ was calculated to be 40–50 nM above the resting level[49]. However, the temporal resolution of the imaging system used in these experiments (5 ratio images/s) is such that a $Ca^{2+}$ wave spreading at a rate of about 10 μm/s will have diffused about 2 μm from its point source (the channel in the plasma membrane) before it can be detected. As $Ca^{2+}$ spreads this distance from its point source, its concentration has been predicted

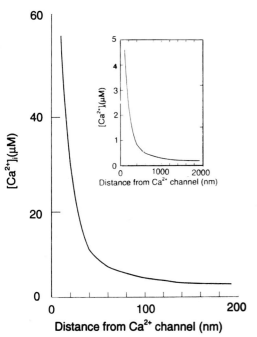

Fig. 1.1. Theoretical $[Ca^{2+}]_i$ at varying distances from the plasma membrane 1ms after the opening of voltage-sensitive $Ca^{2+}$ channels. The inset shows a wider range of distances from the plasma membrane. For comparison, a synaptic vesicle is 50 nm in diameter and a chromaffin granule approximately 200 nm in diameter. The subcortical actin network in chromaffin cells extends about 200 nm from the plasma membrane.

to decay exponentially (Fig. 1.1). Thus, the $Ca^{2+}$ concentration in the vicinity of the mouth of the $Ca^{2+}$ channel is probably more likely to be in the range 10–100 $\mu M$[57]. Recent work has shown the presence of microdomains of calcium in the squid giant synapse, presumably close to $Ca^{2+}$ channels, where $[Ca^{2+}]_i$ can reach 200 to 300 $\mu M$ during stimulation[39]. Unfortunately, such spatially restricted high levels of $[Ca^{2+}]_i$ cannot reliably be visualised with current imaging technology, not only because of the limited temporal and spatial resolution of the imaging systems but also because the majority of dyes currently available to monitor $[Ca^{2+}]_i$ saturate in the range 1–2 $\mu M$.

Recent studies on chromaffin cells using whole cell-attached patches have indicated more directly that these high levels of $Ca^{2+}$ must exist at the sites of exocytosis in stimulated cells: when $[Ca^{2+}]_i$ is raised by dialysis, even 100 $\mu M$ $[Ca^{2+}]$ did not achieve the same rates of secretion as those seen in response to depolarisation. In these experiments, secretion was judged by measuring the change in plasma membrane capacitance[8], which is directly related to membrane area and, thus, detects the insertion of the secretory granule membrane during exocytosis.

The voltage-sensitive $Ca^{2+}$ channels responsible for delivering $Ca^{2+}$ to the sites of exocytosis are probably localised over the entire cell surface[26]. This has been established by visualising the sites of exocytosis, after nicotine-induced depolarisation, using an antibody raised against the chromaffin granule membrane protein dopamine-β-hydroxylase to detect the insertion of the membrane into the plasma membrane.

From studies on neuronal synapses, various experimental approaches have led not only to the idea that $Ca^{2+}$ entry through voltage-sensitive channels is the key trigger for exocytosis but also, more significantly, to the concept that rapid, physiological neurotransmitter release occurs only from synaptic vesicles very close to the $Ca^{2+}$ channels[7].

The extreme specialisation required of fast synapses is such that $Ca^{2+}$ entry and exocytosis must be complete within a few hundred microseconds. This has resulted in the suggestion that the synaptic vesicles that undergo exocytosis must be physically linked to the $Ca^{2+}$ channels to allow a fast response to a $Ca^{2+}$ 'cloud' at the mouth of the channel (Fig. 1.2). Candidates for proteins that link the synaptic vesicle to the $Ca^{2+}$ channel in neurones include synaptic vesicle proteins such as synaptotagmin (p65), as discussed below. It is unlikely that secretory vesicles are docked in this manner in chromaffin cells. Few such vesicles are observed by electron microscopy[12,15] and exocytosis occurs only after a lag of up to 50 ms[31]. This may be the time required for secretory granule docking following the entry of $Ca^{2+}$ and its diffusion

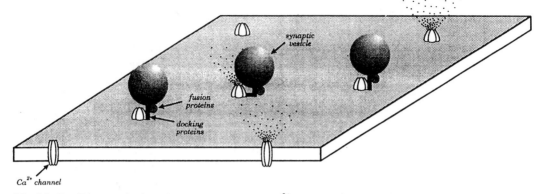

Fig. 1.2. Possible organisation of synaptic vesicle and $Ca^{2+}$ channels at the active zone in a synaptic terminal. The rapid release of a few synaptic vesicles is likely to be the result of exocytosis of those already docked at the plasma membrane and attached to $Ca^{2+}$ channels, where they can sense the $Ca^{2+}$ cloud at the mouth of the channel within a few hundred microseconds, or less, of channel opening. This type of model is required to explain the fast events at the synapse. In other cell types, such as chromaffin cells, the slower rate of exocytosis may be caused by recruitment of secretory granules that are not intimately associated with $Ca^{2+}$ channels, or even docked on the plasma membrane.

over a distance of tens of nanometres from the plasma membrane to the secretory granules.

### 2.1.2   Direct manipulation of intracellular $Ca^{2+}$ concentration

As discussed above, $[Ca^{2+}]_i$ existing within a few nanometres of exocytotic sites cannot yet be directly visualised because of technical limitations, but both theoretical calculations[57] and patch-clamp experiments[8,44] indicate that such $[Ca^{2+}]_i$ probably lies in the range 10–100 μM before dissipating very rapidly (approximately 100–200 ms) into the cytosol. Using the technique of flash photolysis of caged $Ca^{2+}$, Neher and Zucker[46] have elevated average $[Ca^{2+}]_i$ in chromaffin cells to these predicted levels while simultaneously monitoring secretion by measuring plasma membrane capacitance. Elevating $Ca^{2+}$ to $>10$ μM was found to trigger ultrafast ($<50$ ms) exocytosis, possibly resulting from the release of granules already close to the plasma membrane, while elevating $Ca^{2+}$ into the range 70–150 μM was found to trigger, in addition, both a fast (1–2 s) and a slow (10–30 s) exocytotic response, perhaps representing the release of granules that were restrained within the subplasmalemmal

cytoskeleton or were recruited from deep within the cell. Similar findings have been obtained with pituitary melanotrophs[64]. Clearly, experiments such as these in which $[Ca^{2+}]_i$ can be changed rapidly and uniformly in a known manner will be central to unravelling the multiplicity of $Ca^{2+}$-dependent processes that are related to the secretory response in chromaffin cells. It should be noted that even the ultrafast responses in chromaffin cells are considerably slower than the processes in certain synapses, where exocytosis is complete within a few hundred microseconds.

By using video-imaging techniques to visualise stimulus-induced changes in $[Ca^{2+}]_i$[12,20], and whole-cell patch clamp[8,44] and flash photolysis to release caged $Ca^{2+}$ (ref. 46) and, thus, directly manipulate $[Ca^{2+}]_i$ at the single cell level, considerable insight has been gained into why $Ca^{2+}$ influx is so crucial for secretion. It is probable that only entry of $Ca^{2+}$ from the external medium delivers $Ca^{2+}$ in sufficient magnitude to the subplasmalemmal exocytotic sites to activate the fusion process (Fig. 1.3). The difference between $Ca^{2+}$ entry and $Ca^{2+}$ mobilisation as far as exocytosis is concerned perhaps results from the differing $Ca^{2+}$ gradients generated, which

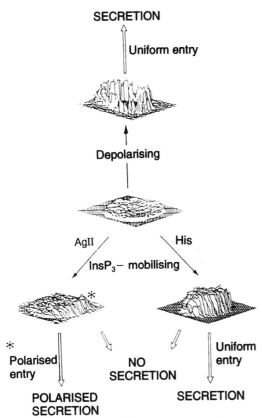

**SECRETION**

↑

**Uniform entry**

**Depolarising**

AgII          His

InsP$_3$– mobilising

\*

\*
Polarised     NO        Uniform
entry      SECRETION     entry

POLARISED          SECRETION
SECRETION

Fig. 1.3. Summary of Ca$^{2+}$ signals generated in adrenal chromaffin cells by various agonists and their relationship to the triggering of exocytotic secretion. The figure shows three-dimensional contour plots of the [Ca$^{2+}$]$_i$ at rest or after stimulation in various ways. The most effective stimuli for exocytosis are those that depolarise the cells, allowing uniform Ca$^{2+}$ entry through voltage-sensitive Ca$^{2+}$ channels in the cell membrane (top). Ins(1,4,5)$P_3$-mobilising agonists such as angiotensin II (AgII) or histamine (His) release Ca$^{2+}$ from internal stores, but it is the subsequent polarised or uniform Ca$^{2+}$ entry that leads to secretion.

can lead to similar average [Ca$^{2+}$]$_i$ within the cell but quite different [Ca$^{2+}$]$_i$ in the subplasmalemmal space (Fig. 1.4).

## 2.2   Intracellular Ca$^{2+}$ stores and exocytosis

Throughout the 1980s, it became clear that, besides the nicotinic cholinergic receptor activation, a number of other cell surface

receptors can either stimulate catecholamine secretion or modulate nicotine-induced secretion[12]. Activation of many of these other receptors leads to activation of phosphoinositidase C with subsequent generation of an intracellular Ca$^{2+}$-mobilising signal, inositol 1,4,5-trisphosphate (Ins(1,4,5)$P_3$).

Nicotine and GABA[34,36] lead to depolarisation and Ca$^{2+}$ entry whereas muscarinic cholinergic, bradykinin, angiotensin II, histamine, prostaglandin E$_2$, vasoactive intestinal peptide (VIP) and ATP receptors are all linked to Ins(1,4,5)$P_3$ and Ca$^{2+}$ mobilisation. Note that these signalling pathways are not necessarily mutually exclusive, because nicotinic stimulation and depolarisation with high K$^+$ levels have been reported to lead in addition to Ins(1,4,5)$P_3$ production through Ca$^{2+}$-dependent activation of phosphoinositidase C[32]. Also, Ins(1,4,5)$P_3$ may itself promote Ca$^{2+}$ entry through non-voltage-sensitive Ca$^{2+}$ channels in the plasma membrane[40].

The various receptor agonists differ in their abilities to trigger secretion, although nicotinic stimulation consistently gives the largest response. Apart from nicotinic agonists, only GABA and histamine produce a substantial secretory response. Little, or even no, secretion is detected in response to the remaining agonists.

Irrespective of the nature of the stimulating agent, secretion from intact cells is abolished by the removal of external Ca$^{2+}$ (ref. 12), a simple demonstration that it is Ca$^{2+}$ entry that is pivotal in triggering exocytosis from these cells. A similar requirement for Ca$^{2+}$ entry has been shown for other neuronal cell types. Consistent with this, it has been found that agents which release internally stored Ca$^{2+}$, such as Ins(1,4,5)$P_3$-generating agonists (see above) or less-specific Ca$^{2+}$-mobilising compounds, such as caffeine and thapsigargin, all fail to promote secretion in the absence of external Ca$^{2+}$. Therefore, the efficacy of a given agonist reflects the degree to which it is able to promote Ca$^{2+}$ entry through either voltage-dependent or voltage-independent pathways rather than its ability to elevate [Ca$^{2+}$]$_i$ *per se*.

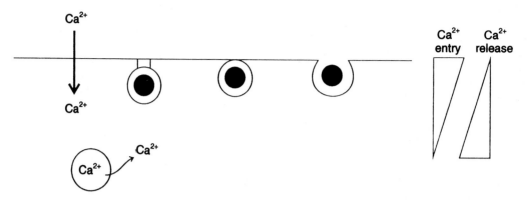

Fig. 1.4. Calcium gradients following $Ca^{2+}$ entry or $Ca^{2+}$ release from internal stores and their relationship to exocytosis. The figure shows that the same average rise in $[Ca^{2+}]_i$ caused by entry or release (shown by the area of the triangles to the right) has different consequences for exocytosis because of the $Ca^{2+}$ gradients generated and the resultant concentration of $[Ca^{2+}]_i$ sensed at the plasma membrane near the sites of exocytosis (see triangles).

### 2.2.1   Ins(1,4,5)$P_3$-mediated $Ca^{2+}$ mobilisation

Muscarinic agonists raise $[Ca^{2+}]_i$ in chromaffin cells by stimulating release from internal stores, but they do not promote secretion from bovine cells[22]. Within a population, not all chromaffin cells respond to muscarinic receptor activation and in those that do, the early subplasmalemmal rise in $[Ca^{2+}]_i$ seen in response to depolarisation does not occur[28]. Instead, the rise in $[Ca^{2+}]_i$ appears initially in a more localised region, presumably as a result of the release of $Ca^{2+}$ from the localised Ins(1,4,5)$P_3$-sensitive store. It is probable that, in intact cells, such an internal release of $Ca^{2+}$ does not result in a sufficient elevation in $[Ca^{2+}]_i$ at the exocytotic sites to activate the fusion process (Fig. 1.4), hence the lack of secretory response. This notion is supported by the findings that non-physiological release of $Ca^{2+}$ from the Ins(1,4,5)$P_3$-sensitive store, using the $Ca^{2+}$-ATPase inhibitor thapsigargin (which prevents reaccumulation of leaked intracellular $Ca^{2+}$), was only capable of activating release if there was a secondary influx of external $Ca^{2+}$ triggered by the $Ca^{2+}$ mobilisation[30].

### 2.2.2   Entry of $Ca^{2+}$ in response to Ins(1,4,5)$P_3$

Histamine and angiotensin II both trigger secretion that depends upon external $Ca^{2+}$, with histamine being much more effective than angiotensin II[12]. This may be because the angiotensin receptor, but not the histamine receptor, desensitises rapidly, thereby shutting off $Ca^{2+}$ entry[60]. Additionally, the localisation of $Ca^{2+}$ entry in response to the two stimuli may differ. Angiotensin II results in an initial local rise in $[Ca^{2+}]_i$, caused by inositol phosphate generation (see below) followed by a polarised entry of external $Ca^{2+}$, as judged by visualising the quenching of fura-2 fluorescence by the $Ca^{2+}$ surrogate $Mn^{2+}$ (ref. 27). This results in a low level of catecholamine release[48] that is also polarised[26]. The more potent secretagogue histamine, at doses optimal for secretion, stimulates $Ca^{2+}$ entry around the whole plasma membrane, explaining its efficacy in stimulating secretion[27] (Fig. 1.3).

The nature of the channels through which angiotensin II and histamine stimulate $Ca^{2+}$ entry and the mechanism of opening these channels are unknown. This remains one of the key unanswered questions in this field.

One possibility is that hormone receptors (for angiotensin II or histamine, for example) directly open a receptor-operated channel (ROC) in the plasma membrane. An alternative possibility is that an intracellular messenger, such as $Ins(1,4,5)P_3$ or inositol tetrabisphosphate $(Ins(1,3,4,5)P_4)$, may promote $Ca^{2+}$ entry through a second-messenger-operated channel. Angiotensin II and histamine both result in a transient generation of $Ins(1,4,5)P_3$ within 10 s in chromaffin cells. In response to histamine, but not angiotensin II, the response is biphasic with a secondary generation of $Ins(1,4,5)P_3$ occurring at 20 s[60]. The secondary increase in $Ins(1,4,5)P_3$ in response to histamine is paralleled by an increase in $Ins(1,3,4)P_3$ that is absent after stimulation with angiotensin II. Since this $Ins(1,3,4)P_3$ could only have originated from dephosphorylation of $Ins(1,3,4,5)P_4$, this suggests that histamine produces more $Ins(1,3,4,5)P_4$, as well as more $Ins(1,4,5)P_3$, than does angiotensin II. With respect to eliciting a secretory response, it may be significant that histamine is more effective than angiotensin II in generating both $Ins(1,4,5)P_3$ and $Ins(1,3,4,5)P_4$, because both of these inositol phosphates have been proposed to trigger $Ca^{2+}$ entry into cells. There is as yet no direct evidence supporting a role for $Ins(1,3,4,5)P_4$ in gating $Ca^{2+}$ entry in chromaffin cells, but Mochizuki-Oda et al.[40] have demonstrated that $Ins(1,4,5)P_3$ is capable of directly opening a plasma membrane channel that gates $Ca^{2+}$ in these cells.

Finally $Ca^{2+}$ entry has been reported to be activated by $Ca^{2+}$-ATPase inhibitors, such as thapsigargin, in the absence of surface receptor stimulation[53], indicating the existence of a *capacitative entry mechanism* in these cells in which $Ca^{2+}$ entry is triggered (in an as yet incompletely understood way) by the emptying of the intracellular stores. Whether or not such a mechanism is responsible for any or all of the $Ca^{2+}$ entry observed after receptor activation remains to be elucidated.

### 2.2.3 Release of $Ca^{2+}$ induced by $Ca^{2+}$

A secondary rise in $[Ca^{2+}]_i$, which follows $Ca^{2+}$ influx, is observed during continued depolarisation of chromaffin cells[49], but not after stimulation with a single action potential[44]. This elevation in $[Ca^{2+}]_i$ could arise in two ways. It could result from either $Ca^{2+}$ release from distinct internal stores that are sensitive to $Ins(1,4,5)P_3$ (see above), or a process of $Ca^{2+}$-induced $Ca^{2+}$ release (CICR) from internal stores[9] that contain caffeine-sensitive ryanodine receptors, related to those present in muscle and which mediate CICR in that tissue. In favour of the first mechanism, it has been shown[32] that both nicotine and membrane depolarisation with high $K^+$ concentrations result in the generation of $Ins(1,4,5)P_3$ in bovine chromaffin cells as the result of $Ca^{2+}$-dependent activation of phosphoinositidase C following the influx of $Ca^{2+}$. With regard to the second mechanism, it has been shown that chromaffin cells contain caffeine-sensitive stores that are evenly distributed throughout the cytoplasm[14,29], and that are, at least in part, $Ins(1,4,5)P_3$ insensitive[21,52]. Several lines of evidence indicate that these stores may contribute to the secondary $Ca^{2+}$ signal. For example, emptying the caffeine-sensitive stores of bovine chromaffin cells reduced the magnitude of a histamine-induced rise in $[Ca^{2+}]_i$[59].

The role that the caffeine-sensitive store plays in $Ca^{2+}$ signalling and bovine chromaffin cell function still has to be fully elucidated, but it may be that the store is involved mainly in $Ca^{2+}$ homeostasis (i.e. the recovery from the $Ca^{2+}$ transient change that triggers exocytosis). Certainly caffeine is unable to trigger significant secretion from intact bovine cells, but the state of filling of the store appears to influence the decay time of a depolarisation-induced $Ca^{2+}$ signal[29].

## 3    The role of the cytoskeleton in the control of exocytosis

In synapses releasing fast-acting neurotransmitters, the initial $Ca^{2+}$-evoked release of neurotransmitter is almost certainly caused by exocytosis of secretory vesicles in a docked, prefusion state at the active zone of the nerve terminal. In the case of slower release processes, such as those in adrenal chromaffin cells or pituitary cells, initial release may involve vesicles close to, but not docked at, the plasma membrane. The cytoskeleton is not likely to be involved in the initial burst of release, but changes in the cytoskeleton, particularly disassembly of the cortical actin network, is necessary for further waves of release in endocrine cells (Fig. 1.5) or recruitment of vesicles in preparation for the next action potential arriving at the nerve terminal[25].

In nerve terminals, synaptic vesicles are located within a cytoskeletal network in which the vesicles are linked to each other and to actin filaments, or fodrin molecules, by the extrinsic synaptic vesicle protein synapsin I. Considerable data have now accumulated that suggest that $Ca^{2+}$-dependent phosphorylation of synapsin I occurs following nerve-terminal depolarisation[65]. The consequent structural reorganisation of the cytoskeleton–vesicle interaction releases vesicles that can enter the presynaptic active zone. Synapsin I is a substrate for calmodulin-dependent protein kinase II, an enzyme that is activated following $Ca^{2+}$ entry into the nerve terminal. Phosphorylated synapsin I is less effective in vesicle binding than the non-phosphorylated form and will dissociate from the vesicles, freeing them from their cytoskeletal restraints and allowing them to move to the presynaptic membrane[65]. Following recovery from the depolarisation-induced $Ca^{2+}$ transient, synapsin I is dephosphorylated and the vesicles are once again frozen within the cytoskeletal network. This model can explain how the recruitment of new vesicles could be related to depolarisation, but clearly the changes in synapsin I phosphorylation and vesicle movement are unlikely to be fast enough to account for the immediate exocytotic fusion of synaptic vesicles. Nevertheless, changes in synapsin I phosphorylation could be an important regulatory mechanism that would determine the subsequent efficiency of the neurotransmitter release process.

Data in support of these ideas about the function of synapsin I and calmodulin-dependent protein kinase II have come from work on the squid giant synapse[38] and mammalian brain synaptosomes[47]. In both systems, introduction of calmodulin-dependent protein kinase II or the dephospho form of synapsin I have the effects predicted by the model described above. Thus, calmodulin-dependent protein kinase II stimulates and dephospho-synapsin I inhibits the extent of neurotransmitter release in these preparations. Synapsin I phosphorylation could, therefore, be a key element in presynaptic modulation of neurotransmitter release.

Synapsin I is not present in non-neuronal cells; therefore, in these cells the situation is rather different. In adrenal chromaffin cells, for example, more extensive release of stored neurotransmitters/hormones can be activated. This involves the rapid release[48] of vesicles close to the plasma membrane (1–5% of secretory vesicles[12,15]) and a slower, sustained release of a substantial proportion (up to 30%) of total secretory vesicles recruited from deep within the cell. The sustained release requires reorganisation of the cortical actin network that is found beneath the plasma membrane and which normally acts as a barrier to exocytosis of these vesicles[13]. Reversible disassembly of cortical actin can be detected following stimulation of chromaffin cells, which leaves regions of the cell cortex free of actin filaments[17,23,66]. These are then the sites of extensive exocytosis. Changes in cortical actin have been detected by fluorescence imaging using rhodamine–phalloidin[23,66] and by use of biochemical assays that allow quantitative assessment of the amount of assembled actin present[17,23]. In chromaffin cells, actin

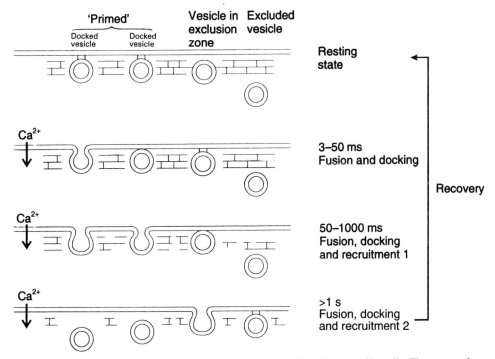

Fig. 1.5. Stages in exocytosis and secretory granule recruitment in adrenal chromaffin cells. The range of possible states of secretory vesicles in the resting state, is shown, but the first phase of release from chromaffin cells may be mainly of those in a docked state or, more likely, in the exclusion zone formed by cortical actin filaments. The subsequent phases of release as described by Neher and Zucker[46] would involve recruitment of further pools of vesicles (by $Ca^{2+}$-dependent processes) following cortical actin disassembly and vesicle movement to the plasma membrane.

disassembly can be activated by $Ca^{2+}$ or by protein kinase C and is inhibited by elevated cyclic AMP (cAMP)[24]. The cortical actin network could, therefore, act as an important target for regulation of the extent of exocytosis, particularly when exocytosis is prolonged over seconds or minutes. In this respect, it may be a target for known modulators of $Ca^{2+}$-dependent exocytosis, such as protein kinase C and cAMP-dependent protein kinase (see also Chapter 9).

## 4    Identification of $Ca^{2+}$-sensitive proteins involved in exocytosis

Over the years, a variety of pharmacological agents have been used in attempts to identify proteins, including $Ca^{2+}$-binding proteins, that may be involved in exocytosis. This type of approach has not been successful because of the lack of specificity of the drugs used. From a variety of such studies, the only finding that has been substantiated is that protein kinase C is a widespread stimulator of the exocytotic machinery. It should be noted, however, that protein kinase C may not be essential for exocytosis. In contrast, more recent protein chemical studies have begun to identify secretory vesicle and cytosolic proteins that may be part of the exocytotic machinery and it is clear that this sort of approach will facilitate further progress[16].

One major experimental approach has been the characterisation of integral synaptic vesicle proteins, based on the assumption that one or more of these is likely to be important in the neurotransmitter-release process[62]. Many synaptic vesicle proteins have now been identified and sequenced and, apart from those that function as neurotransmitter transporters, three are known that are of interest here. These have been named synaptophysin, synaptotagmin (p65) and synaptobrevin and all three have been suggested to play a role in exocytosis.

### 4.1    Synaptophysin

Synaptophysin is a very abundant synaptic vesicle protein[61]. It has the characteristics of a transmembrane channel protein and it has been suggested, on the basis of its behaviour following reconstitution in lipid bilayers[63], that it could form part of the fusion pore that precedes exocytosis. There is no functional evidence yet for this precise role in exocytosis, but work on *Xenopus* oocytes, in which neurotransmitter release occurs after assembly of vesicles encoded by injected brain mRNA, has shown that disruption of synaptophysin using antibodies or antisense oligonucleotides does lead to a reduction in neurotransmitter release[1]. This study, however, could not exclude a purely structural role for synaptophysin in the assembly and organisation of synaptic vesicle proteins. Note also that synaptophysin is not present in many exocrine or endocrine secretory vesicles, such as chromaffin granules.

### 4.2    Synaptotagmin

Synaptotagmin is a lipid- and $Ca^{2+}$-binding protein[11,50], which suggests that it could possibly link vesicles to the plasma membrane at elevated $[Ca^{2+}]_i$. More particularly, it has been suggested that synaptotagmin interacts with $Ca^{2+}$ channels and could dock synaptic vesicles at release sites[37] to allow rapid exocytosis of neurotransmitters[3] (Fig. 1.2). Against this suggestion is the finding that selected variants of the rat pheochromocytoma cell line PC12 that express undetectable levels of this protein secrete perfectly well and, in fact, secrete to a higher extent than does the parent cell line[56]. Recent genetic studies also suggest that synaptotagmin is not essential for neurotransmitter release[51]: synaptotagmin mutants of *Caenorhabditis elegans* and *Drosophila* could still release neurotransmitter though in an aberrant fashion. The significance of synaptotagmin to exocytosis is still the subject of much debate.

### 4.3    Synaptobrevin

The synaptic vesicle protein synaptobrevin has been relatively little studied but recently more attention has been focused on it. Synaptobrevin is present as two isoforms. These are small transmembrane proteins most of which project into the cytosol where they could interact with other proteins. Synaptobrevin could also interact with other elements of the plasma membrane[4]. Functional evidence for this protein being involved in neurotransmitter release has come from the use of neurotoxins. It has been known for a long time that neurotransmitter release can be effectively blocked by tetanus and botulinum neurotoxins if they gain entry to the nerve terminal. It has now been found that tetanus and botulinum-B toxins have zinc-dependent protease activity and that they specifically cleave one of the rat synaptobrevin isoforms called synaptobrevin-2[55]. These findings, if correct, would mean that synaptobrevin-2 plays an essential role in neurotransmitter release. Such a role for synaptobrevin-2 may not be universal in exocytosis, since this protein is apparently not found on secretory vesicles of endocrine or exocrine cells. Nevertheless, this is a potentially significant advance in the identification of proteins involved in exocytosis. Recent work[58] has suggested that synaptobrevin and the plasma-membrane proteins syntaxin and SNAP-25 (soluble *N*-ethylmaleimide-sensitive fusion protein (NSF)-attachment protein (SNAP)) may interact through the NSF and

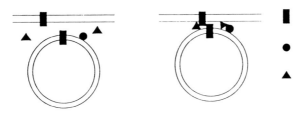

Fig. 1.6. Hypothetical assembly of a protein fusion machine for exocytosis. Exocytosis appears to involve multiple proteins that may act in concert to form a fusion machine involving integral plasma and vesicle membrane proteins (■), extrinsic membrane proteins (●) and cytosolic proteins (▲).

SNAP proteins previously implicated in other vesicular transport steps, such as those in the Golgi apparatus. The work suggests that this group of proteins forms a key part of the docking/fusion machinery in the synapse. This idea is supported by the recent finding that the two plasma membrane proteins are also cleaved by clostridial neurotoxins.

## 4.4   Soluble proteins

An alternative approach to the study of exocytotic mechanisms has been the use of various permeabilised cell preparations to examine the role of soluble rather than vesicular membrane proteins. In the case of several of these preparations, including adrenal chromaffin cells, PC12 cells, $GH_3$ cells, mast cells and brain synaptosomes, an essential requirement for soluble cytosolic proteins can be demonstrated[16]. Work on adrenal chromaffin cells and PC12 cells has resulted in the identification of some of these soluble proteins. The approach was to use digitonin-permeabilised cells, which leak essential soluble proteins slowly, and 'cracked' PC12 cells in which all soluble proteins are rapidly washed away. The different permeabilisation protocols for the two cell types probably explains why different proteins have been identified with each assay. In work on PC12 cells, a pro-

tein called p145 was identified[67]. This 145 kDa protein exists as a dimer in the native state, is not related to any known protein and is required for $Ca^{2+}$-dependent triggering of exocytosis. Because of its large native size, p145 leaks only slowly from digitonin-permeabilised chromaffin cells and, therefore, in the chromaffin cell assay would not be a rate-limiting factor. However, three other proteins have been identified as candidates for mediators of exocytosis in permeabilised chromaffin cells[2,42]. These are annexin II, a $Ca^{2+}$- and phospholipid-binding protein[2], Exo1, which is a set of polypeptides also known as the 14-3-3 family[43], and Exo2, which is the catalytic subunit of cAMP-dependent protein kinase $C^{[42]}$. Interestingly, the stimulatory effects of both p145 and Exo1 are enhanced by protein kinase C activation, which is known to increase the extent of exocytosis (see also Chapter 9). Exo1 (14-3-3 proteins) and annexin II share a conserved 16 residue domain that is present at the C-terminus of the annexins. A synthetic peptide based on this domain partially inhibited secretion from permeabilised chromaffin cells, demonstrating that this sequence has a key role in exocytosis[54]. Both p145 and Exo1 are present in brain and Exo1 is known to be axonally transported to the nerve terminal. However, the function of these proteins in neurotransmitter release from synapses is not yet known. Studies of this sort should continue to identify soluble proteins that are required for, or regulate, exocytosis.

It seems certain that multiple proteins are required for exocytosis and that these will include cytosolic and both intrinsic and extrinsic membrane proteins (Fig. 1.6). Further work will be required to determine the nature of the interactions between the soluble and membrane proteins and to determine which proteins are the essential components of the exocytotic fusion machine.

## 5   Summary

Much is now known about the nature of the $Ca^{2+}$ signal that activates exocytosis. Some insights into the protein machinery leading to membrane fusion have begun to appear and it seems likely that multiple proteins are involved. Three major questions remain to be answered in this field. First, what is the exact role of the intracellular $Ca^{2+}$ stores in regulating and modulating the $Ca^{2+}$ signal caused by $Ca^{2+}$ entry? One possibility here is that the major role of the $Ca^{2+}$ stores is in the recovery phase. Alternatively, $Ca^{2+}$ release from stores may regulate intracellular events associated with neurotransmitter supply, for example for protein synthesis by post-translational (e.g. phosphorylation of tyrosine hydroxylase) or transcriptional (e.g. increase in peptide precursor mRNA) mechanisms. Second, what is the nature of the $Ca^{2+}$ entry pathways activated by the $Ins(1,4,5)P_3$-mobilising agonists that do not activate voltage-sensitive $Ca^{2+}$ channels? Third, which proteins are the essential components of the membrane-fusion machinery and how does membrane fusion occur? Progress is being rapidly made in all of these areas and the study of proteins involved in exocytosis is currently moving ahead at an exciting rate. In addition, studies of exocytosis with the patch-clamp capacitance method have allowed direct measurement of individual fusion events[45]. This method monitors directly the increase in plasma membrane capacitance

resulting from secretory vesicle membrane insertion at the time of single exocytotic fusion events. An early event appears to be the formation of a transient, reversible fusion pore[10,41]. Further application of this technique will allow more direct investigation of the mechanisms involved and, hopefully, a full understanding of $Ca^{2+}$-dependent exocytosis will emerge within the next few years.

## References

1. Alder J, Lu B, Valtorta F, Greengard P and Poo M (1992) Calcium-dependent transmitter secretion reconstituted in Xenopus oocytes: requirement for synaptophysin. *Science* **257:** 657–661
2. Ali SM, Geisow MJ and Burgoyne RD (1989) A role for calpactin in calcium-dependent exocytosis in adrenal chromaffin cells. *Nature* **340:** 313–315
3. Almers W (1990) Exocytosis. *Annual Reviews of Physiology* **52:** 607–624
4. Archer BT, Ozcelik T, Jahn R, Francke U and Sudhof TC (1990) Structures and chromosomal localizations of two human genes encoding synaptobrevins 1 and 2. *Journal of Biological Chemistry* **265:** 17267–17273
5. Artalejo CR, Garcia AG and Aunis D (1987) Chromaffin cell calcium channel kinetics measured isotopically through fast calcium, strontium and barium fluxes. *Journal of Biological Chemistry* **262:** 915–926
6. Artalejo CR, Mogul DJ, Perlman RL and Fox AP (1991) Three types of bovine chromaffin cell $Ca^{2+}$ channels: facilitation increases the opening probability of a 27 pS channel. *Journal of Physiology* **444:** 213–240
7. Augustine GJ, Adler EM and Charlton MP (1991) The calcium signal for transmitter secretion from presynaptic nerve terminals. *Annals of the New York Academy of Sciences* **635:** 365–381
8. Augustine GJ and Neher E (1992) Calcium requirements for secretion in bovine adrenal chromaffin cells. *Journal of Physiology* **450:** 247–271
9. Berridge MJ (1993) Inositol trisphosphate and calcium signalling. *Nature* **361:** 315–325
10. Breckenridge LJ and Almers W (1987) Currents through the fusion pore that forms

during exocytosis of a secretory vesicle. *Nature* **328:** 814–817

11. Brose N, Petrenko AG, Sudhof TC and Jahn R (1992) Synaptotagmin: a calcium sensor on the synaptic vesicle surface. *Science* **256:** 1021–1025

12. Burgoyne RD (1991) Control of exocytosis in adrenal chromaffin cells. *Biochimica et Biophysica Acta* **1071:** 174–202

13. Burgoyne RD and Cheek TR (1987) Reorganisation of peripheral actin filaments as a prelude to exocytosis. *Bioscience Reports* **7:** 281–288

14. Burgoyne RD, Cheek TR, Morgan A *et al.* (1989) Distribution of two distinct $Ca^{2+}$-ATPase-like proteins and their relationship to the agonist-sensitive calcium store in bovine adrenal chromaffin cells. *Nature* **342:** 72–74

15. Burgoyne RD, Geisow MJ and Barron J (1982) Dissection of stages in exocytosis in adrenal chromaffin cells with the use of trifluoperazine. *Proceedings of the Royal Society of London, Series B* **216:** 111–115

16. Burgoyne RD and Morgan A (1993) Regulated exocytosis. *Biochemical Journal* **293:** 305–316

17. Burgoyne RD, Morgan A and O'Sullivan AJ (1989) The control of cytoskeletal actin and exocytosis in intact and permeabilized chromaffin cells: role of calcium and protein kinase C. *Cell Signalling* **1:** 323–334

18. Cena V, Stutzin A and Rojas E (1989) Effects of calcium and Bay K-8644 on calcium currents in adrenal medullary chromaffin cells. *Journal of Membrane Biology* **112:** 255–265

19. Cheek TR (1991) Calcium regulation and homeostasis. *Current Opinion in Cell Biology* **3:** 199–205

20. Cheek TR (1992) Calcium signalling and the triggering of secretion in adrenal chromaffin cells. *Pharmacological Therapeutics* **52:** 173–189

21. Cheek TR, Barry VA, Berridge MJ and Missiaen L (1991) Bovine adrenal chromaffin cells contain an inositol 1,4,5-trisphosphate-insensitive but caffeine-sensitive $Ca^{2+}$ store that can be regulated by intraluminal free $Ca^{2+}$. *Biochemical Journal* **275:** 697–701

22. Cheek TR and Burgoyne RD (1985) Effect of activation of muscarinic receptors on intracellular free calcium and secretion in bovine adrenal chromaffin cells. *Biochimica et Biophysica Acta* **846:** 167–174

23. Cheek TR and Burgoyne RD (1986) Nicotine evoked disassembly of cortical actin filaments in bovine adrenal chromaffin cells. *FEBS Letters* **207:** 110–113

24. Cheek TR and Burgoyne RD (1987) Cyclic AMP inhibits both nicotine stimulated actin dissassembly and catecholamine secretion from bovine adrenal chromaffin cells. *Journal of Biological Chemistry* **262:** 11663–11666

25. Cheek TR and Burgoyne RD (1992) The cytoskeleton in secretion and neurotransmitter release. In: Burgoyne RD (ed), *The Neuronal Cytoskeleton.* pp 309–325, Wiley-Liss, New York,

26. Cheek TR, Jackson TR, O'Sullivan AJ, Moreton RB, Berridge MJ and Burgoyne RD (1989) Simultaneous measurement of cytosolic calcium and secretion in single bovine adrenal chromaffin cells by fluorescent imaging of fura-2 in co-cultured cells. *Journal of Cell Biology* **109:** 1219–1227

27. Cheek TR, Morgan A, O'Sullivan AJ, Moreton RB, Berridge MJ and Burgoyne RD (1993) Spatial localization of agonist-induced $Ca^{2+}$ entry in bovine adrenal chromaffin cells: different patterns induced by histamine and angiotensin II and relationship to catecholamine release. *Journal of Cell Science* **105:** 913–921

28. Cheek TR, O'Sullivan AJ, Moreton RB, Berridge MJ and Burgoyne RD (1989) Spatial localization of the stimulus-induced rise in cytosolic $Ca^{2+}$ in bovine adrenal chromaffin cells: distinct nicotinic and muscarinic patterns. *FEBS Letters* **247:** 429–434

29. Cheek TR, O'Sullivan AJ, Moreton RB, Berridge MJ and Burgoyne RD (1990) The caffeine-sensitive store in bovine adrenal chromaffin cells: An examination of its role in triggering secretion and $Ca^{2+}$ homeostasis. *FEBS Letters* **266:** 91–95

30. Cheek TR and Thastrup O (1989) Internal $Ca^{2+}$ mobilization and secretion in bovine adrenal chromaffin cells. *Cell Calcium* **10:** 213–221

31. Chow RH, von Ruden L and Neher E (1992) Delay in vesicle fusion revealed by electrochemical monitoring of single secretory events in adrenal chromaffin cells. *Nature* **356:** 60–63

32. Eberhard DA and Holz RW (1987) Cholinergic stimulation of inositol phosphate formation in bovine adrenal chromaffin cells: distinct nicotinic and muscarinic mechanisms. *Journal of Neurochemistry* **49:** 1634–1643

33. Ito S, Mochizuki-Oda N, Hori K, Ozaki K, Miyakawa A and Negishi M (1991) Characterization of prostaglandin $E_2$-induced $Ca^{2+}$ mobilization in single bovine adrenal chromaffin cells by digital image microscopy. *Journal of Neurochemistry* **56:** 531–540

34. Katoaka Y, Ohara-Imaizumi M, Ueki S and Kumakura K (1988) Stimulatory action of gamma-aminobutyric acid on catecholamine secretion from bovine adrenal chromaffin cells measured by a real time monitoring system. *Journal of Neurochemistry* **50:** 1765–1768

35. Kim KT and Westhead EW (1989) Cellular responses to $Ca^{2+}$ from extracellular and intracellular sources are different, as shown by simultaneous measurements of cytosolic $Ca^{2+}$ and secretion from bovine chromaffin cells. *Proceedings of the National Academy of Sciences, USA* **86:** 9881–9885

36. Kitayama S, Ohtsuki H, Morita K, Dohi T and Tsujimoto A (1990) Bis-oxonol experiment of plasma membrane potentials of bovine adrenal chromaffin cells: depolarizing stimuli and their possible interaction. *Neuroscience Letters* **116:** 275–279

37. Leveque C, Hoshino T, David P *et al.* (1992) The synaptic vesicle protein synaptotagmin associates with calcium channels and is a putative Lambert–Eaton myasthenic syndrome antigen. *Proceedings of the National Academy of Sciences, USA* **89:** 3625–3629

38. Llinas R, McGuiness TL, Leonard CS, Sugimori M and Greengard P (1985) Intraterminal injection of synapsin I or calcium/calmodulin-dependent protein kinase II alters neurotransmitter release at the squid giant synapse. *Proceedings of the National Academy of Sciences, USA* **82:** 3035–3039

39. Llinas R, Sugimori M and Silver RB (1992) Microdomains of high calcium concentration in a presynaptic terminal. *Science* **256:** 677–679

40. Mochizuki-Oda N, Mori K, Negishi M and Ito S (1991) Prostaglandin $E_2$ activates $Ca^{2+}$ channels in bovine adrenal chromaffin cells. *Journal of Neurochemistry* **56:** 541–547

41. Monck JR and Fernandez JM (1992) The exocytotic fusion pore. *Journal of Cell Biology* **119:** 1395–1404

42. Morgan A and Burgoyne RD (1992) Exo1 and Exo2 proteins stimulate calcium-dependent exocytosis in permeabilized adrenal chromaffin cells. *Nature* **355:** 833–835

43. Morgan A, Wilkinson M and Burgoyne RD (1993) Identification of Exo2 as the catalytic subunit of protein kinase A reveals a role for cyclic AMP in $Ca^{2+}$-dependent exocytosis in chromaffin cells. *EMBO Journal* **10:** 3747–3752

44. Neher E and Augustine GJ (1992) Calcium gradients and buffers in bovine chromaffin cells. *Journal of Physiology* **450:** 273–301

45. Neher E and Marty A (1982) Discrete change of cell membrane capacitance observed under conditions of enhanced secretion in bovine adrenal chromaffin cells. *Proceedings of the National Academy of Sciences, USA* **79:** 6712–6716

46. Neher E and Zucker S (1993) Multiple calcium-dependent processes related to secretion in bovine chromaffin cells. *Neuron* **10:** 21–30

47. Nichols RA, Sihra TS, Czernik AJ, Nairn A and Greengard P (1990) Calcium/calmodulin-dependent protein kinase II increase glutamate and noradrenaline release from synaptosomes. *Nature* **343:** 647–651

48. O'Sullivan AJ and Burgoyne RD (1989) A comparison of bradykinin angiotensin II and muscarinic stimulation of cultured bovine adrenal chromaffin cells. *Bioscience Reports* **9:** 243–252

49. O'Sullivan AJ, Cheek TR, Moreton RB, Berridge MJ and Burgoyne RD (1989) Localization and heterogeneity of agonist-induced changes in cytosolic calcium concentration in single bovine adrenal chromaffin cell from video-imaging of fura-2. *EMBO Journal* **8:** 401–411

50. Perin MS, Fried VA, Mignery GA, Jahn R and Sudhof TC (1990) Phospholipid binding by a synaptic vesicle protein homologous to the regulatory region of protein kinase C. *Nature* **345:** 260–263

51. Popov SV and Poo M-m (1993) Synaptotagmin: a calcium sensitive inhibitor of exocytosis. *Cell* **73:** 1247–1249

52. Robinson IM and Burgoyne RD (1991) Characterisation of inositol 1,4,5-trisphosphate-sensitive and caffeine-sensitive calcium stores in digitonin-permeabilised adrenal chromaffin cells. *Journal of Neurochem*istry **56:** 1587–1593

53. Robinson IM, Cheek TR and Burgoyne RD (1992) $Ca^{2+}$ influx induced by the $Ca^{2+}$-ATPase inhibitors 2,5-di-(*tert*-butyl)-1,4-benzohydroquinone and thapsigargin in bovine adrenal chromaffin cells. *Biochemical Journal* **288:** 457–463

54. Roth D, Morgan A and Burgoyne RD (1993) Identification of a key domain in annexin and 14-3-3 proteins that stimulate calcium-dependent exocytosis in permeabilized adrenal chromaffin cells. *FEBS Letters* **302:** 207–210

55. Schiavo G, Benfenati F, Poulain B *et al.* (1992) Tetanus and botulinum-B neurotoxins block neurotransmitter release by proteolytic cleavage of synaptobrevin. *Nature* **359:** 832–835

56. Shoji-Kasai Y, Yoshida A, Sato K *et al.* (1992) Neurotransmitter release from synaptotagmin-deficient clonal variants of PC12 cells. *Science* **256:** 1820–1823

57. Smith SJ and Augustine GJ (1988) Calcium ions, active zones and synaptic transmitter release. *Trends in Neuroscience* **11:** 458–464

58. Sollner T, Whiteheart SW, Brunner M, Erdjument-Bromage H, Geromanos S, Tempst P and Rothman JE (1993) SNAP receptors implicated in vesicle targeting and fusion. *Nature* **362:** 318–324

59. Stauderman KA and Murawsky MM (1991) The inositol 1,4,5-triphosphate- forming agonist histamine activates a ryanodine-sensitive $Ca^{2+}$ release mechanism in bovine adrenal chromaffin cells. *Journal of Biological Chemistry* **266:** 19150–19153

60. Stauderman KA and Pruss RM. (1990) Different patterns of agonist-stimulated increase of $^3H$-inositol phosphate isomers and cytosolic $Ca^{2+}$ in bovine adrenal chromaffin cells: comparison of the effects of histamine and angiotensin II. *Journal of Neurochemistry* **45:** 946-953

61. Sudhof TC, Czernik AJ, Kao H-T *et al.* (1989) Synapsins: mosaics of shared and individual domains in a family of synaptic vesicle phosphoproteins. *Science* **245:** 1474–1479

62. Sudhof TC and Jahn R (1991) Proteins of synaptic vesicles involved in exocytosis and membrane recycling. *Neuron* **6:** 665–677

63. Thomas L, Hartung K, Langosch D *et al.* (1988) Identification of synatophysin as a hexameric channel protein of the synaptic vesicle membrane. *Science* **242:** 1050–1053

64. Thomas P, Wong JG and Almers W (1993) Millisecond studies of secretion in single rat pituitary cells stimulated by flash photolysis of caged $Ca^{2+}$. *EMBO Journal* **12:** 303–306

65. Valtorta F, Benfenati F and Greengard P (1992) Structure and function of the synapsins. *Journal of Biological Chemistry* **267:** 7195–7198

66. Vitale ML, Rodriguez Del Castillo A, Tchakarov L and Trifaro J-M (1991) Cortical filamentous actin disassembly and scinderin redistribution during chromaffin cell stimulation precede exocytosis, a phenomenon not exhibited by gelsolin. *Journal of Cell Biology* **113:** 1057–1067

67. Walent JH, Porter BW and Martin TFJ (1992) A novel 145 kd brain cytosolic protein reconstitutes $Ca^{2+}$-regulated secretion in permeable neuroendocrine cells. *Cell* **70:** 765–775

# 2 Co-transmission

Peter Sneddon

For many years, it was thought that each neurone released but one transmitter substance at its terminals. This view prevailed even in the 1970s, but since that time it has become abundantly clear that single-substance neurotransmission is the exception rather than the rule. Most neurones release multiple transmitter substances – known collectively as co-transmitters – ranging from simple organic compounds, such as monoamines or amino acids, to relatively large polypeptides. In this chapter Peter Sneddon considers the classes of compound that have been found to be co-released from nerve terminals along with the classical neurotransmitters and describes their effects, individually and together, on the innervated effector tissue. Important in the context of this book, the possible role of the released co-transmitters in modulating their own release or release of other transmitters is considered.

## 1 Introduction

Fundamental to a proper understanding of the mechanisms and control of transmitter release is the identification of the substance or substances that act as neurotransmitters at the nerve terminal. Most of the experimental analyses that have led to our understanding of neurotransmitter-release mechanisms were performed with the underlying assumption that a single transmitter was released from the nerve. The purpose of this chapter is to draw the reader's attention to the many recent studies which indicate that in a wide variety of nerve types there is more than one neurotransmitter. In some instances, this has important implications for our understanding of the physiological and pharmacological properties of the process of neurotransmission and its modulation.

## 1.1 Historical perspective of the co-transmitter hypothesis

As recently as the early 1980s, co-transmission was regarded by most researchers as an interesting curiosity and a phenomenon which could account for the unusual responses to nerve stimulation seen in a few autonomically innervated smooth muscles. Now, most researchers in the field are coming round to the view that co-transmission is the rule rather than the exception in neurotransmission. The purpose of this historical review is to chart the main ideas that have brought about this important change in our understanding of neuronal function.

### 1.1.1 Classical autonomic pharmacology

The pioneering studies of neurotransmission, performed chiefly by Sir Henry Dale and his colleagues in the 1930s[8] firmly established the simple axiom of autonomic neurotransmission, i.e. that sympathetic nerves use noradrenaline and parasympathetic nerves use acetylcholine as their sole neurotransmitter substance. Dale proposed that, in view of the metabolic unity of a given neurone, all the terminals of that nerve would release the same transmitter. Whilst this does not preclude the involvement of several co-transmitters in autonomic nerves, subsequent influential texts (see, for example, ref. 9) adopted the idea that only a single transmitter was involved. In retrospect, whilst this was a reasonable interpretation of the data available in Dale's era, it seems to have become a dogma that perhaps hindered the interpretation of subsequent experimental findings. Examination of physiology and pharmacology textbooks shows that the simple principle of one nerve using one transmitter was almost universally accepted for almost half a century, and even today, most of the popular textbooks give an account of peripheral and central neurotransmission based on the single-transmitter hypothesis.

There were several strands of investigation that established co-transmission as an important concept. These can broadly be divided into (i) functional studies, in which responses of certain isolated smooth muscle preparations were found not to show the responses that would be expected of classical noradrenergic or cholinergic nerves, and (ii) (immuno) histochemical studies that showed co-localisation of two or more transmitters in the same nerve terminal.

### 1.1.2   Early evidence for co-transmission

In the late 1950s, the work of Burn and Rand[2,3] provided a stimulating 'false start' to the concept of co-transmission in autonomic nerves. They suggested that noradrenergic neurones release acetylcholine, which then acts prejunctionally to promote noradrenaline release. Even though this 'cholinergic link' hypothesis in noradrenergic nerves is no longer considered tenable, it did provide a considerable challenge to the idea that autonomic neurotransmission is a simple, single transmitter process.

In the 1960s, as new and more selective drugs became available, the pharmacology of autonomic neurotransmission was intensely investigated. Burnstock and his colleagues in Australia found that the responses of many isolated smooth muscle preparations could not be explained in terms of classical noradrenergic and cholinergic mechanisms. They adopted the term 'non-adrenergic, non-cholinergic' (NANC) nerves to indicate this new class of autonomic nerves and set about trying to establish the identity of the NANC neurotransmitter. By the early 1970s, evidence had been accumulated to support the proposal that the endogenous purine adenosine 5'-triphosphate (ATP) was the NANC neurotransmitter. The evidence supporting what Burnstock called 'purinergic nerves' was presented in his landmark review of this topic in 1972[4].

At this point, it should be stated clearly, particularly in view of what is to be said below about ATP, that the purinergic nerve hypothesis is also a single-transmitter hypothesis, i.e. it envisaged that a separate set of nerves exists that are analogous to noradrenergic or cholinergic nerves but use ATP as the single transmitter. The fact that ATP has subsequently been proposed as a co-transmitter in sympathetic nerves with noradrenaline and in parasympathetic nerves with acetylcholine has sometimes led to confusion about purinergic nerves. For example, later in this chapter it will be shown how stimulation of sympathetic nerves in the vas deferens produces a response which has 'purinergic' and 'noradrenergic' components, but these nerves should not be referred to as purinergic nerves (nor, in fact, should they strictly be called noradrenergic nerves!). A detailed description of the role of ATP as a neurotransmitter in vas deferens is given below. Since the advent of the idea of purinergic nerves in the early 1970s, few hypotheses have generated as much heated debate and intense investigation, and today there are still some researchers who are sceptical of their existence. Whatever the merits of the purinergic nerve hypothesis, it has certainly been one of the main factors that has stimulated investigation into the idea of co-transmission in autonomic nerves.

### 1.1.3  Establishing the co-transmitter hypothesis

In retrospect, we can now see that there was considerable evidence for co-transmission accumulating throughout the 1970s, but the idea was given its first real impetus by the review by Burnstock[5] in 1976 in which he posed the question, 'Do some nerve cells release more than one transmitter?' The review answered the question in the affirmative, although the experimental evidence available at the time was far from conclusive and was open to a variety of interpretations. The early evidence for co-transmission emerged when studies investigating mechanical responses of isolated smooth muscles to stimulation of NANC nerves began to be reassessed in terms of the possibility of co-transmission. Chief amongst these preparations was the isolated vas deferens of rodents, which, for such a simple preparation, seems to have played an extraordinarily important role in the unravelling of the co-transmitter story. The result of a variety of studies on the vas deferens, looking in detail at mechanical responses, release of neurotransmitter and electrophysiological responses, all combined to provide strong evidence that ATP and noradrenaline act as co-transmitters to mediate the complex mechanical response of the muscle to stimulation of its sympathetic innervation. This evidence is summarised in considerable detail below, since it was not only the first, but still by far the most complete set of data that provides evidence for the functional significance of co-transmitters. Similar evidence has subsequently supported the idea of ATP as a co-transmitter with noradrenaline in sympathetic nerves or with acetylcholine in parasympathetic nerves in a wide variety of autonomically innervated tissues, such as the smooth muscle of the urinary bladder, and in vascular smooth muscle.

In parallel with these functional studies

came a series of biochemical and histological studies indicating that nerve terminal varicosities contain several putative neurotransmitters. ATP was found to co-exist with noradrenaline in chromaffin granules of the adrenal medulla and in vesicles isolated from sympathetic neurones, whilst the emergence of immunohistochemical techniques enabled the identification of putative peptide co-transmitters. Since the survey of the localisation of neuropeptides began in the mid 1970s, the field has expanded from a handful of putative neuropeptides to what is now a catalogue of around 40 different peptides. These have been co-localised in various combinations in almost every type of neuronal tissue. In contrast to the co-transmitter evidence involving ATP, there have been few studies that have clarified the functional significance of the co-localised peptides. Notable exceptions are the studies by Lundberg and his colleagues on VIP as a co-transmitter with acetylcholine in the salivary glands of the cat, which neatly combined histological and functional experimental investigations[14]. In this case, the main role of VIP seems to be to produce vasodilatation and modulate the release of acetylcholine. However, in most instances, the role of co-localised peptides as co-transmitters is unclear, and this is obviously an important area for future investigation.

## 1.2  Definition of co-transmission

A host of substances are released by nerve stimulation, including glycoproteins, enzymes, inorganic ions, metal ions, phospholipids, purines, amines, peptides, etc. Amongst this cocktail of chemicals will be one or more substances that are accepted as neurotransmitters. Deciding which chemicals should be awarded the status of transmitter or co-transmitter is not as obvious as might be supposed. The broadest definition of a co-transmitter would be any substance that, when released from the nerve, transmits a message, either to surrounding cells or back to the nerve, and thereby modulates their function. However, these chemicals are usually subdivided into the various categories of neurotransmitter, neuromodulator or trophic factor, often in a somewhat arbitrary fashion. Indeed, many of the released substances are accorded no function or status and are just regarded as by-products of the neurotransmission process. Any definition of co-transmission is bound to be influenced by our knowledge of how conventional neurotransmitters are expected to act. Therefore, based on our knowledge of acetylcholine and noradrenaline, a putative transmitter should be synthesised in the nerve terminal, stored in vesicles, released as quantal packets upon nerve stimulation, act on specific receptors on the effector cells to produce a rapid response and then be inactivated by a combination of enzymes and uptake mechanisms. These criteria may also be applied to putative co-transmitters, and substances such as ATP, 5-hydroxytryptamine (5-HT) and dopamine fulfil the criteria. Substances that are released from the nerve, but do not fulfil these criteria, may fit the definitions of neuromodulator or trophic factor. A neuromodulator is generally considered to be a substance that does not itself act directly on the effector cell to elicit a response but acts to modify the function of the primary transmitter, either by influencing how it interacts with the effector cell, or by acting back on the nerve to modify the release of the primary transmitter. Trophic factors are thought of as substances which elicit no direct response in the effector tissue and do not directly modify the neurotransmission process. However, they do promote some long-term metabolic or regulatory change within the nerve or effector tissue that, over a longer period, will alter the responsiveness of the system to nerve activity. Neuromodulators and trophic factors may also be released from non-neuronal sites and act to modify the neurotransmission process.

Throughout the 1980s, the number of different combinations of putative (co-) transmitters steadily grew, and by 1987, the term 'chemical coding' was introduced to describe subpopulations of neurones, each with a specific set of transmitters that perform different functions. The term 'plurichemical transmission' has also been used to describe neurotransmission involving several substances[11]. This term seems to be entirely synonymous with the word co-transmission. In many nerves, it seems clear that one substance can be regarded as a primary transmitter, and other substances co-released act in a supporting role as co-transmitters.

The section below, which details some of the experimental evidence supporting co-transmission, concentrates on mammalian efferent autonomic peripheral neurones from which the strongest evidence for co-transmission has been accumulated. However, it should be noted that considerable evidence now exists for co-localisation of putative co-transmitters in the central nervous system (CNS), peripheral autonomic ganglia, sensory neurones and somatic motor nerves, not only in mammals but also in invertebrates, crustaceans, insects, amphibians and birds. (For details see the recent review by Kupferman[13].)

## 2  Co-transmitter synthesis, storage and release

The early work of Blaschko and his colleagues in the 1950s not only established the synthetic pathway for noradrenaline but also established that ATP exists in high concentrations and is stored with noradrenaline in chromaffin granules of the adrenal medulla. It was subsequently shown that isolated noradrenergic nerve vesicles could also store and release ATP, together with noradrenaline. Although this is now seen as early evidence for co-transmission, it was not regarded as such at the time, and most researchers explained the presence of ATP as a substance involved in the storage and packaging of noradrenaline in the sympathetic vesicle. There are a wide variety of biochemical estimates of the relative amounts of noradrenaline to ATP stored in sympathetic vesicles, ranging from the original estimate of 4:1, to more recent, and probably more reliable, estimates of 20:1 to 50:1. Soon after ATP was identified as a constituent of noradrenergic nerve terminal vesicles, it was found that it was also stored together with acetylcholine in cholinergic nerve terminals.

Considerable impetus has been given to the co-transmitter hypothesis by histological studies investigating the distribution of peptides in neurones. Particular advances were made in the late 1970s as immunohistochemical techniques were used to localise an ever increasing number of putative peptide neurotransmitters. There is now a vast literature that documents thousands of examples of co-localisation of peptides in all kinds of neurones. (For review see ref. 11). A survey of this literature presents a bewildering variety of combinations of peptides that have been shown to be co-localised. Unfortunately, there is no consistent pattern that would provide some insight into the functional significance of the co-existence of the various peptides. In some neurones, as many as four or five peptides have been shown to be co-localised. For example, the secretomotor neurones in the guinea-pig small intestine show immunoreactivity to CCK (cholecystokinin), CGRP (calcitonin gene-related peptide), GAL (galanin), NPY (neuropeptide Y) and somatostatin, whilst sensory neurones in the guinea-pig skin stain positively for CCK, CGRP, DYN (dynorphin) and substance P. In guinea-pig uterine arteries, vasodilator neurones have been shown to contain VIP, DYN, NPY and somatostatin.

An important combination seems to be the co-storage of one or more peptides along with non-peptide neurotransmitters. A particularly good example of this is NPY, which is one of the most abundant neuropeptides found in the CNS and peripheral neurones, where it is often found in combination with noradrenaline (see review in ref. 15). In the case of the guinea-pig vas deferens, NPY co-exists with two non-peptide neurotransmitters: ATP and noradrenaline. In the CNS, neocortical neurones contain both VIP and acetylcholine.

One relevant point, which probably has functional significance, is that while the non-peptide transmitters such as ATP, noradrenaline and acetylcholine are synthesised locally within the nerve terminal, neuropeptide production is usually restricted to the ribosomes within the nerve cell body. The peptide must then be transported in vesicles from the cell soma to the nerve terminals by the relatively slow process of axonal transport. This means that relatively small amounts of peptide are available for release, and stores would be slow to replenish after a burst of nerve activity. Biochemical estimates indicate that the concentration of peptides stored in the nerves is usually several orders of magnitude less than the concentration of the classical co-transmitter. In general, however, the peptides tend to have high affinity for their receptors and therefore act at much lower concentrations than the conventional neurotransmitters, often being active in the nanomolar range, compared with the micromolar concentrations associated with non-peptide transmitters.

## 2.1  Subpopulations of storage vesicles

An important aspect of co-transmission, which has functional ramifications, is whether co-transmitters occur packaged together in a homogeneous population of synaptic vesicles, or whether different transmitters occur in separate subpopulations of vesicles. There is some indication that the latter is more likely. Subpopulations of neurotransmitter vesicles can be analysed biochemically after subcellular fractionation of homogenised tissues. Notwithstanding the possibility of cross contamination of vesicle subpopulations, which makes this technique open to criticism, a fairly clear pattern has emerged from these experiments in which peptide neurotransmitters are stored only in large dense-cored vesicles, whilst non-peptides, such as acetylcholine, noradrenaline, 5-HT and ATP, are found both in small vesicles and sometimes in the larger vesicles with the peptide.

Differential storage of co-transmitters opens up the possibility that different proportions of the various co-transmitters are released during a period of nerve activity. Also, if different co-transmitters are mobilised or replenished at different rates, then the response to nerve stimulation might change during a period of prolonged nerve activity. For example, it is often found that higher frequencies of stimulation are required to release co-transmitter peptides than to release conventional transmitters, such as noradrenaline and acetylcholine.

Unfortunately, conventional light microscopy does not have sufficient spatial resolution to allow immunocytochemical techniques to be used to identify in which vesicles transmitters are localised, but the higher resolution of the electron microscope, in conjunction with double-labelling studies, has been used to identify more precisely the localisation of neurotransmitters. These studies have confirmed the co-storage in the same large, dense-cored vesicle of noradrenaline with opioid peptides, substance P with 5-HT, and CGRP with substance P in various types of nerve terminal. However, it bears repeating that, although there is a wealth of experimental evidence demonstrating co-localisation of several neuropeptides in a single neurone and even in single vesicles, this is not sufficient evidence to assume that the substances are co-transmitters. In many studies, the putative transmitters have been shown to be present in the soma of the neurone, but not necessarily in the nerve terminals. Even when the substance is shown to be released from the nerve, there are few studies that demonstrate how it contributes to neurotransmission. Obviously this is an area that requires much more investigation to establish the functional significance of the plethora of co-existing neuronal peptides.

## 2.2 Co-release of transmitters

Data from experiments in which the efflux of putative co-transmitters into the perfusate was measured by biochemical analysis have also been put forward to support the co-transmitter hypothesis. In the late 1970s, experiments in which the efflux of radiolabelled noradrenaline and adenosine was measured provided evidence to support a role for ATP as a co-transmitter in sympathetic nerves. Exogenously added [$^3$H]-adenosine was presumed to be taken up by nerves and converted to [$^3$H]-ATP, which was subsequently released upon nerve stimulation. However, this type of study was criticised on the basis that the released purine might have come from other pools that could have become loaded with exogenous adenosine, such as those in muscle cells. More recent studies in which the release of endogenous ATP was measured by high-pressure liquid chromatography (HPLC) or by luciferin–luciferase assays appear to confirm that only some of the measured ATP is being released from nerves. In guinea-pig vas deferens, it has been estimated that about 32% of the nerve stimulation-evoked efflux of ATP actually comes from the sympathetic nerve, the majority probably originates from smooth muscle cells when they are stimulated by noradrenaline acting on $\alpha_1$-adrenoceptors[28]. It has been shown that stimulation of the sympathetic nerves to the guinea-pig vas deferens co-releases noradrenaline, ATP and NPY into the perfusate[12]. It has been proposed that noradrenaline and ATP packaged in small synaptic vesicles are released at low stimulation rates, whilst NPY, which only occurs in large vesicles, is only released during periods of higher frequency bursts of nerve activity.

In summary, there is an abundance of evidence to show that many types of nerve synthesise, store and release several putative neurotransmitter substances. What is much less clear is what role these various substances play in the neurotransmission process. In the next section, consideration is given to experimental data concerning the actions of putative co-transmitters on their effector tissues, and also to evidence concerning co-transmitter action prejunctionally to modulate transmitter release.

## 3 Functional significance of co-transmission

A consideration of how the nervous systems of animals have evolved suggests that neurones containing several transmitters were common even in the earliest and simplest creatures. Many invertebrates have been shown to have neurones with multiple transmitters. For example, studies on the cholinergic neurones innervating the body wall of the leech and cholinergic neurones in the giant neurones of the mollusc *Aplysia* have shown that these not only contain acetylcholine but also contain peptide co-transmitters including FMRF amide (Phe-Met-Arg-Phe-amide). The large size of these neurones has enabled the combination of co-transmitter peptides to be identified in individual cells and it has also allowed this to be related to the function of the nerve cell, for example in the control of buccal muscle responses to motor nerve stimulation in *Aplysia*[7]. An inspection of neurones from various species across different stages of the evolutionary tree, from crustaceans, insects, amphibians, birds and mammals, shows that co-transmission is a feature common to all the groups, but there is no clear indication whether co-transmission is an evolutionarily more primitive or advanced trait in neuronal development.

### 3.1 Why have more than one transmitter?

Given the wide variety of examples of co-transmission, it is likely that there is no one explanation for why multiple transmitters occur that covers all the different situations. The most plausible explanations are considered below. First, it is worth considering the evolution of the nervous system in relation to multiple transmitters. Since the complex organisation of nerves in higher animals is thought to have evolved from the primitive nervous systems of the lower orders, it may be that there has been selection of a single or dominant transmitter for specialised functions as an adaptation to provide a more efficient form of neurotransmission, while the other co-transmitters were selected against. For example, in sympathetic nerves where both dopamine and noradrenaline are synthesised and released, noradrenaline might have won the evolutionary battle for selection because it was a more effective agonist at the α-adrenoceptors that were evolving on the effector tissues. Also, the suggestion that nervous and endocrine tissues evolved from common origins raises the possibility that nerves have retained the ability to synthesise several potential transmitter substances as a relic of their previous neuroendocrine roles.

From the above, it follows that some substances that are co-released from nerves may be 'non-transmitters' performing no functional role and simply exist as evolutionary relics, which continue to exist simply because they were never selected against. However, it is also clear that, in some cases, co-transmitters could have important functional roles, in terms of the function of both the nerve and the target tissues. In the nerves, the co-transmitters might act to assist in the storage of the main transmitter, perhaps to maintain its stability. For example, in noradrenergic nerve terminal varicosities, it was originally proposed that ATP was stored together with noradrenaline in order to balance the ionic charges within the storage vesicle. The co-transmitters might also act to modulate the release of the main transmitter by stimulating prejunctional receptors to enhance or inhibit subsequent release of neurotransmitters. Furthermore, if there is more than one transmitter available for release, then the nerve's capacity to respond to different patterns of stimulation might be enhanced. For example, if the nerve can only store and release a small amount of transmitter A, then during periods of prolonged activity, transmitters B or C could be released as reserves. In some circumstances, the physiological function of an organ might require a short burst of high-frequency nerve activity that releases one transmitter, while during other periods it might require a slow tonic release of another transmitter.

Postjunctionally, having more than one transmitter could enhance the flexibility of the effector tissue's response. Obviously several different transmitters can simultaneously pass on several different messages to the effector tissues. The most common pattern is where different substances act synergistically to enhance the other's actions. However, note that co-released substances may act not only on the same target cells in the tissues but also on different target cells. For example, the dual action of acetylcholine and VIP in salivary glands produces vasodilation and secretory cell stimulation. This was one of the earliest examples of functional synergism of co-transmitters in parasympathetic nerves[14].

Since each transmitter could activate a different effector pathway within the cell, then desensitisation or tachyphylaxis, which might be incurred if a single pathway were involved, might be avoided as a consequence of co-transmission. For example, contraction of vascular smooth muscle can be produced by release of $Ca^{2+}$ from an intracellular store by a transmitter which stimulates inositol trisphosphate production, or by $Ca^{2+}$ influx through ion channels opened following receptor activation by a different transmitter.

One of the most extensively investigated examples of the postjunctional actions of co-transmitters is that of ATP and noradrenaline released from the sympathetic nerves innervating the rodent vas deferens. This will be described in some detail since it exemplifies many of the features that demonstrate the physiological relevance of co-transmission and the potential pharmacological significance of the variety of receptor subtypes that are involved.

### 3.2 The rodent vas deferens as a model in which to distinguish postjunctional actions of co-transmitters

In rat vas deferens a single stimulus to the sympathetic nerves produces a biphasic contraction of the smooth muscle (Fig. 2.1). The initial peak is thought to be mediated by

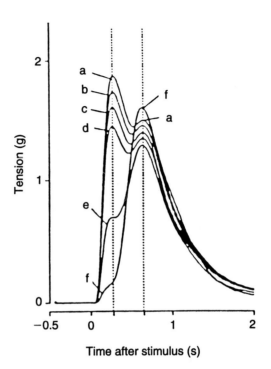

Fig. 2.1. Co-transmission in rat vas deferens. The contractile response of rat vas deferens to a single stimulus to the sympathetic nerves is biphasic, as shown in the control trace (a). The first phase of the contraction is reduced by increasing concentrations of the putative $P_2$ purinoceptor antagonist suramin (b, 0.1 μM; c, 1 μM; d, 10 μM; e, 100 μM; and f, 1 mM). The second component is not inhibited by suramin but is readily abolished by α-adrenoceptor antagonists, not shown. (From ref. 17.)

ATP, and the second by noradrenaline. The most compelling arguments in favour of this interpretation have come from pharmacological investigations using selective antagonists (see ref. 27). The initial phase of the response is selectively reduced by agents which inhibit the action of ATP on $P_2$ purinoceptors, such as suramin, whilst the second phase is selectively reduced by $α_1$-adrenoceptor antagonists. In guinea-pig and rabbit vas deferens, a single stimulus of the sympathetic nerves produces little or no mechanical response, and, therefore, trains of pulses, usually from

2–32 Hz applied for 10–30 s, are used to investigate the neurogenic response. As with the rat, in these tissues the response to trains of pulses is biphasic, with an initial peak occurring after 3–4 s, which then subsides before a second phase occurs that reaches a plateau after about 10 s. Again, antagonist studies have provided convincing evidence that the initial phasic component of this sympathetic response is mediated by ATP and the second component by noradrenaline (see Fig. 2.2). The first clear pharmacological evidence for ATP as a co-transmitter came from studies using the photo-affinity label arylazidoaminopropionyl-ATP (ANAPP$_3$), which was shown to inhibit the initial phase of the sympathetic contraction in vas deferens and also the contraction to exogenous ATP. However, it had no effect on the second phase of the neurogenic response or on the contractions produced by noradrenaline or other agonists. This result was confirmed by using the stable ATP analogue $\alpha,\beta$-methylene-ATP ($\alpha,\beta$-mATP) to produce selective desensitisation of P$_2$ purinoceptors in the tissue. All components of the mechanical response are abolished by guanethidine and 6-hydroxydopamine, which selectively destroy noradrenergic nerves, indicating that the ATP is not released from a separate population of purinergic nerves. Conversely, reserpine, which depletes noradrenaline from noradrenergic nerves, inhibits the second component of the response but not the initial phasic contraction.

An important feature relevant to the function of the vas deferens is that the smooth muscle cells in different regions of the tissue seem to have different relative sensitivities to ATP and noradrenaline. It has been shown recently that segments of vas deferens taken from the prostatic (distal) region of the rat, rabbit or guinea-pig vas deferens are approximately ten times more sensitive than epididymal (proximal) segments to exogenous ATP (or the stable analogue $\alpha,\beta$-mATP) whilst segments from the epididymal region are at least ten times more sensitive than prostatic segments to application of exogenous $\alpha$-

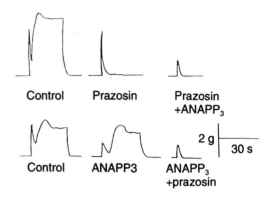

Fig. 2.2. The effect of selective antagonists on the biphasic contraction in rabbit isolated vas deferens. Trains of pulses at 16 Hz for 30 s produced a biphasic contraction (control panels). The initial phasic component was selectively reduced by the P$_2$ purinoceptor antagonist ANAPP$_3$, whereas the secondary, tonic contraction was selectively blocked by $\alpha_1$-adrenoceptor antagonists, such as prazosin. (From ref. 25.)

adrenoceptor agonists such as noradrenaline[23]. This implies that, even if the sympathetic nerves release constant amounts of noradrenaline and ATP throughout a train of pulses, the purinergic and noradrenergic contribution to the neurogenic response will vary considerably from one region of the organ to another. The physiological function of the vas deferens is to propel sperm from the epididymis to the urethra. Therefore, the slow maintained contraction at the epididymal end could help to direct the sperm toward the urethra during the rapid expulsion produced by the phasic contraction at the prostatic end.

### 3.2.1  Electrophysiological evidence for co-transmission in the vas deferens

In vas deferens, ATP and noradrenaline appear to activate separate transduction mechanisms to produce contraction. Activation of P$_2$ purinoceptors by ATP produces depolarisation of the muscle, manifested as an excitatory junction potential, or EJP.

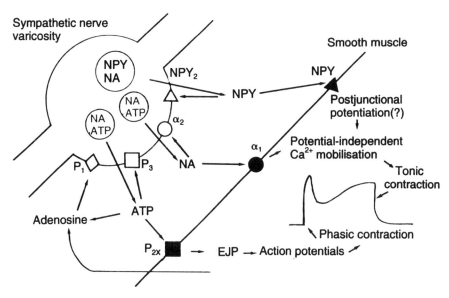

Fig. 2.3. Neurotransmission in sympathetic nerves involving ATP, noradrenaline (NA) and NPY as co-transmitters. There may be subpopulations of vesicles within the nerve terminal varicosities, which could allow for different ratios of release of ATP:noradrenaline:NPY at different stimulation durations and intensities. Each transmitter produces a different effect on the smooth muscle cells: ATP mediating rapid depolarisation (EJPs) and phasic contraction, whilst noradrenaline produces a slow, maintained contraction, possibly caused by release of internal $Ca^{2+}$ stores. NPY at the concentrations achieved during low-frequency nerve stimulation probably has a predominantly prejunctional action, but it may also act postjunctionally to enhance the action of both ATP and noradrenaline by a mechanism that is not yet clear. ATP may act on $P_3$ purinoceptors to inhibit transmitter release. Adenosine, either from the smooth muscle or from degradation of neuronal ATP, may act on $P_1$ purinoceptors to inhibit release. Prejunctional $\alpha_2$-adrenoceptors, stimulated by released noradrenaline, appear to be the most important modulator of transmitter release and mediate inhibition.

Trains of EJPs will summate to produce action potentials that result in an influx of $Ca^{2+}$ through voltage-sensitive channels, leading to the initial, rapid contraction. Noradrenaline, however, does not appear to contribute significantly to the nerve-mediated membrane depolarisation; $\alpha_1$-adrenoceptor stimulation probably mediates the slow phase of the neurogenic contraction by generation of the second messenger $Ins(1,4,5)P_3$, which is able to release $Ca^{2+}$ stored in the sarcoplasmic reticulum (see Chapter 1). When EJPs were first recorded in vas deferens in the early 1960s, it was assumed that they were mediated by noradrenaline, which was the

established transmitter in sympathetic nerves. This view prevailed for about 20 years until selective antagonists of ATP became available. It could then be shown that EJPs in guinea-pig vas deferens were almost abolished by the $P_2$ purinoceptor antagonist $ANAPP_3$ but were not reduced by selectively low concentrations of $\alpha$-adrenoceptor antagonists[24]. It was shown subsequently in reserpinised animals, in which almost all neuronal noradrenaline was depleted but ATP release continued, that the magnitude of EJPs was not reduced from that seen under control conditions. By comparison, the unexpected action of cocaine

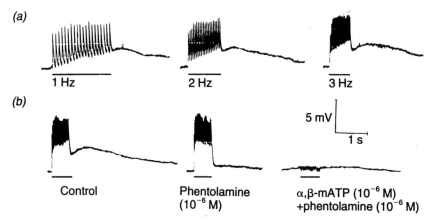

Fig. 2.4. Intracellular microelectrode recordings from individual smooth muscle cells in rat tail artery, illustrating that each stimulus to the sympathetic nerves produced a rapid EJP of about 5 mV. (*a*) Trains of stimuli (20 pulses from 1–3 Hz) also induced a slow, maintained depolarisation of the cell. (*b*) The slow depolarisation at 4 Hz (control) was abolished by the α-adrenoceptor antagonist phentolamine but the rapid EJPs were not altered. The EJPs were abolished after desensitisation of $P_{2x}$ purinoceptors with α,β-mATP. (For further details see ref. 22.)

(which increases synaptic noradrenaline concentrations by preventing its inactivation by reuptake) was to depress the magnitude of EJPs. Subsequent electrophysiological studies using $P_2$ purinoceptor desensitisation by α,β-mATP and the $P_2$ purinoceptor antagonist suramin[21] have supported the proposal that EJPs are mediated by ATP. The $P_2$ purinoceptors in the vas deferens are now defined as $P_{2x}$, in contrast to $P_{2y}$ purinoceptors, which often mediate hyperpolarisation and relaxation of smooth muscles.

The sympathetic nerves in vas deferens also release NPY, which may act both postjunctionally to enhance the action of the other co-transmitters and prejunctionally on $NPY_2$ receptors, which mediate a negative feedback mechanism for modulating neurotransmitter release. These studies, combined with other work, led to the proposal of the model for sympathetic neurotransmission that is depicted in Fig. 2.3. Many of the features of this model of co-transmission also appear to apply to a variety of autonomically innervated smooth muscles, particularly arteries.

## 3.3   Co-transmission in arteries

Sympathetic neurotransmission in many arteries seems to involve ATP, noradrenaline and various peptides including NPY. In arteries, the electrical response of the muscle to the co-transmitters is more complex than in vas deferens. Each stimulus to the sympathetic nerves produces a rapid EJP similar in magnitude, time course and pharmacological profile to that in the vas deferens, but in arteries a train of pulses produces a slow depolarisation, which is mediated by noradrenaline (see Fig. 2.4). The figure shows that the α-adrenoceptor antagonist phentolamine blocks the slow depolarisation produced by a train of pulses, but the rapid EJPs are blocked by $P_2$ purinoceptor desensitisation with α,β-mATP. The contribution that ATP and noradrenaline make to sympathetic vasoconstriction varies enormously from one artery to another[26]. For example, in rat tail artery and rabbit pulmonary artery, ATP seems to make little or no contribution to sympathetic vasoconstriction. In rat and dog mesenteric arteries and rabbit ileocolonic arteries, there is often a biphasic response with purinergic and noradrenergic phases analogous to those seen in vas deferens, while in rabbit saphenous artery and small jejunal arteries the sympathetic vasoconstriction is largely mediated by ATP.

As well as releasing ATP and noradrenaline, the sympathetic nerves in vas deferens and in some blood vessels also release NPY. At present, it is not clear what functional role NPY plays in the neurotransmission process. In some arteries NPY is a potent vasoconstrictor, but in the low concentrations released its predominant action may be to potentiate the constrictor effects of noradrenaline. Alternatively, it might inhibit noradrenaline release by a prejunctional action. Electrophysiological investigations in vas deferens have shown that NPY can reduce the magnitude of EJPs by prejunctional inhibition of ATP release (see below). The lack of a selective NPY antagonist makes it difficult to confirm the role it plays in sympathetic vasoconstriction[19].

In some human arteries, it has been found recently that vasoactive peptides are released not only from sympathetic nerves (NPY with noradrenaline) but also from parasympathetic nerves (VIP with histidine isoleucine and acetylcholine) and sensory nerves (CGRP with tachykinins). The peptides appear to serve as co-transmitters in the sympathetic and parasympathetic nerves only at high stimulation frequencies but are released from sensory nerves during low-frequency stimulation[16].

## 4 Prejunctional modulation of co-transmitter release

### 4.1 Modulation of their own release by co-transmitters

The idea that a neurotransmitter can act not only postjunctionally on the effector cell but also prejunctionally on autoreceptors to modulate its own release was first established in sympathetic nerves. Here noradrenaline was shown to be able to promote its own release via prejunctional β-adrenoceptors and then, at higher concentrations, inhibit its own release via prejunctional α-adrenoceptors (see Chapters 5 and 14). Physiologically, the β-adrenoceptors probably respond to circulating adrenaline, which is a far more potent β-adrenoceptor agonist than noradrenaline.

The fact that several co-transmitters are released from some nerves could imply that each transmitter individually plays a role in the modulation of transmitter release. In turn, this raises the possibility that several different mechanisms are involved in the modulation process. The additional fact that different transmitters are often stored in different subpopulations of neurotransmitter vesicles raises the possibility that modulatory mechanisms operate to modify the relative amounts of each transmitter being released. Furthermore, presynaptic modulation of transmitter release is known to be dependent upon stimulation frequency (see Chapter 5), and the relative amounts of co-transmitter released also depends upon stimulation frequency. For example, in those neurones in which a peptide acts as a co-transmitter with ATP, noradrenaline or acetylcholine, it has been found that release of the peptide often occurs at higher frequencies of stimulation than those required for the non-peptide.

As an example of some of the above concepts, consider Fig. 2.3. This figure shows the situation that exists in sympathetic nerves in the rodent vas deferens and arteries, which have been extensively studied to determine the role of the three putative co-transmitters, ATP, noradrenaline and NPY, in modulation of transmitter release. Noradrenaline acts on prejunctional $\alpha_2$-adrenoceptors to modulate its own release and the release of ATP and NPY. The important role of noradrenaline-mediated autoinhibition of (co-) transmitter release can be demonstrated by the use of $\alpha_2$-adrenoceptor antagonists, such as yohimbine, which greatly enhance both phases of the sympathetic contractile response and also enhance the EJPs, which are purely purinergic. There is also clear evidence that stimulation

Table 2.1. *Examples of prejunctional receptors that regulate the release of putative co-transmitters*

| Nerve / tissue type | Putative co-transmitters | Prejunctional receptor | Role in modulation of release |
|---|---|---|---|
| Sympathetic nerves in vas deferens, some arteries, etc. in various species | ATP | $P_1$ purinoceptor ($A_1$-subclass) | Possible inhibition |
| | | $P_3$ purinoceptor (?) | Possible inhibition |
| | NA | $\alpha_2$-Adrenoceptor | Inhibition |
| | NPY | $NPY_2$ | Inhibition (at high stimulation rates |
| Cholinergic nerves of cat submandibular gland | ACh | Muscarinic | Inhibition |
| | VIP | VIP | Inhibition |
| Some cholinergic cortical neurones | PHI | ? | ? |
| Ventral spinal cord in rat CNS | 5-HT | $5\text{-}HT_1$ | Inhibition |
| | | $5\text{-}HT_2$ | Enhancement |
| | SP | SP | Inhibition |
| | TRH | ? | No effect |
| Cholinergic projection nerves to rat ventral hippocampus | ACh | Muscarinic | Inhibition |
| | Galanin | Galanin | Inhibition |

For details see ref. 1.
NA, noradrenaline; ACh, acetylcholine; PHI, peptide histidine isoleucine; TRH, thyrotrophin releasing hormone

of prejunctional purinoceptors inhibits both phases of the neurogenic contraction and reduces EJP magnitude. The prejunctional purinoceptors are stimulated by adenosine and its analogues, and, since they are selectively blocked by compounds such as 8-sulphonylphenyltheophylline, they are classified as $P_1$ purinoceptors. These receptors could respond to adenosine coming from the breakdown of neuronally released ATP, or adenosine from other sources, such as the effector smooth muscle (see Chapter 7). It has been proposed that, in vas deferens and some arteries, ATP *per se* can inhibit transmitter release by acting on a novel class of purinoceptors[20] designated $P_3$.

Besides noradrenaline and ATP, the release of transmitters from vas deferens is probably also inhibited by the third co-transmitter released from sympathetic nerves, NPY, acting at the $NPY_2$ subclass of receptor (at least it has been shown that exogenous NPY can reduce transmitter release). Since NPY is thought to be released only during higher-frequency bursts of nerve stimulation, this putative negative feedback mechanism may complement the $\alpha_2$-adrenoceptor mediated autoinhibition mechanism that can be demonstrated at stimulation frequencies as low as 0.5 Hz. Therefore, during stimulation with a prolonged train of pulses, the regulation of transmitter release would change as a function of the concentrations of the various transmitters present. (For a detailed discussion of this topic see ref. 1).

Analogous co-transmitter-mediated auto

regulatory mechanisms seem to operate in peripheral parasympathetic nerves and in cholinergic nerves in the CNS. For example, in cat salivary gland, the release of the co-transmitters acetylcholine and VIP is reduced by negative feedback of acetylcholine acting on prejunctional muscarinic receptors; VIP also inhibits transmitter release. A comparable mechanism has also been found in those cholinergic neurones of the cerebral cortex which utilise VIP as a co-transmitter. Table 2.1 gives some examples of autoreceptors that are thought to modulate transmitter release in nerves in which co-transmission has been established.

## 4.2  Modulation of co-transmitter release by other endogenous substances

Circulating hormones and autacoids can modulate co-transmitter release. One interesting recent example is the finding that in guinea-pig vas deferens angiotensin II enhances ATP-mediated EJPs in normal tissues, but after noradrenaline depletion by reserpine, angiotensin II inhibits EJPs, possibly as the result of the generation of prostaglandins[29]. Prostaglandin $E_2$ ($PGE_2$) has been shown to reduce EJP magnitude in vas deferens. Conversely, it has also been reported that $PGE_2$ enhances ATP efflux (estimated biochemically) but reduces the efflux of [³H]-noradrenaline from guinea-pig vas deferens[10]. A further example of modulation of the release of co-transmitters is illustrated by the action of somatostatin in the rabbit ear artery[18], where noradrenaline and ATP are thought to act as co-transmitters. When applied to the artery, the polypeptide somatostatin had no direct effect, but it did inhibit the vasoconstriction produced by sympathetic nerve stimulation. Somatostatin appeared to produce this effect by a prejunctional action to inhibit transmitter release (as indicated by reduced efflux of [³H]-noradrenaline) and by a postjunctional action to inhibit the constrictor effect of noradrenaline, but not of ATP. The fact that

somatostatin-like immunoreactivity has been found in perivascular nerves implies that somatostatin could play a physiological role in modulating sympathetic vasoconstriction.

## 5  Summary

The original concept of defining neurones in the central or peripheral nervous system in terms of a single transmitter, as either cholinergic, noradrenergic or dopaminergic, now seems to be outdated and simplistic. As our knowledge of neurotransmission has improved, the general pattern which has emerged is that, while in some cases one substance is the principal neurotransmitter in a nerve, most nerves also release several other substances that act as co-transmitters. The detailed examples given in this chapter illustrate some important principles of co-transmission.

- Most nerves are able to synthesise and store more than one neurotransmitter, often within subpopulations of storage vesicles.
- Neuropeptides are often stored with noradrenaline, acetylcholine, ATP, etc. but only appear to contribute to neurotransmission during intense stimulation.
- The relative contribution which each co-transmitter makes to the response of the effector tissue varies with the frequency and duration of the nerve activity.
- Co-transmitters act on their own receptors on the effector tissue, which are generally coupled to a separate signal transduction mechanism, allowing different types of response (e.g. phasic or tonic contractions) to occur in the tissue.
- The co-transmitters (or their metabolites) can act on prejunctional autoreceptors to modulate their own release or that of other co-transmitters. The prejunctional autoreceptors are often pharmacologically distinct from the postjunctional receptor.
- The contribution that each co-transmitter makes to a presynaptic or postsynaptic

response varies with the local concentration of co-transmitter, which in turn will vary with the duration and intensity of nerve activity.

It should also be borne in mind that the co-transmitters that a particular nerve utilises may not be fixed but may vary during the development of the animal, perhaps as a result of ageing or disease processes[6].

Finally, while the physiological relevance of co-transmitters is now beginning to be appreciated, the pharmacological significance of the possible pre- and postjunctional interactions between drugs and the different neurotransmitter systems at nerve endings is rarely considered. For example, how will a drug that depletes one co-transmitter, (removing not only its postjunctional effects but also abolishing its prejunctional autoregulatory functions) modify the pattern of release and responsiveness to the other co-transmitters? Specifically, how would the action of reserpine, which depletes sympathetic nerves of noradrenaline but not of ATP or NPY, change the pattern of response in the tissues innervated? Noradrenaline would no longer produce its postjunctional excitatory action, or its prejunctional inhibitory action to modulate the release of ATP. Alternatively, how would a drug that inhibits the inactivation of one co-transmitter affect the release and effects of the others? Specifically, cocaine, by inhibiting neuronal uptake of noradrenaline, would lead to an increased synaptic concentration of noradrenaline. The noradrenaline-dependent postjunctional effects would be increased but so would its prejunctional negative feedback effect, which would reduce the release of ATP and NPY. Whilst the complex interactions of several co-transmitters activating multiple pre- and postjunctional mechanisms certainly make pharmacological investigations more complex, they also present wider opportunities for more subtle modification of the neurotransmission process, which could ultimately be exploited to therapeutic advantage.

## References

1. Bartfai T, Iverfeldt K and Fisone G (1988) Regulation of the release of co-existing neurotransmitters. *Annual Reviews of Pharmacology and Toxicology* **28**: 285–310
2. Burn JH and Rand MJ (1959) Sympathetic postganglionic mechanisms. *Nature* **184**: 163–165
3. Burn JH and Rand MJ (1965) Acetylcholine in noradrenergic transmission. *Annual Reviews of Pharmacology and Toxicology* **5**: 163–182
4. Burnstock G (1972) Purinergic nerves. *Pharmacological Reviews* **24**: 509–581
5. Burnstock G (1976) Do some nerve cells release more than one transmitter? *Neuroscience* **1**: 239–248
6. Burnstock G (1990) Changes in expression of autonomic nerves in aging and disease. *Journal of the Autonomic Nervous System* **30**: S25–S34
7. Church PJ and Lloyd PE (1991) Expression of diverse neuropeptide cotransmission by identified motor neurons in Aplysia. *Journal of Neuroscience* **11**: 618–625
8. Dale HH (1935) Pharmacology and nerve endings. *Proceedings of the Royal Society of Medicine* **28**: 319–322
9. Eccles JC (1957) *The Physiology of Nerve Cells*. Johns Hopkins University Press, Baltimore, MD
10. Ellis JL and Burnstock G (1990) Modulation by prostaglandin $E_2$ of ATP and noradrenaline cotransmission in guinea-pig vas deferens. *Journal of Autonomic Pharmacology* **10**: 363–372
11. Furness JB, Morris JL, Gibbins IL and Costa M (1989) Chemical coding of neurons and plurichemical transmission. *Annual Reviews of Pharmacology and Toxicology* **29**: 389–406
12. Kasakov L, Ellis J, Kirkpatrick K, Milner P and Burnstock G (1988) Direct evidence for concomitant release of noradrenaline, adenosine 5′-triphosphate and neuropeptide Y from sympathetic nerve supplying the guinea-pig vas deferens. *Journal of the Autonomic Nervous System* **22**: 75–82
13. Kupferman I (1991) Functional studies of cotransmission. *Physiological Reviews* **71**: 683–732
14. Lundberg JM (1981) Evidence for coexistence of vasoactive intestinal polypeptide (VIP) and

acetylcholine in neurons of cat exocrine glands. *Acta Physiologica Scandinavica* **112:** 1–57

15. Lundberg JM, Franco-Cereceda A, Hemsen A, Lacroix JS and Pernow J (1990) Pharmacology of noradrenaline- and neuropeptide tyrosine (NPY)-mediated sympathetic cotransmission. *Fundamental Clinical Pharmacology* **4:** 373–391

16. Lundberg JM, Franco-Cereceda Lacroix JS and Pernow J (1991) Release of vasoactive peptides from autonomic and sensory nerves. *Blood Vessels* **28:** 27–34

17. Mallard NJ, Marshall RW, Sithers AJ and Spriggs TLB (1992) Suramin: a selective inhibitor of purinergic neurotransmission in the isolated rat vas deferens. *European Journal of Pharmacology* **220:** 1–10

18. Maynard KI, Saville VL and Burnstock G (1991) Somatostatin modulates vascular sympathetic neurotransmission in the rabbit ear artery. *European Journal of Pharmacology* **196:** 125–131

19. Pernow J, Modin A and Lundberg JM (1992) No effect of D-myo-inositol-1,2,6-trisphosphate on vasoactive constriction evoked by neuropeptide Y and non-noradrenergic sympathetic nerve stimulation. *European Journal of Pharmacology* **222:** 171–174

20. Shinozuka K, Bjur RA and Westfall DP (1988) Characterization of prejunctional purinoceptors on noradrenergic nerves of the rat caudal artery. *Naunyn-Schmiedeberg's Archives of Pharmacology* **338:** 221–227

21. Sneddon P (1992) Suramin inhibits excitatory junction potentials in guinea-pig vas deferens.

*British Journal of Pharmacology* **107:** 101–103

22. Sneddon P and Burnstock G (1984) ATP as a cotransmitter in rat tail artery. *European Journal of Pharmacology* **106:** 149–152

23. Sneddon P and Machaly M (1992) Regional variation in purinergic and noradrenergic responses in isolated vas deferens of rat, rabbit and guinea-pig. *Journal of Autonomic Pharmacology* **12:** 421–428

24. Sneddon P and Westfall DP (1984) Pharmacological evidence that adenosine triphosphate and noradrenaline are co-transmitters in the guinea-pig vas deferens. *Journal of Physiology* **347:** 561–580

25. Sneddon P, Westfall DP, Colby J and Fedan JS (1984) A pharmacological investigation of the biphasic nature of the contractile response of rabbit and rat vas deferens to field stimulation. *Life Science* **35:** 1903–1912

26. Starke K, von Kügelgen I, Bulloch JM and Illes P (1991) Nucleotides as cotransmitters in vascular neuroeffector transmission. *Blood Vessels* **28:** 19–26

27. von Kügelgen I and Starke K (1991) Noradrenaline and ATP cotransmission in the sympathetic nervous system. *Trends in Pharmacological Sciences* **12:** 319–324

28. von Kügelgen I and Starke K (1991) Release of noradrenaline and ATP by electrical stimulation and nicotine in guinea-pig vas deferens. *Naunyn Schmiedeberg's Archives of Pharmacology* **344:** 419–429

29. Ziogas J and Cunnane TC (1991) An electrophysiological study of angiotensin II at the sympathetic neuroeffector junction in the guinea-pig vas deferens. *British Journal of Pharmacology* **103:** 1196–1202

# 3 Models and mechanisms of neurotransmission

Maxwell R. Bennett

It would not be unreasonable to presume from the preceding chapters, or from the study of elementary accounts elsewhere of neurotransmission, that an action potential passing down the axon inevitably and invariably results in an episode of neurotransmitter release from every vesicle-containing varicosity or nerve terminal. In this chapter, Maxwell Bennett shows that this is not so: indeed the probability of any one potential release site actually releasing neurotransmitter during the passage of an action potential is extremely low. Here, the concept of quanta – minimal packets of neurotransmitter molecules – and quantised release is considered in some detail together with the statistical principles that best describe such release.

## 1 Chemical theory of neurotransmission

In his landmark paper of 1905, which founded the chemical theory of synaptic transmission, Elliott[16] commented that 'In all vertebrates the reaction of any plain muscle to adrenalin is of a similar character to that following excitation of the sympathetic (thoracico-lumbar) visceral nerves supplying that muscle'. He also wrote 'that adrenalin excites not the muscle fibre directly, but a substance developed out of it, and in consequence of the union of the sympathetic axon with it'. These prescient statements were ultimately confirmed by experimentation that led to the establishment of the idea that transmission at neuro-effector junctions involves the secretion of a chemical substance that acts on a 'receptive substance' in the muscle fibres[38]. By the outbreak of the First World War, adrenaline was recognised as the most likely transmitter for sympathetic nerves and a muscarine-like substance for parasympathet-ic nerves. However, it was not until some twenty years later that acetylcholine was shown definitively to be the transmitter at the somatic neuromuscular junction. Now it is well accepted that with very few exceptions all communication between neurones and other neurones or effector organs is chemical and is achieved by the release of stored neurotransmitter that diffuses through the synapse to affect the postsynaptic elements.

With the introduction of electrophysiological techniques to study neuro-effector transmission by Bremer[7] in 1932, the attempt was made to identify the electrical signs of the action of the chemical transmitter on the effector cell membrane. The unequivocal demonstration that acetylcholine mediated transmission from the vagus nerve to the heart, by Loewi and his colleagues[30], made this a particularly attractive preparation to begin an electrophysiological investigation of neuro-effector transmission. In 1934, Brown and Eccles[9] discovered that if the vagal volley is set up late in a cardiac cycle then that

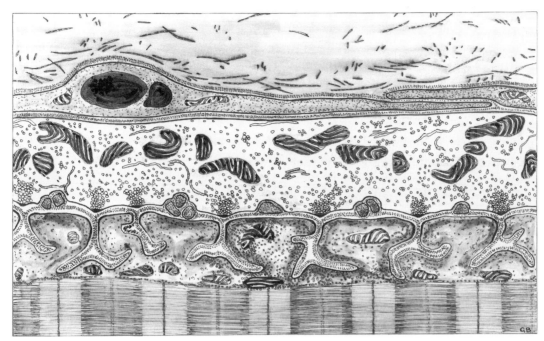

Fig. 3.1. A diagrammatic representation of the single motor nerve terminal synapse on an amphibian muscle cell. A longitudinal section through a portion of a nerve terminal branch is shown on the muscle fibre. Individual neurotransmitter-release sites are present, delineated by the high density of synaptic vesicles, with active zones at which quantal secretion occurs. Length of figure: approximately 8 μm.

cardiac cycle is not inhibited, the latent period of the inhibition being usually 100 ms to 160 ms. Of this period, the conduction time to the region of the pacemaker probably only accounted for about 10 ms, i.e. the greater part of the latent period appears to occur after the arrival of the inhibitory impulses at the nerve fibres of the pacemaker. It is probable that most of this time is occupied by the liberation of the acetylcholine and with its diffusion to the point of its action. This time course of action of acetylcholine came to be regarded as the bench-mark for determining the action of chemical transmitters.

## 2   Release of neurotransmitter measured by intracellular recording

The study of synaptic transmission was revolutionised by the introduction of intracellular recording techniques, which were applied to the neuromuscular synapse by Fatt and Katz[17]. They confirmed that the synaptic potential at motor nerve terminals (called the endplate potential, EPP) had all the appropriate characteristics for the initiation of the muscle fibre action potential: it was suprathreshold for the initiation of the muscle action potential in normal Ringer's solution. Furthermore, the endplate potential was a passive potential that propagated electrotonically from the site of its origin at the endplate (Fig. 3.1). The following year, they reported the exciting discovery of subthreshold EPPs[18]. These potentials had all the characteristics of the EPP except that they were much smaller in amplitude, therefore subthreshold for the initiation of the muscle action potential, and occurred independently of the nerve impulse. It was soon shown, using a statistical analysis described below,

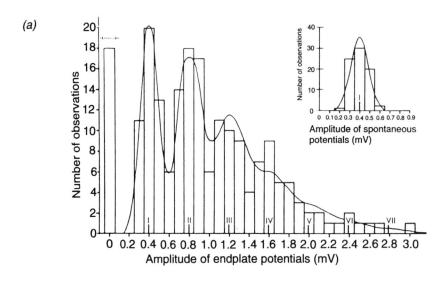

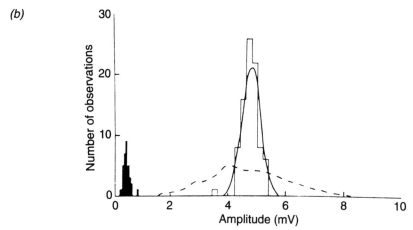

Fig. 3.2. Amplitude–frequency histograms of synaptic potentials at the neuromuscular synapse showing the extent to which they can be predicted by Poisson or binomial statistics, statistics that are used to determine the average probability of secretion of a quantum from the release sites. (*a*) A histogram of EPPs and spontaneous EPPs (inset) from a mature mammalian motor nerve terminal; the peaks of the EPP amplitude distribution tend to occur at integral multiples of the mean amplitude of the spontaneous EPPs; the continuous line gives the predictions of Poisson statistics (from ref. 6, with permission). (*b*) Histograms of EPPs and spontaneous EPPs (filled histogram) from an immature mammalian motor nerve terminal; the amplitude distribution of EPPs is approximately Gaussian; the continuous line gives the predictions of binomial statistics (in which the average probability for secretion $p = 1$ and $n = 12$) and the broken line gives the predictions of Poisson statistics which do not fit the observations at all. (From ref. 2, with permission.)

that the evoked EPP was composed of units equivalent in size to these miniature EPPs[12]. Within ten years of these discoveries on the somatic neuromuscular junction, similar observations were made with intracellular microelectrodes on the autonomic neuromuscular junction. Burnstock and Holman[10] first showed that the synaptic potential (here called the excitatory junction potential, EJP) could be graded in height, this depending on the number of nerves stimulated, as expected given the multiple innervation of the tissue. In addition, spontaneous potentials occurred independently of the nerve impulse and these were taken to be analogous to the spontaneous (miniature) EPPs recorded at the somatic neuromuscular junction[11]. The discovery of EPPs, junction potentials and their miniature equivalents at neuro-effector junctions by the beginning of the 1960s laid the foundations for the analysis of transmitter secretion by electrophysiological means that is described below.

## 3   Is neurotransmitter release quantised?

If motor nerves are stimulated at low frequency in the presence of a $Ca^{2+}$ concentration sufficiently small to ensure that the EPP is subthreshold for initiation of the muscle action potential, then these potentials fluctuate in amplitude from impulse to impulse. These fluctuations are the result of release of neurotransmitter. The smallest potentials have an amplitude similar to that of the spontaneous potentials[13]. If the frequency of occurrence of the evoked potentials that possess a particular amplitude is plotted, then the amplitude distribution has peaks that are integer multiples of the mean size of the spontaneous potentials (Fig. 3.2a).

This observation led to the idea that the spontaneous potentials are the result of leakage of packets of transmitter of fairly uniform size, called quanta, and that the evoked potentials consist of multiples of these quanta[13]. If quanta are drawn from a pool in the nerve terminal, within which all the quanta have equal low probabilities of release on arrival of the nerve impulse, then the frequency distribution of the number of quanta released by each impulse over a large number of impulses should follow Poisson statistics. These statistics are used when studying independent events that are very improbable

but for which a large number of observations can be made, as in traffic accidents or in radioactive emissions. In the present context, the event of a particular quantum being released is very improbable, but large numbers of impulse trials can be used to analyse the process. When applied to neurotransmitter release, Poisson's law states that the probability of $x$ quanta being released over a large number of impulses is

$$p_x = (m^x/x!)e^{-m} \qquad (3.1)$$

where $m$ is the mean number of quanta released over all the trials. The variance (or square of the standard deviation) of this distribution predicted by Poisson statistics is very large, being equal to the mean of the distribution. If there are $N$ impulses, then the Poisson prediction is that $Npx$ of these will contain $x$ quanta, where $p$ is the probability of release occurring. In order to apply this idea to a motor nerve terminal, allowance has to be made for the fact that the quantal size as given by the spontaneous potentials is not invariant but is distributed as a random normal variable with mean $q$ and variance $s$. It follows then that, if Poisson statistics predict that there will be $Np$ occasions on which $x$ quanta will be released, these will follow a normal distribution of amplitude $qx$ and variance $sx$. Under conditions of low release, the predictions of Poisson statistics are good. Therefore, the prediction of a pool of available quanta in the nerve terminal, quanta that are independent and so do not interact and that have a low probability of being released, is likely to be true under these conditions.

However, this prediction that the nerve terminal contains a large pool of non-interacting quanta, each with a low probability of being released on arrival of the nerve impulse, does not always hold for motor nerve terminals. Therefore, it is of interest to enquire into the kind of statistics that do describe quantal release, as this can suggest appropriate models that illustrate the characteristics of the storage and secretion of quanta of neurotransmitter. Poisson statistics fail to describe secretion adequately during development and regeneration of motor nerve terminals (Fig. 3.2*b*); Poisson statistics also do not hold if the rate of quantal release is raised towards physiological levels at mature terminals by increasing the external $Ca^{2+}$ concentration. Under these circumstances, the variance of the distribution of the number of quanta released over many trials is much smaller than that predicted by Poisson statistics but approximates that predicted by binomial statistics[2]. The assumptions of binomial statistics are that there is a relatively small pool of non-interacting quanta, each with a relatively *high* probability of being released on the arrival of the nerve impulse. In this case, the probability can be estimated by consideration of the variance ($s^2$) and the mean ($m$) of the distribution of the number of quanta secreted by each impulse over many trials by

$$p = 1 - s^2/m \qquad (3.2)$$

and the number of non-interacting quanta in the small pool of quanta available for release by the nerve impulse is given by $n = m/p$. There is a reasonably good fit of the binomial prediction to observed quantal releases at normal motor nerve terminals in relatively physiological $Ca^{2+}$ conditions. This suggests that under these conditions the nerve terminals have only a limited supply of quanta available for release.

The fact that a particular statistical distribution gives a reasonable prediction from a set of observations does not mean that the assumptions underlying the theoretical distribution always hold for the system being analysed. Other statistical distributions with different assumptions may also give good predictions. The formulation of these distributions may accord more nearly with other criteria, such as the structure of the nerve terminal and its organelles.

## 4   Are there specialised neurotransmitter-release sites on the nerve terminal?

Some time after Fatt and Katz[18] discovered the quantum of transmitter release, de Robertis[14] identified large numbers of small spherical organelles in nerve terminals with the electron microscope. These organelles (synaptic vesicles) were subsequently shown to contain transmitter substances. It was then natural to suppose that the synaptic vesicles constituted the morphological equivalent of the transmitter quanta, and there is now much evidence to support this idea.

The correlation between the amount of transmitter that gives rise to the spontaneous EPPs, i.e. quanta, with the transmitter in a synaptic vesicle then led to a search for the release sites on the motor nerve terminal from which the quanta are released. Active zones, each consisting of a raised presynaptic membrane passing at right-angles to the longitudinal axis of the motor nerve terminal and possessing large numbers of synaptic vesicles, were identified at about 1 μm intervals along the length of terminal branches. As these active zones possess at least ten synaptic vesicles in close apposition to the terminal membrane, and there are at least 200 active zones at an amphibian motor nerve terminal, then it was deduced that these terminals have several thousand synaptic vesicles available for release by the nerve impulse. It is very difficult to reconcile the occurrence of thousands of vesicles in the motor nerve terminal with the assumption of binomial statistics that there are only a few quanta available for release from the nerve terminal (see Section 3 above). The resolution of this paradox is given below, in which it is shown that neither the assumption that each quantum has the same probability of being secreted nor the assumption that the quanta do not interact is likely to be true.

## 5  Quantal release from sympathetic nerve terminals

Spontaneous subthreshold potentials occur in the smooth muscle of the guinea-pig iris, which has a dense sympathetic innervation[11] (Fig. 3.3). However, the discovery that the temporal characteristics of these spontaneous potentials are very different to those of evoked junction potentials indicated that an analogy could not be drawn between the kinds of potential observed at motor nerve terminals and those at sympathetic nerve terminals. An experimental difficulty is encountered with the study of sympathetic nerve terminals, as the amplitude–frequency distribution of the spontaneous potentials is skewed, with the highest frequency occurring for the smallest potentials, just above the noise level of the recording system[11]. It is not then possible to use the mean and variance of the spontaneous potentials to give a measure of the quantal size of sympathetic neurotransmitter release, as it is possible to do at the neuromuscular junction. The problem of whether there is quantal transmission at sympathetic nerve terminals can only be resolved by methods that circumvent the electrical syncytial properties of smooth muscle. This is necessary because the secretion of transmitter onto a smooth muscle cell gives rise to a potential which propagates with diminution into adjoining muscle cells through the electrical syncytial connections between the cells. The result is that recordings from a single smooth muscle cell include the electrical signs of transmission to that cell as well as the attenuated signs of transmission to adjoining cells that are electrically coupled to the cell in question. Notwithstanding, if transmission from sympathetic nerves is quantal, then a skewed amplitude–frequency distribution of spontaneous potentials would be recorded, and this is what is observed[11]. The quantitative basis of this has been described in a number of theoretical works[1].

Two approaches have been used to determine if there is indeed quantal transmission

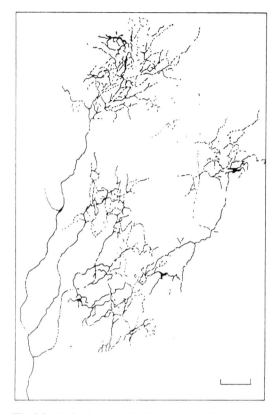

Fig. 3.3. A single sympathetic nerve terminal field on a mammalian iris smooth muscle. The terminal consists of four systems of branches emanating from a single axon in the lower left-hand corner. Each of these branches is composed of strings of varicosities; each varicosity may secrete a quantum of transmitter. Scale bar: 100 μm.

at sympathetic nerve terminals. In the first of these, Hirst and Neild[21] greatly reduced the extent to which the electrical events originating in one muscle cell could propagate into adjacent cells by cutting the muscle under investigation (an arteriole) into very short lengths. Under these conditions, the amplitude–frequency distribution of the spontaneous potentials is unimodal with the smallest potentials much larger than the noise level of the recording, although the distribution is still skewed. An entirely different approach to the problem involves recording from single release sites of sympathetic nerve terminals. In this case, sympathetic nerve terminals on the surface of a muscle are caused to fluoresce with a vital dye ($DiOC_2$), which allows for the clear delineation of the terminal together with its varicosities; the dye can also be used to show living motor nerve terminals on skeletal muscles. This visualisation of individual varicosities and, therefore, release sites that are confined to the varicosities allows for the positioning of an external microelectrode over a single release site. In this way, recordings can be made of the kind already shown for the neuromuscular junction, described above. An advantage of the sympathetic nerve terminals over the motor nerve terminals is that the varicosities of the former are about 4 μm apart[31] whereas the release sites of the latter are immediately adjacent to each other, perhaps only 1 μm apart. This greater separation allows for the relative isolation of the electrical signs of secretion from a single sympathetic varicosity, which can be compared to that from a release site of a motor nerve terminal[19]. Under conditions of electrical isolation, the amplitude–frequency distribution of the spontaneous potentials recorded with an external microelectrode over a varicosity is frequently unimodal (Fig. 3.4).

The amplitude–frequency distribution of the evoked potentials that occur during hundreds of impulses in sympathetic nerve terminals can be well predicted in those cases in which the amplitude–frequency distribution of spontaneous potentials is unimodal. The prediction takes the form of treating the mean and variance of the spontaneous potential distribution as giving a measure of quantal size, as for the motor nerve terminals, and allocating different frequencies to the number of single, double, triple, etc. quantal releases. Hirst and Neild[21] did this for their intracellular recordings from arterioles so as to optimise the fit to the evoked potential distribution. Lavidis and Bennett[29] were able to obtain a good fit to the observed distribution of evoked currents recorded with an extracellular electrode by allocating the different

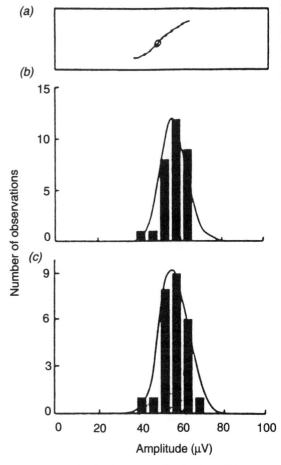

Fig. 3.4. Amplitude–frequency distribution of spontaneous excitatory junctional currents (b) and evoked excitatory junctional currents (c) recorded with a very small diameter electrode (4 μm) from a single visualised varicosity of a sympathetic nerve terminal on the mouse vas deferens. The position of this varicosity and the recording electrode tip are shown in the drawing in (a). Binomial statistics gave the predicted distribution in (c) with a probability for secretion of $p = 0.13$ (From ref. 29, with permission.)

frequencies of single, double, triple, etc. quantal releases according to a binomial distribution. These observations indicate that quantal transmission is likely to occur at sympathetic nerve terminals as it does at motor nerve terminals.

# 6   Is the quantum of transmitter merely an artefact?

It is possible that the electrical manifestation or definition of transmitter quanta arise as a consequence of the saturation of a restricted patch of postsynaptic receptors by the secreted neurotransmitter. Direct experimental evidence against the idea that the acetylcholine molecules that give rise to spontaneous miniature EPPs saturate the postsynaptic receptors at motor nerve terminals was obtained by Hartzell, Kuffler and Yoshikami[20] using the snake neuromuscular junction. They showed that the peak of the response to spontaneous or evoked units of transmitter release adds linearly to the response produced by an appropriate background concentration of acetylcholine from a micropipette. Thus, the amount of transmitter giving rise to spontaneous or unit-evoked potentials does not saturate the receptors, or else the size of these potentials would decrease in the presence of the background concentration of acetylcholine. It should also be noted that inhibition of acetylcholinesterase at these junctions increased the peak amplitude of the spontaneous or evoked potentials by about 25%; this is not the result to be expected if the amount of acetylcholine giving rise to these potentials saturated the receptors beneath the nerve terminal. Further evidence that quantisation is not an artefact arising through saturation of postsynaptic receptors at the endplate comes from experiments in which the quantal size is increased using hypertonic solutions. Solutions made hypertonic with 200 mM sodium gluconate more than double, and sometimes quadruple, the size of spontaneous endplate currents (EPCs) in both the amphibian and mouse neuromuscular junctions. The acetylcholine receptors themselves are not affected by this treatment, but the effect is blocked by vesamicol, which blocks the uptake of acetylcholine into synaptic vesicles, indicating that the hypertonic solutions act presynaptically. Hypertonic solutions appear to ensure that the maximum number of acetylcholine molecules that could be packed into a synaptic vesicle, about 45 000, or about four times the number of molecules normally found in a vesicle, are indeed concentrated in the vesicles. If vesamicol is used in normal solutions and the terminals stimulated, spontaneous potentials immediately decline in amplitude, indicating again that quantal size is determined presynaptically at the endplate.

# 7   Is only one quantum secreted per release site?

Several theoretical studies have argued that the number and distribution of the $Ca^{2+}$ channels at a release site determines the probability of secretion of a quantum from that site (see, for example Zucker and Fogelson[37]). In support of this idea are the observations which show that the extent of transmitter release per unit length of motor nerve terminal is well correlated with the extent of active zone size. In amphibia, for example, more strongly secreting cutaneous pectoris motor nerve terminals have significantly longer active zones on average than the relatively weakly secreting nerve terminals in the sartorius or the cutaneous dorsi muscles. More recently Pawson and Grinnell[32] have succeeded in obtaining freeze–fracture replicas of extensive lengths of single nerve-terminal branches, allowing detailed studies to be made of the distributions of active zone particles along the length of these branches. Their results show that the average length of the double rows of particles at the active zones per 10 μm length of terminal branch does not change much along 100 μm lengths of branch, except at the very ends of the terminals. It is interesting in this context that Ko[27] has shown that, during the competition between motor nerve terminals for muscle fibres that accompanies development, a motor nerve terminal on a fibre may possess mature active zones with vesicle openings whilst an adjoining motor nerve terminal may possess disorganised active zones without vesicle openings. These observations correlate with the finding that during synapse elimination on amphibian muscles one motor nerve terminal may retain its integrity but fail to secrete quanta on arrival of a nerve impulse whilst an adjoining terminal secretes successfully. Opposed to these views that stress the uniformity of the average length of active zones per unit length of nerve terminal are observations that indicate the existence of correlations between the differences in probability of quantal secretion at different release sites along a terminal branch and the length of active zones. For example, the measurement of the largest width of nerve terminal (probably correlated with active zone length) per 10 μm length of nerve terminal along a terminal branch correlates with the maximum probability for secretion of a quantum within that 10 μm length.

As there are many small synaptic vesicles at each of the active zones on motor nerve terminals, it might be anticipated that several quanta could be secreted from an active zone on arrival of the nerve impulse. As the secretion of quanta is dependent on the influx of $Ca^{2+,}$ then raising the external $Ca^{2+}$ concentration to very high levels should saturate the secretory process. When this is done at amphibian motor nerve terminals, the number of quanta secreted in a saturating concentration of 10 mM $Ca^{2+}$ is about 300 to 400. This is of the same order as the number of active zones (about 700 or so) rather than of the number of synaptic vesicles (which is about 35 000 if there are 50 synaptic vesicles at the presynaptic membrane of each active zone). A similar study has been carried out for preganglionic nerve terminals on sympathetic ganglia, for which the maximum number of quanta secreted in relatively high $Ca^{2+}$ levels was about 10. This is about the same as the number of preganglionic nerve terminal varicosities per ganglion cell estimated by Elfvin[15] for cat superior cervical ganglion, rather than the number of synaptic vesicles. More recently, recordings have been made of quantal secretion from small numbers of visualised sympathetic nerve terminal varicosities in the presence of high concentrations of $Ca^{2+}$ (4 mM)[29]. In this case, there is an almost linear correlation between the

maximum number of quanta secreted during a train of nerve impulses and the number of varicosities beneath the recording electrode. These observations on the relationship between the number of quanta secreted and the number of release sites at nerve terminals in the somatic and autonomic nervous systems suggest that each release site secretes at most a single quantum on arrival of the nerve impulse; this seems to be the case even in high $Ca^{2+}$ concentrations. If a quantum of transmitter is contained within a synaptic vesicle, then these results indicate that only one synaptic vesicle participates in secretion at a release site out of the tens that are apparently available there. This argument that only one quantum is secreted per release site implies that some kind of inhibitory mechanism must operate at the site. This would determine that when one vesicle secretes its contents the remaining vesicles at the site are inhibited from secreting during the period of raised probability for secretion, which lasts for a few milliseconds.

At motor nerve terminals, there is a strong negative correlation between the number of small synaptic vesicles remaining in the nerve terminal following treatment with black widow spider venom and the number of quanta secreted[22]. A similar negative correlation exists between the number of remaining synaptic vesicles following treatment with purified α-latrotoxin, which greatly accelerates quantal secretion in a $Ca^{2+}$-free medium, and the number of quanta secreted[22]. The slope of the regression line in each case is −1.1 vesicles per quantum, indicating that it is very unlikely that a quantum arises from the secretion of several vesicles at the one active zone (for a review of this possibility see ref. 35).

The argument that the largest number of quanta secreted by a nerve terminal during a normal nerve impulse is limited by the ability of single release sites to secrete a single quantum does not imply that this is the case under all conditions. Katz and Miledi[25] have shown that if the nerve impulse is greatly extended in duration by blocking the rate of repolarisation of the impulse, with the voltage-dependent $K^+$ channel blocker tetraethylammonium, then the number of quanta secreted is very much in excess of the number of release sites in the terminal (see also Chapter 4). At the amphibian motor nerve terminal, the number of quanta released is raised to over 10 000 by this procedure[25]. This is of the same order as the number of available synaptic vesicles at all the release sites of the terminal (see above). The greatly increased duration of the nerve terminal action potential can, therefore, release many more quanta than a normal action potential. These observations can be reconciled with those above if it is supposed that the secretion of a quantum leaves the release site membrane momentarily refractory to the release of another quantum; this refractory period is longer than that of the normal raised probability for secretion that lasts for only a few milliseconds. If, however, the action potential is greatly prolonged in duration, then, as the end of the refractory period is reached during the plateau phase of the extended action potential, another quantum may be secreted. In this way many quanta may be secreted during a single, long-duration action potential. It remains to be seen whether such a refractory mechanism for secretion exists in the sympathetic nerve terminal.

## 8   Do all release sites have the same probability to secrete a quantum?

Somatic motor nerve terminals consist of hundreds of release sites at which tens of vesicles are in close apposition with the specialised active zones. The question arises as to whether the thousands of synaptic vesicles available for release at the release sites of a nerve terminal all have the same probability for secretion on arrival of the nerve impulse? A variety of different technical approaches to this problem show that release sites in the more proximal part of the nerve terminal, near the last node of Ranvier, have much larger probabilities for the secretion of a quantum than do release sites situated near the ends of terminal branches[3,4,12].

It has been shown in studies on the $Ca^{2+}$ dependence of secretion at different release sites, determined with an extracellular microelectrode, that sites which have a very low capacity for evoked secretion occur amongst sites that have a comparatively high capacity for spontaneous secretion. The findings are as follows: if the extracellular $Ca^{2+}$ concentration is increased from very low levels while recording evoked quantal secretion, then the average number of quanta secreted increases as the fourth power of the $Ca^{2+}$ concentration (see also Chapter 1). It is sometimes observed that, as the $Ca^{2+}$ concentration is increased, more than a single quantum is secreted in response to the nerve impulse. On the assumption that a release site can secrete at most a single quantum in response to a nerve impulse, it can be concluded that a previously silent release site, with, therefore, a very low probability for secreting a quantum, is now participating in secretion. Thus, low-probability release sites must exist amongst relatively high-probability release sites.

What are the implications of these observations on the lack of uniformity of the secretory mechanism within the amphibian neuromuscular junction, especially given the central place of this junction as a paradigm for other synapses[23]? One implication is that the binomial statistical description of transmitter release cannot be correct. This assumes that there is a uniform probability of secretion from a small pool of available quanta, and the observations described above show that this probability is not uniform. One consequence of this is that equation (3.2) should contain a term for the variance in $p$ itself. When this is included, it can be shown that '$n$' is grossly under-estimated. An elegant illustration of this derives from an investigation of crab neuromuscular junctions, which showed that the number of release sites contributing to secretion exceeded the binomial estimate of '$n$' by a wide margin.

It has been suggested that the existence of relatively high-probability sites at the amphibian neuromuscular junction, amongst large numbers of low-probability sites, would explain why binomial statistics gives a reasonable description of evoked quantal secretion at these synapses. Indeed del Castillo and Katz[13] suggested, in their original description of the statistics of quantal secretion, that deviations of evoked quantal secretion from the predictions of Poisson statistics could occur because 'different members of the population may not have the same chances of success, and that for large values of "$m$" some individual units have a high probability and respond almost every time, whilst others have a low probability and contribute to the endplate potential only occasionally. The presence of some units which respond regularly is bound to diminish the statistical fluctuation of the endplate potential.' It has now been shown that this argument only holds if, amongst the hundreds of active zones at the amphibian neuromuscular junction, only a few active zones release quanta during the hundreds of nerve impulse trials over which data is collected, while the remainder do not[5]. If, however, there is a continuous distribution of probabilities for secretion over all the release sites, such as a beta distribution, then Poisson statistics will still describe the evoked release. This will be the case even if the beta distribution has a spatial element to it, such that high probabilities are found on proximal parts of terminal branches and low probabilities on distal parts[5].

The inability of Poisson statistics to predict accurately quantal secretion at reasonably high levels of release means that at least one of the assumptions underlying this statistic, namely that there are a very large number of non-interacting quanta each available for release at a low probability, is wrong. The fact that release probability is not uniform but graded over release sites means that one of the assumptions of binomial statistics is also incorrect. The question then arises as to why binomial statistics gives such a reasonable fit to the observed distributions. At present there is only one theory that provides an explanation for the observations at this stage,

and this requires that the assumption that quanta do not interact is abandoned. There is a period of a few milliseconds following an impulse in a nerve terminal during which there is a raised probability for the secretion of a quantum of transmitter from a release site[26]. If, following an impulse, the secretion of a quantum from a release site leads immediately to a decrease in the probability of secretion from surrounding release sites for a few milliseconds, then binomial statistics will give a very good fit to the observed distributions of quantal releases over many trials[5]. Abandoning the assumption that there is no interaction of quanta leads to a sufficient decrease in the variance of the release for the observed distributions to follow much more nearly binomial statistics than Poisson statistics. However, the question remains as to whether a model is realistic in which the secretion of a quantum at a release site leads to a series of reactions that decrease the probability of secretion at surrounding release sites, at least over a micrometre away, within a few milliseconds.

There are several different ways of studying the probability of quantal secretion at the release sites of autonomic postganglionic nerve terminals. One is to record the EJP in the smooth muscle cells during sympathetic nerve stimulation and then differentiate the rising phase. This allows isolation of the individual contributions of different varicosities to the current that gives rise to the junction potential. Theoretical studies have shown that this approach gives a reliable account of the number of varicosities that contribute quanta to the junction potential. Furthermore, the number of times that a particular varicosity releases a quantum of transmitter over a large number of trials can be determined. According to these criteria, the probability of secretion of a quantum from any varicosity is shown to be very low, of the order of 0.01. In addition, it is clear that there are preferred varicosities from which evoked quanta are secreted, although many more varicosities contribute to the spontaneous secretion of quanta. This description of

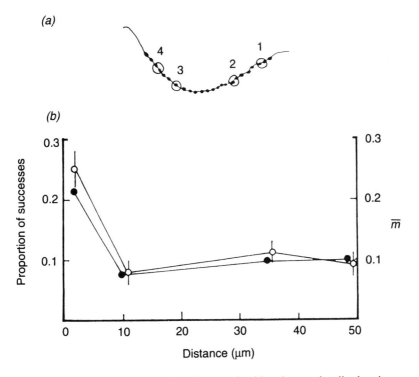

Fig. 3.5. Changes in the secretion of neurotransmitter from varicosities along a visualised varicose sympathetic axon on the surface of the mouse vas deferens, recorded with a small diameter (4 μ) microelectrode. (a) Diagram to show the varicose axon on which ellipses show the outline of the recording electrode tip and numbers indicate the sequence in which the recordings were made. (b) The proportion of stimuli that gave a response at the different recording positions (○) and the average quantal secretion $\bar{m}$ (●) plotted in the direction along the axon branch that gives a decreasing proportion of successes. (From ref. 29, with permission.)

the probability of quantal secretion from sympathetic nerve terminals is similar to that given above for somatic motor nerve terminals.

Another approach to the problem of analysing the probability of quantal secretion at sympathetic nerve terminals has been introduced by Brock and Cunnane[8]. Using external recording electrodes with tip diameters of about 50 μm, they recorded the electrical signs of quantal secretion from sympathetic nerve terminals on the surface of the mouse vas deferens. Some of the excitatory junctional currents they recorded had identical amplitudes and time courses and were, therefore, taken to arise from the same varicosity[8]. On this assumption, the probability of

quantal secretion was observed to vary between 0.005 and 0.8 for different varicosities. Given the occurrence of junctional currents of like amplitude, they concluded also that a single varicosity could release at most a quantum on arrival on the nerve impulse. The more direct method of recording from sympathetic nerve terminals[29], involving the placement of small diameter electrodes (about 4 μm) over the surface of visualised varicosities that have been caused to fluoresce with $DiOC_2$ has also been used. This showed that different varicosities along a single sympathetic nerve terminal have different probabilities for the secretion of a quantum, as is the case for somatic motor nerve terminals (Fig. 3.5).

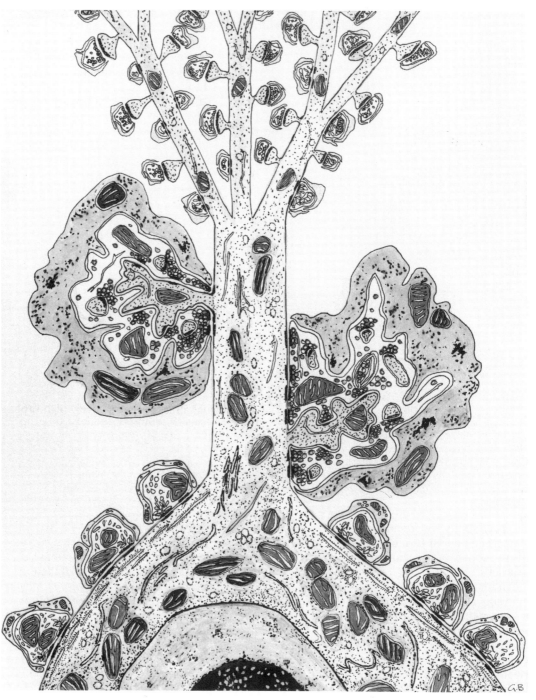

Fig. 3.6.  A single mossy fibre nerve terminal forms a synapse on the apical dendrite of a hippocampal CA3 pyramidal neurone, near the neurone soma, whereas a single recurrent collateral nerve terminal forms a synapse on the distal processes of the dendrite. The mossy fibre synapse consists of the largest bouton in the brain, whereas the recurrent collateral synapse consists of a typical bouton, about 1 μm in diameter, which ends on a dendritic spine. The diameter of the neurone soma is approximately 20 μm.

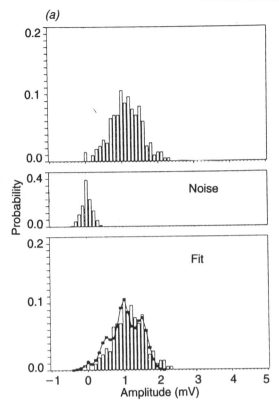

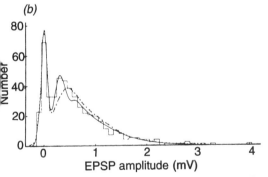

# 9 The probability of neurotransmitter release in the CNS

The probability for the secretion of a quantum has also been examined for boutons in the CNS (for a review of this literature, see ref. 33). It has been shown for group 1A synapses on motoneurones that some boutons of a single axon have very low probabilities (about 0 under the stimulus regimen used) whereas others have probabilities near 1. The same is true of group 1 synapses on dorso-spinal cerebellar tract neurones, in which the release sites of some boutons have a probability for secretion of 1 whereas others have much lower probabilities. The probability of quantal secretion from single mossy fibre synapses and recurrent collaterals to CA3 pyramidal neurones in the hippocampus have also been investigated (Fig. 3.6).

Interestingly, the giant mossy fibre bouton has a low probability for secretion, the amplitude–frequency distributions of the secretions being well fitted by Poisson statistics (Fig. 3.7b). This is in contrast to the relatively high probability for secretion observed at the boutons of recurrent collaterals; the amplitude–frequency distribution of the synaptic potentials here are well fitted by binomial statistics (with an average probability of 0.6). Taken together, it seems very likely that there is a non-uniform probability for the secretion of quanta at different release sites of single axons in the CNS.

Fig. 3.7. The amplitude–frequency distribution of synaptic potentials at synapses formed by (a) a recurrent collateral fibre on a hippocampal CA3 pyramidal cell and (b) a mossy fibre on a CA3 pyramidal cell in the hippocampus. (a) The top rectangle shows the amplitude–frequency distribution of synaptic potentials resulting from stimulation of a single recurrent collateral terminal. The middle rectangle indicates the noise level; and the lower rectangle gives the fit of a binomial distribution (continuous line through filled circles) in which the average probability for secretion is 0.69 and the average quantal secretion is 2.07 (the amplitude of the quantal size was distributed normally with mean 0.51 mV and standard deviation 0.05 mV). (b) The amplitude–frequency distribution of synaptic potentials resulting from stimulation of a single mossy fibre terminal. The broken line gives the predictions of Poisson statistics in which the mean quantal content was 1.6 (number of failures to give a synaptic potential on stimulation is given by the number distributed around zero, the amplitude of the quantal size was 0.39 mV); the continuous line gives the predictions of Pascal statistics for which the mean quantal content was 2.0 (and the amplitude of the quantal size was 0.30 mV). ((a) From ref. 34, (b) from ref. 36, with permission.)

## 10　Does the facilitated secretion of transmitter during trains of impulses involve the recruitment of low-probability release sites?

At the neuromuscular junction, there is an enhanced level of quantal secretion by a test impulse following a conditioning impulse within about 100 ms. This facilitation of transmitter release has been quantitatively predicted in terms of the increased level of $Ca^{2+}$ in the nerve terminal that occurs following a conditioning impulse. The $Ca^{2+}$ concentration does not return to normal for about 100 ms, so that $Ca^{2+}$ entry during a subsequent test impulse adds onto an existing elevated $Ca^{2+}$ level giving an enhanced transmitter release[19]. This 'residual $Ca^{2+}$' hypothesis can be used to predict the increase in quantal secretion during short trains of impulses if the absolute level of quantal release is kept low[19]. However, there is no direct evidence that residual $Ca^{2+}$ does remain at the active zone after an impulse; the spatial and temporal resolution of $Ca^{2+}$-imaging techniques is not yet adequate to detect the small temporal rise in $Ca^{2+}$ concentration at the active zone that has been hypothesised to occur.

If a high-frequency train of impulses is used to stimulate a terminal for a relatively short period of time, transmitter release is elevated for any subsequent impulse that occurs within about 2 min after the train; this is known as post-tetanic potentiation. Calcium-imaging techniques are adequate to detect the rise in $Ca^{2+}$ concentration that occurs throughout a nerve terminal during and after a high-frequency train of impulses that leads to post-tetanic potentiation. At the crayfish neuromuscular junction, the $Ca^{2+}$ concentration is elevated in the varicosities following such a tetanus for the entire period of post-tetanic potentiation; the $Ca^{2+}$ concentration and post-tetanic potentiation then decay at the same rate. This linear relationship is not that expected on the basis of the power relationship that is known to exist between transmitter release by a single nerve impulse and the $Ca^{2+}$ flux into the nerve terminal. Such a power rela-tionship is required to successfully predict facilitation of transmitter release during a short train of impulses. If facilitation is caused by the accumulation of residual $Ca^{2+}$ in the terminal, then this $Ca^{2+}$ must be acting on a different mechanism to that which is acted upon by $Ca^{2+}$ during post-tetanic potentiation. One possibility is that facilitation involves the action of residual $Ca^{2+}$ on the fusion protein at the active zone, which binds the synaptic vesicles to the terminal membrane (see Chapter 1). It is possible that this fusion protein only allows exocytosis to proceed if four $Ca^{2+}$ ions are bound to it at strategic sites, so that exocytosis involves a fourth power relationship between $Ca^{2+}$ influx and secretion. By comparison, potentiation requires a general increase in $Ca^{2+}$ throughout the terminal, where it acts on $Ca^{2+}$-calmodulin-dependent protein kinase II. This kinase leads to the phosphorylation of synapsin I on synaptic vesicles so that they are released from the terminal cytoskeleton to participate in secretion. Such a mechanism may explain why there is a linear relationship between potentiation and $Ca^{2+}$ levels in the nerve terminal.

The above description of the 'residual $Ca^{2+}$' hypothesis for facilitation does not take into account the differences in the probability for secretion of a quantum of transmitter that occur between different release sites within the same nerve terminal. Extracellular recordings of quantal secretion at relatively high probability for secretion sites at amphibian motor nerve terminals show that the probability for secretion is elevated at these sites following a nerve impulse. The very low probability for release sites that exist amongst these relatively high-probability sites are also facilitated following a nerve impulse. If a release site can secrete at most a single quantum of transmitter on arrival of the nerve impulse, then it is the low-probability sites that mostly contribute to facilitation at a nerve terminal during a train of impulses. This occurs because the high-probability sites are soon secreting their maximum number of quanta during a train, namely one, leaving the low-probability sites alone to contribute to an increase. Facilitation may then be thought of as primarily involving the recruitment of low-probability sites during a train of impulses. Since these occur predominantly towards the ends of terminal branches, then facilitation has a spatial element associated with it: release sites towards the ends of terminals will be recruited into the secretory process during a train of impulses. These considerations are dependent on the probability for secretion at all release sites having the same sensitivity to $Ca^{2+}$, whether they are of low or high probability, and this seems to be the case.

## 11   The probability of quantal secretion is most likely determined by $Ca^{2+}$ influx levels at release sites

The idea that transmitter is secreted as quanta is reasonably well established at the somatic neuromuscular junction, but it is not at all clear that this is the case at the autonomic neuromuscular junction. It might be that the size of the spontaneous potentials is determined by transmitter acting on a restricted number of postsynaptic receptors rather than by the nature of prepacking of the transmitter within the nerve terminal and the nature of its release. Nevertheless, the probabilistic nature of transmitter secretion at both somatic and autonomic neuromuscular junctions seems to be well established. Less clearly established is the idea that a single release site within a nerve terminal can secrete at most a single quantum on arrival of the nerve impulse, although evidence is presented that this is probably the case. These release sites within a nerve terminal do not all have the same capacity to secrete transmitter. Some sites have particularly low probabilities for secretion on arrival of the nerve impulse, and this is especially the case at autonomic neuromuscular junctions. These low probabilities do not arise as a consequence of the presynaptic modulation of transmitter release via receptors on nerves of the kind described in following chapters. Indeed the rates of stimulation of nerves used to determine the probabilities

of secretion are much lower than those at which presynaptic receptor mechanisms are operational, about 0.1 Hz (see Chapter 5). Rather, the different probabilities for secretion found amongst the release sites within a nerve terminal are most likely to be determined by variations in $Ca^{2+}$ influx into these release sites on arrival of the nerve impulse.

## References

1. Bennett MR (1972) Autonomic Neuromuscular Transmission. *Monograph of the Physiological Society, No. 30.* Cambridge University Press, Cambridge
2. Bennett MR and Florin T (1974) A statistical analysis of the release acetylcholine at newly formed synapses in striated muscle. *Journal of Physiology* **238:** 93–107
3. Bennett MR, Jones P and Lavidis NA (1986) The probability of quantal secretion along visualised terminal branches at amphibian (*Bufo marinus*) neuromuscular synapses. *Journal of Physiology* **379:** 257–274
4. Bennett MR and Lavidis NA (1979) The effect of $Ca^{2+}$ ions on the secretion of quanta evoked by an impulse at nerve terminal release sites. *Journal of General Physiology* **74:** 429–456
5. Bennett MR and Robinson J (1990) Probabilistic secretion of quanta from nerve terminals at synaptic sites on muscle cells: non-uniformity, autoinhibition and the binomial hypothesis. *Proceedings of the Royal Society of London, Series B* **239:** 329–358
6. Boyd IA and Martin AR (1956) The end-plate potential in mammalian muscle. *Journal of Physiology* **132:** 74–91
7. Bremer F (1932) Researches on the contracture of skeletal muscle. *Journal of Physiology* **76:** 65–94
8. Brock JA and Cunnane TC (1988) Electrical activity at the sympathetic neuroeffector junction in the guinea-pig vas deferens. *Journal of Physiology* **399:** 607–632
9. Brown GL and Eccles JC (1934) The action of a single vagal volley on the rhythm of the heart beat. *Journal of Physiology* **82:** 211–241
10. Burnstock G and Holman ME (1961) The transmission of excitation from autonomic nerve to smooth muscle. *Journal of Physiology* **155:** 115–133

54 MR Bennett

11. Burnstock G and Holman ME (1962) Spontaneous potentials at sympathetic nerve endings in the smooth muscle. *Journal of Physiology* **160**: 446-460

12. d'Alonzo AJ and Grinnell AD (1985) Profiles of evoked release along the length of frog motor nerve terminals. *Journal of Physiology* **359**: 235-258

13. del Castillo J and Katz B (1954) Quantal components of the end-plate potential. *Journal of Physiology* **125**: 560–573

14. de Robertis E (1962) Fine structure of synapses in the CNS. *International Congress of Neuropathology* **2**: 35–38

15. Elfvin LG (1963) The ultrastructure of the superior cervical sympathetic ganglion of the cat. I. The structure of the ganglion cell processes as studied by serial sections. *Journal of Ultrastructure Research* **8**: 403–440

16. Elliott TR (1905) The action of adrenalin. *Journal of Physiology* **32**: 401–467

17. Fatt P and Katz B (1951) An analysis of the end-plate potential recorded with an intracellular electrode. *Journal of Physiology* **115**: 320–370

18. Fatt P and Katz B (1952) Spontaneous subthreshold activity at motor nerve endings. *Journal of Physiology* **117**: 109–128

19. Fogelson AL and Zucker RS (1985) Presynaptic $Ca^{2+}$ diffusion from various arrays of single channels. *Biophysics Journal* **48**: 1003–1017

20. Hartzell HC, Kuffler SW and Yoshikami D (1975) Postsynaptic potentiation and interaction between quanta of acetylcholine at the skeletal neuromuscular junction. *Journal of Physiology* **251**: 427–463

21. Hirst GDS and Neild TO (1980) Some properties of spontaneous excitatory junction potentials recorded from arterioles of guinea-pigs. *Journal of Physiology* **303**: 43–60

22. Hurlbut WP, Lezzi N, Fesce R and Ceccarelli B (1990) Correlation between quantal secretion and vesicle loss at the frog neuromuscular junction. *Journal of Physiology* **425**: 501–526

23. Katz B (1969) The release of neural transmitter substances. *The Sherrington Lectures, X*. Liverpool University Press, Liverpool

24. Katz B and Kuffler SW (1941) Multiple motor innervation of the frog's sartorius muscle. *Journal of Neurophysiology* **4**: 207–223

25. Katz B and Miledi R (1979) Estimates of the quantal content during 'chemical potentiation' of transmitter release. *Proceedings of the Royal Society of London, Series B* **205**: 369–378

26. Katz B and Miledi R (1965) The measurement of synaptic delay, and the time course of acetylcholine release at the neuromuscular junction. *Proceedings of the Royal Society of London, Series B* **161**: 483–495

27. Ko CP (1985) Regeneration of the active zone at the developing neuromuscular junctions in larval and adult bullfrogs. *Journal of Neurocytology* **14**: 487–512

28. Langley JN (1906) On the reaction of cells and of nerve-endings to certain poisons, chiefly as regards the reaction of striated muscle to nicotine and to curare. *Journal of Physiology* **33**: 374–413

29. Lavidis NA and Bennett MR (1992) Probabilistic secretion of quanta from visualized sympathetic nerve varicosities in mouse vas deferens. *Journal of Physiology* **454**: 9–26

30. Loewi O (1921) Uber humorale Ubertragsbarkeit der Herznervenwirkung. *Pflugers Archiv gesellschaft für Physiologie* **189**: 239–242

31. Merrillees NCR (1967) The nervous environment of individual smooth muscle cells of the guinea pig vas deferens. *Journal of Cell Biology* **37**: 794–817

32. Pawson PA and Grinnell AD (1990) Freeze-fracture ultrastructure of the frog neuromuscular junction active zone reveals no marked proximal–distal gradient in synaptic structure. *Society for Neuroscience, Abstracts* **16**: 673 (no. 282–2)

33. Redman SJ (1990) Quantal analysis of synaptic potentials in neurons of the central nervous system. *Physiological Reviews* **70**: 165–198

34. Traub RD and Miles R (1991) *Neuronal Networks of the Hippocampus*. Cambridge University Press, Cambridge

35. Tremblay JP, Laurie RF and Collonnier M (1983) Is the MEPP due to the release of one vesicle or to the simultaneous release of several vesicles at one active zone. *Brain Research Reviews* **6**: 299–314

36. Yamamoto C, Higashima M, Sawada S and Kamiya H (1991) Quantal components of the synaptic potential induced in hippocampal neurons by activation of granule cells, and the effect of 2-amino-4-phosphonobutyric acid. *Hippocampus* **1**: 93–106

37. Zucker RS and Fogelson AL (1986) Relationship between transmitter release and presynaptic $Ca^{2+}$ influx when $Ca^{2+}$ enters through discrete channels. *Proceedings of the National Academy of Sciences, USA* **83**: 3032–3036

# 2 Modulation of neurotransmitter release: basic principles and key players

# 4 Modulation of neurotransmitter release

Lennart Stjärne

Despite the fact that neurotransmitter release from any one release site occurs with extremely low probability during the passage of an action potential, Lennart Stjärne shows in this chapter that this probability is clearly subject to further adjustment. The concept of modulation of neurotransmitter release is introduced here and can be described thus: the site that will on this occasion release quanta of neurotransmitter is subject to external modulatory influences that increase or reduce the amounts of neurotransmitter released. Also in this chapter is an analysis of where, in principle, these modulatory influences could be acting, and the possibility is raised that such modulatory sites in any one neurone can be remote from, as well as close to or at, the actual release site. This chapter and the three which precede it describe the context and set the scene for the subsequent detailed analyses of the phenomenon of modulation of neurotransmitter release, the biochemical mechanisms involved and the physiological relevance and possible pathophysiological significance of altered neuro-effector transmission.

## 1 Theoretically possible sites for modulatory influences to act

The purpose of this chapter is to describe the possible sites at which chemical agents, both endogenous and exogenous, may modulate the nerve impulse-induced exocytosis of neurotransmitters. The basic features and molecular and cellular mechanisms of exocytosis of the transmitter contents of small and large vesicles, and the evidence that individual neurones often utilise more than one transmitter, have been described already (see Chapters 1, 2 and 3). Here it will be assumed that (i) both small and large vesicles release their transmitters in quanta, i.e. as multimolecular packets of preset size; (ii) large vesicles release their contents from random sites while small vesicles release theirs from specialised sites, the active zones; (iii) even

those nerve terminals in which active zones have not yet been demonstrated by morphological techniques possess functional active zones, although small and perhaps dispersed; and (iv) individual active zones behave as binary units, i.e. respond to the nerve impulse by releasing 0 or 1 quantum. The discussion will deal mainly with what at present is best known, the modulation of the probability of release of single small quanta from individual active zones, and it will deal to a lesser extent with the less well-known control of the release of big quanta from random sites.

### 1.1 Modulation of neurotransmitter release at cellular level

Neurones are morphologically elongated, functionally highly polarised and secretory,

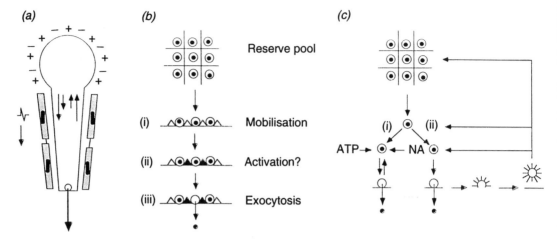

Fig. 4.1. (*a*) Possible levels at which release modulation can occur in a standard neurone. (*b*) The steps that determine the release probability at a potential release site at the active zone. (*c*) The mode of exocytosis (in this example, in a sympathetic varicosity) (i) at low and (ii) at high frequency of stimulation. For comments, see text.

i.e. gland-like cells (Fig. 4.1*a*). Basically, transmitter release is a function of the number and frequency of nerve impulses propagated to the terminals. This in turn is a function of the integrated excitatory (+) and inhibitory (−) afferent input to the soma-dendritic region of the neurone. In the nerve terminals, the impulse travels at 0.1–0.5 m/s, and in many (but not all) neurones invades all regions actively, triggering a regenerative, mainly or exclusively $Na^+$-channel-dependent all-or-none action potential in all varicosities and boutons[1,5,15,20]. However, it is important to keep in mind that the ability of nerve impulses to evoke transmitter release is dependent not only on this surface traffic but also on movement inside the axon. The latter involves a variety of 'particles' (including transmitter and transport vesicles) and associated substances and soluble material, which move towards terminals and/or back to the soma by 'fast' or 'slow' intra-axonal transport, at 0.5–5 μm/s or 0.01–0.05 μm/s, respectively[4]. Furthermore, the evidence is growing that the transmitter release capability of neurones may be highly dependent on the properties of the Schwann (or in the CNS, glial) cells, coupled by gap junctions, in which the

nerve terminals are wrapped except at release sites where there is a 'window' in the sheath[12]. Briefly, the following possibilities should be considered.

### 1.1.1 Schwann or glial cell activity may be a target for some release modulators

The cells in this sheath may modulate neurotransmission in several ways[12]. For example, nerve activity may reduce the mechanical encroachment of Schwann or glial cell processes between nerve and effector membranes and, thus, increase the area of synaptic contact. Furthermore, the Schwann or glial cells communicate with the axon by bidirectional signals (e.g. acetylcholine, glutamate, glycine, arachidonic acid, nitric oxide, etc. passing between support cell and neurone) and possess receptors to various neurotransmitters, transporters for uptake of various transmitters, and ion channels (to $Na^+$, $K^+$, $Ca^{2+}$ or $Cl^-$) similar to those that occur in neurones. The supporting cells, which, therefore, may act as ion sensors, may control the $Ca^{2+}$ and $K^+$ level in the narrow perineuronal space[12,15,17]. Certain transmitters (e.g. glutamate) trigger $Ca^{2+}$ transients, which spread as waves both within and between the electrically coupled Schwann or glial cells and hence may act as longitudinal signals along the terminal regions of neurones. Activity in these cells may, thus, influence both the release and inactivation of transmitters and thereby synaptic strength. The possibility that some release modulators may exert their effects via these cells should, therefore, not be overlooked[12].

### 1.1.2   Intra-axonally transported factors may influence neurotransmitter release probability

That the logistic and regulatory material carried intra-axonally by fast and slow, antero- and/or retrograde transport influences the long-term transmitter release capability of nerve terminals is obvious. In addition, however, particle-associated regulatory factors, such as calmodulin, carried to the terminals by fast intra-axonal transport may, for example by influencing the phosphorylation of substrates (ion channels, vesicle or active zone-docking proteins, etc.), exert short-term effects on $Ca^{2+}$ entry, the availability of 'releasable transmitter' and, ultimately, neurotransmitter release. It is interesting, therefore, that the rate of fast axonal transport has been shown to vary with the fluctuations in the $Ca^{2+}$ level in the perineuronal space, which in turn are associated with nerve activity. This indicates that the supply of regulatory factors to the nerve terminals may itself be regulated by nerve impulses[4,15,16].

### 1.1.3   Modulation of the nerve-terminal action potential may modulate release

Nerve impulses induce release by opening voltage-sensitive $Na^+$ channels that admit $Na^+$ to depolarise the terminals. This causes the opening of voltage-sensitive $Ca^{2+}$ channels allowing the influx of $Ca^{2+}$ which triggers exocytosis of transmitter vesicles[1,5,15,20]. The $Na^+$ influx is not essential: passive depolarisation of nerve terminals by current injection, or by raising the external $K^+$ level, releases transmitter even in $Na^+$-free media or when $Na^+$ channels are blocked by tetrodotoxin.

Nor is a change in membrane potential essential: intra-terminal injection of $Ca^{2+}$, or ionophore-induced $Ca^{2+}$ influx, induces exocytosis 'artificially' without depolarising the nerve terminals. However, both the 'voltage' effect of the nerve impulse and the evoked $Na^+$ influx into the terminals may modulate the release and/or inactivation of transmitters and thereby affect neurotransmission.

The action potential is generated by activation of local regenerative $Na^+$ channels. Local changes in the action potential probably do not (except when they result in conduction failure) change the action potential in other regions of the same terminal branch[17]. In general, changes in the amplitude of the action potential, i.e. the degree of its 'overshoot', either have little effect on transmitter release or do not change it in the expected direction. In some systems, maintained resting depolarisation of nerve terminals (which reduces the amplitude of a superimposed action potential) enhances nerve impulse-evoked transmitter release, while resting hyperpolarisation (which increases the amplitude of the action potential) reduces release[15]. The reasons why transmitter release is poorly correlated with the amplitude of the action potential are probably that (i) $Ca^{2+}$ channels open more slowly than $Na^+$ channels and, therefore, $Ca^{2+}$ influx would occur mainly during the falling limb of the action potential; and (ii) the reversal of charge during the peak of the action potential slows $Ca^{2+}$ entry. However, changes in the duration of the action potential strongly modulate transmitter release locally (see Section 4.1).

### 1.2   Modulators may influence the probability of monoquantal release at several points

Fig. 4.1b shows two of the conditions that must be fulfilled to enable the action potential to release a quantum from an active zone (see Chapter 1). The first is that a synaptic vesicle must be mobilised from the reserve pool and docked at the active zone. This step depends, at least in part, on the intra-terminal $Ca^{2+}$ concentration and the degree of phosphorylation of synapsin I induced by $Ca^{2+}$-calmodulin-dependent protein kinase II. Synapsin I in its dephosphorylated state cross-links the vesicle to actin filaments in the cytoskeleton[7]. The docking mechanism is not considered here (but see Section 5). The second condition is that the docked vesicle must be 'activated' by a mechanism that may involve a small-molecular-weight GTP-binding protein[8]. This is indicated by the finding that intra-terminal injection of a non-hydrolysable GTP analogue, GTPγS, blocked release of vesicles (in squid giant synapse) without changing the $Ca^{2+}$ signals or the number of vesicles apparently docked at active zones. 'Activation' of the release mechanisms, therefore, seems to require hydrolysis of GTP[8]. The 'activation' step is highly restricted; the nerve-terminal action potential normally releases the contents of only one out of the > 50 vesicles (e.g. in frog neuromuscular junction) that, by morphological criteria, are docked at an active zone[15]. The restriction is disrupted by the $K^+$-channel blockers tetraethylammonium (TEA) or 4-aminopyridine (4-AP), which enable a single action potential to induce exocytosis of all vesicles at individual active zones (see Section 4.1). These findings suggest that (i) the restriction of the 'activation' of docked vesicles may involve $K^+$-channel activity; and (ii) all docked vesicles may be 'potentially releasable' and all docking sites are 'potential release sites'.

The probability that a nerve impulse will release a quantum from an individual potential release site appears to be a function of (i) the probability ($p_a$) that a synaptic vesicle has been mobilised from the reserve pool, i.e. moved to the active zone; (ii) the probability ($p_b$) that this vesicle has become 'activated', i.e. made 'releasable'; and (iii) the probability ($p_c$) that the depolarisation-induced $Ca^{2+}$ influx will cause exocytosis of the quantum in this vesicle[1,11,20.] The 'compound probability' ($p$) for release of a quantum from this site is thus $p_a \times p_b \times p_c$. In most active zones, $p_c$ may approach unity; the rate-limiting step at low frequency in the absence of drugs may be $p_b$,

and during a high-frequency train $p_a$ becomes increasingly important. Each step is likely to be separately regulated and a potential target for modulators of release (see Section 5).

### 1.3 Impulse frequency may 'modulate' the mode of exocytosis

The nerve-impulse frequency modulates the mode of transmitter exocytosis in at least two ways. First, impulses at low frequency release preferentially the transmitters in small vesicles docked at active zones, while high-frequency bursts promote release of the contents (neuropeptides) of large vesicles from random sites[15]. Second, the nerve impulse frequency may even control the mode of exocytosis at active zones. This feature is illustrated in Fig. 4.1c. Nerve impulses at low frequency may induce transient fusion of the vesicle and plasma membranes and, after releasing their contents, empty vesicles are refilled by uptake of transmitters (in sympathetic nerves: ATP and noradrenaline) from the cytosol and reused locally. In the exocytosis induced by nerve impulses at high frequency, the vesicle membrane is fully incorporated into the plasma membrane, retrieved by endocytosis, re-entered at various levels in the total pool of vesicles and reused. It is suggested that the explanation is that nerve impulses at low frequency cause incomplete dissociation, and at high frequency complete dissociation, of synapsin I from the vesicle[7].

## 2   To what extent do present experimental methods resolve neurotransmitter release?

The most fundamental problem in this area of research is that no current method measures transmitter release directly. Estimates of transmitter release are based on inferences from the overflow of transmitter from the release sites, or from the electrical or mechanical responses of the effector. In either case, what is actually measured is the concentration of transmitter at the detection point, in turn a function of transmitter release *minus* clearance. This is a source of error, as clearance may be a physiological variable (see Section 2.6). Another important caveat to consider when analysing the release of any neurotransmitter and its modulation is that tissue differences preclude generalisation from one tissue to the next.

## 2.1  Sympathetic neurotransmitter release is useful as a model

The mechanisms of transmitter release and its prejunctional modulation are probably different in detail but similar in principle in most neurones[1,15,20]. Sympathetic nerves are particularly suitable as models to study transmitter release and its regulation at the level of single 'boutons' (varicosities). One reason is that sympathetic varicosities, each probably with a single small active zone, are more widely separated than active zones in other neurones used for such analysis (5 μm between varicosities versus 1 μm between active zones in frog motor nerve terminals), which facilitates resolution of events in individual active zones[10,15]. Furthermore, the average sympathetic varicosity contains a much smaller number of transmitter vesicles (approximately 500, in rodents ≥ 95% small and ≤ 5% large vesicles; in large animals and man ≤ 80% small and ≥ 20% large vesicles) than, for example, cholinergic motor terminals and, therefore, is useful for study of the necessary parsimony of quantal release[15]. An added advantage is that these nerves release both a 'fast' ionotropic transmitter, ATP, and one or more 'slow' metabotropic transmitter(s), noradrenaline and often, in addition, a neuropeptide, e.g. neuropeptide Y. In sympathetic nerves, the noradrenaline and ATP in single small vesicles may represent the small quantum, and the noradrenaline, ATP and neuropeptide in single large vesicles the big quantum[15]; however, this view is debated[19.]

The excitatory junction current (EJC) and the 'discrete event', the d$V$/d$t$ of the rising phase of the EJP, in smooth muscle in certain rodent tissues may be used to study the release of (the ATP component of) quanta from small vesicles at the active zones[5,15]. The overflow of neuropeptide (at least in large laboratory animals and man) may be used as a marker of release from large vesicles, probably from random sites[15,18]. It is important to keep in mind that sympathetic co-transmitters, although released together, differ greatly in clearance. The ATP component of the quantum is metabolised by ecto-ATPase and completely eliminated within 50–100 ms[5], while the noradrenaline component, which is metabolically stable extracellularly, is eliminated from the receptor area[2] only after ≥ 2–3 s, mainly by neuronal uptake and diffusion into the effluent[15]. Some sympathetic neuropeptide transmitters may be metabolised by ecto-enzymes, but others, e.g. neuropeptide Y, are relatively stable and leave the receptor area slowly by diffusion to the effluent.

## 2.2  Factors which modulate transmitter release and clearance

As a background for the discussion, consider Fig. 4.2. This schematic diagram shows the complexity of the pre- and postsynaptic factors which modulate the input–output relationship in the synapse between a model neurone A and its effector B. All of these factors have to be considered when analysing the presynaptic modulation of transmitter release from A. The diagram shows first that the efficacy of transmission from A to B depends on two factors: the concentration of transmitters at the receptors driving the response of B (in turn a function of their release and clearance) and the responsiveness of B. An illustrative example of the technical difficulties in the analysis of transmitter release and its prejunctional modulation is that the stimulus employed to release transmitters from A (e.g. field stimulation or depolarisation with high $K^+$ concentrations) in addition may release modulating transmitters from a second neurone C. Another example is that each endogenous or exogenous release-modulating factor (e.g. agonists or antagonists at

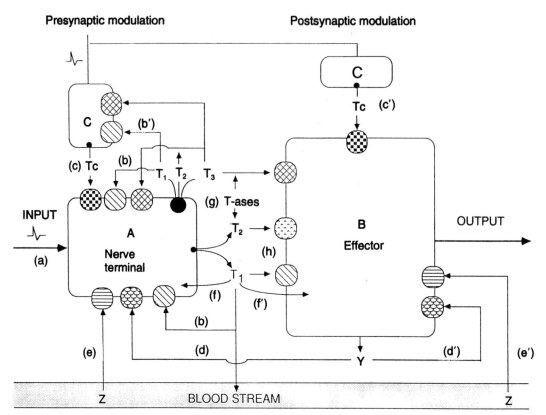

Fig. 4.2. Schematic diagram of the pre- and postsynaptic modulation of the input–output relationship in a synapse between a nerve terminal A and its effector B, to indicate its probable complexity. A utilises three transmitters, $T_1$–$T_3$, stored in different combinations in small and large vesicles. The action potential may release a small quantum (e.g. the $T_1$ and $T_2$ contents of a small vesicle docked at the active zone) and, more rarely, a big quantum (e.g. the $T_1$, $T_2$ and $T_3$ contents of a large vesicle, from a random site). $T_1$ is eliminated by neuronal and extraneuronal uptake and diffusion to the effluent, $T_2$ and $T_3$ by ecto-enzymes (T-ases) and/or diffusion. Transmission from A to B may be modulated prejunctionally by the following factors, which alter the per pulse release: (a) the number and frequency of nerve impulses; (b) feedback by $T_1$ and $T_3$ via prejunctional autoreceptors; (c) effects of a transmitter $T_C$ from a nerve terminal C, via prejunctional heteroreceptors on A; the activity in C is in turn influenced (b') by $T_1$ and $T_3$ via prejunctional heteroreceptors; (d) effects of substance(s) Y released from non-neuronal cells ('trans-synaptic feedback'); and (e) effects of substance(s) Z derived from the circulation, acting via humoral heteroreceptors. The effect on B of a given release from A may be altered by activity-induced changes in the clearance of released $T_1$ (f, f') as well as that of $T_2$ and $T_3$ (g). The responsiveness of B may be modulated postjunctionally both (h) by changes in the sensitivity (e.g. desensitisation) of the receptors to $T_1$–$T_3$, and (c'–e') by postreceptor effects caused by several of the aforementioned factors ('receptor–receptor interaction'). For further comments and a concrete example, see text.

presynaptic receptors, or $Ca^{2+}$ or $K^+$ channel-blocking agents) may affect several sites on A–C. Above all, however, the diagram emphasises that available methods (i.e. overflow of transmitters or the electrical or mechanical effector responses) do not measure transmitter release as such, but release minus clearance (by enzymatic degradation, neuronal and extraneuronal uptake, or by diffusion).

The general scheme in Fig. 4.2 summarises the numerous factors which may modulate, for example, sympathetic neuromuscular transmission. In that case, the transmitters ($T_1$, $T_2$ and $T_3$) in varicosity A are noradrenaline, ATP and one or several neuropeptides, respectively. The response of B, often a smooth muscle cell, is modulated both pre- and postjunctionally by factors that alter the release and clearance of these transmitters as well as by the responsiveness of the muscle cell. The probability of release of small quanta from preferred release sites and of big quanta from random sites in A is basically determined by the number and frequency of nerve impulses. The already low release probability may be further depressed by released noradrenaline and neuropeptides (but probably not ATP) via prejunctional autoreceptors. Furthermore, the probability of release from A may be depressed or enhanced by other transmitters (e.g. acetylcholine, sensory neuropeptides or even noradrenaline) released from other neurones and acting via prejunctional heteroreceptors, by substances (e.g. adenosine, arachidonic acid, prostaglandins, nitric oxide, etc.) released from smooth muscle or other cells ('trans-synaptic feedback') and by substances (e.g. adrenaline, angiotensin II) derived from the circulation. At a given level of release, the concentration of these transmitters at the receptors is determined by the rate of clearance, which, as explained below (see Section 2.6), may be a physiological variable[2,16]. Postjunctionally the effector response may be further modulated both by factors which alter the receptor sensitivity and by postreceptor effects, resulting from positive or negative interaction between noradrenaline acting on adrenoceptors and ATP on purinoceptors (and probably often neuropeptides acting on their specific receptors)[2].

## 2.3   A debated issue: parallel or dissociated release of co-transmitters?

Electrochemical and electrophysiological studies of neurotransmission in rat tail artery are compatible with the model in Fig. 4.2, according to which sympathetic nerves release $T_1$ and $T_2$, i.e. noradrenaline and ATP, in parallel[11]. In contrast, results based on study of the overflow of noradrenaline and ATP (and/or its metabolites) or of the 'noradrenergic' and 'purinergic' neurogenic contractions of a number of other preparations from different species suggest that the release of noradrenaline from sympathetic nerves is often dissociated from that of ATP[19]. Three possible explanations for the discrepancy arise: (i) noradrenaline and ATP are released in parallel in all sympathetic nerves; the observed dissociation is caused by inadequacies of the methods; (ii) noradrenaline and ATP are released in parallel in some but not all sympathetic nerves; and (iii) the release of noradrenaline is always dissociated from that of ATP and observations of parallel release are fortuitous. The issue is extremely important because it relates to the fundamental problem of how to correctly assess transmitter release *per se* (see also Chapter 2). Subsequent discussion will focus mainly on one concrete example, transmitter release from sympathetic nerves.

## 2.4   How trustworthy are the methods used to measure release?

Three main methods are currently used to study the release of ATP and/or noradrenaline from sympathetic nerves. The most reliable method to measure the quantal release of ATP is extracellular or intracellular recording of the electrical responses in smooth muscle, the EJC and EJP, respectively[5,15]. These responses may reflect relatively accurately the pulse by pulse release of ATP (not of noradrenaline, as its electrical effects are too inconstant and/or slow for this purpose). The EJCs and the 'discrete events' (the $dV/dt$ of the rising phase of the EJPs) may resolve the release of single ATP quanta from individual varicosities[5]. The time course of EJCs (but not of evoked EJPs, since they are slowed by electrical coupling between the smooth muscle cells) reflects that of the rise

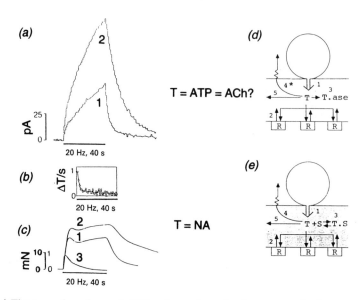

Fig. 4.3. (a–c) The per pulse release of ATP and noradrenaline from sympathetic nerves in rat tail artery, the noradrenaline level at the receptors and the neurogenic contractile responses during a tetanus (800 pulses at 20 Hz). (a) The concentration of released noradrenaline at a carbon-fibre electrode, as reflected by the noradrenaline oxidation current (pA) measured by differential pulse amperometry. Trace 1 is without drug; 2 is in the presence of the noradrenaline-uptake blocker cocaine (3 $\mu$M). (b) The relative increments in noradrenaline concentration in consecutive measurements used as a rough measure of the per second neural release of both noradrenaline and ATP (T) and referred to as $\Delta$T/s. (c) The neurogenic contractile responses. Traces 1 and 2 are the (mainly) noradrenaline-induced contractions in the absence and presence of cocaine, respectively (vertical calibration bar: 10 mN). Trace 3 is the ATP-induced, $P_{2x}$ purinoceptor-mediated contraction (vertical calibration: 1 mN). (d) Release and clearance of a quantum of a 'fast' ionotropic transmitter T, e.g. acetylcholine (ACh), in the endplate. The neuromuscular gap (width < 50 nm) is filled with basal lamina rich in T-ase, the enzyme which destroys T. (1) Exocytotic release of a quantum of T. (2) T shoots through the basal lamina and binds reversibly to the ionophore receptor R. (3) 30% of the T in the quantum is destroyed by T-ase during this passage; most of the remainder is destroyed after dissociating from the receptors. (4) Neuronal uptake of the metabolite (choline). (5) Only a small fraction of the released T escapes to the effluent. (e) The release and clearance of a quantum of a 'slow' metabotropic transmitter T, e.g. noradrenaline (NA), in a junction between a sympathetic varicosity and a smooth muscle cell. The neuromuscular gap (width < 100 nm) is filled with basal lamina rich in S, a hypothetical low-affinity noradrenaline-binding site. (1) Exocytotic release of a quantum of T. (2) T shoots through the basal lamina and binds reversibly to the metabotropic receptor(s) R inside the junction. (3) Free T is buffered by reversible binding to S and slowly eliminated by neuronal reuptake (4) and diffusion to the surroundings (5). For further comments see text.

and fall in the ATP concentration at the postjunctional receptors[2,5]. It should be noted, however, that EJCs and 'discrete events' probably reflect the ATP component only of small quanta and only when these are released from varicosities junctionally related to smooth muscle. This would not include the ATP component of big quanta released from random sites, nor the molecular leakage of ATP from all excitable cells[15].

A less reliable approach is to use the 'purinergic' and 'noradrenergic' components of the contractile response as measures of the release of ATP and noradrenaline[19]. This is hazardous, first, because the contractile responses to ATP and noradrenaline are not necessarily proportional to the release of ATP and noradrenaline (see Fig. 4.3a–c), and, second, because the responses are often distorted by positive or negative interaction between ATP- and noradrenaline-induced effects ('receptor–receptor interaction')[2].

A third approach is to use the overflow of endogenous or tracer-labelled noradrenaline and ATP (and/or ATP metabolites) into the effluent from the examined tissue as a measure of the neural release of noradrenaline and ATP. Data by this much-used method should be interpreted with great caution, first because the method does not measure transmitter release but release minus clearance (see above), second, because the overflow of labelled transmitter(s) does not necessarily reflect that of endogenous transmitter(s), and third, because the method does not distinguish between quantal and non-quantal release or, for ATP, between release from neural and non-neural sources. Furthermore, the spatial and temporal resolution of the method is insufficient to reveal the spatial distribution of the released transmitters or the kinetics of the rise and fall in their concentration at the receptors which drive the contraction[2].

Far superior in most respects is focal electrochemical recording of the noradrenaline oxidation current, using a small carbon-fibre electrode[2,11]. This is a very useful tool to study the kinetics of neural release and clearance of endogenous noradrenaline both in the brain and in peripheral tissues. However, even this signal measures only the local overflow of noradrenaline from the release site, i.e. release minus clearance. As a consequence (see Fig. 4.3a–c), it does not always reflect the quantal release of noradrenaline or the noradrenaline concentration driving the contraction[2].

## 2.5 Release of sympathetic co-transmitters during a tetanus: tissue differences

Many neurones have been reported to differ in quantal release, especially during a high-frequency train of stimuli ('tetanus')[1,20]. In some, transmitter release is first facilitated then depressed during the tetanus and afterwards recovers within 10 s. In others, release is predominantly facilitated; in yet others it is predominantly depressed during the tetanus. As shown by comparison of the EJC responses (i.e. the per pulse quantal release of ATP) in mouse vas deferens and rat tail artery, the sympathetic nerves in these tissues differ in quantal release and its prejunctional modulation[11]. In mouse vas deferens, the amplitude of the EJCs increased by approximately 3-fold during the first part of the tetanus (700 pulses at 20 Hz); later the EJCs were moderately reduced in size but rarely declined to levels much below that of the first EJC. The facilitation was enhanced and the depression partially offset by an $\alpha_2$-adrenoceptor antagonist. The depression, therefore, resulted partly from $\alpha_2$-adrenoceptor-mediated inhibition of the release mechanisms. Strikingly different results were obtained in rat tail artery during similar nerve stimulation. Here the EJCs caused by the first pulses were modestly enhanced (by $\leq 30\%$) and those caused by later pulses increasingly depressed, often to barely detectable levels. When switching the stimulation frequency from 20 Hz to 0.1 Hz, the EJCs recovered within 10 s. Control experiments indicated that the depression of EJCs in this preparation were not caused by desensitisation of $P_{2x}$ purinoceptors but by a reduced per pulse quantal release of ATP[11].

The per pulse release of noradrenaline during the tetanus in rat tail artery was assessed electrochemically. The noradrenaline oxidation current was measured by differential pulse amperometry once per second, using an extracellular carbon-fibre electrode (diameter, 8 μm; length, 30–50 μm) apposed to the innervated outer surface of the tunica media. The increments in this current caused by trains of 4, 8, 12, 16, or 20, 40, 60, 80, 100 pulses at 20 Hz indicated that the per pulse release of noradrenaline, similarly to that of ATP, increased during the first few pulses of a 20 Hz train and then declined profoundly. Both the depression of the EJCs and the noradrenaline oxidation current responses were unaffected by addition of $\alpha_2$-adrenoceptor antagonists or noradrenaline-uptake blockers. In rat tail artery, ATP and noradrenaline are probably released in parallel; during a tetanus the depression of the pulse release of both is apparently independent of $\alpha_2$-adrenoceptor-mediated control and unaffected by noradrenaline reuptake[11].

## 2.6 Mismatch between release, overflow and effector response: 'plasticity' of clearance

The results of the experiments with rat tail artery shown in Fig. 4.3*a–c* give a concrete example both of the hazards involved in using either the overflow of transmitter or the effector response as measures of the per pulse release and of what appears to be nerve stimulation-induced 'plasticity' of clearance of some released transmitters.

Figure 4.3*a* trace 1, shows the 'cumulative' noradrenaline oxidation current, i.e. the concentration of released noradrenaline in the 'pocket' surrounding the carbon-fibre electrode, during nerve stimulation with 800 pulses at 20 Hz in the absence of drugs. Compare this and trace 1 in Fig. 4.3*c*, the (mainly) noradrenaline-induced neurogenic contractile response, with Fig. 4.3*b*, which shows the per second neural release of noradrenaline[2,11,16]. It can be seen that both the noradrenaline overflow and the contractile response are extremely poorly correlated with the release of noradrenaline, under these conditions.

The issue was further analysed by studying the effects of cocaine, added to block the neuronal reuptake of released noradrenaline. As mentioned above, in this preparation, the drug does not alter the per pulse release of noradrenaline (or ATP) during 20 Hz trains[11]. The finding that cocaine enhanced both the noradrenaline oxidation current (Fig. 4.3*a*, trace 2) and the noradrenaline-induced contraction (Fig. 4.3*c*, trace 2) and strongly slowed the relaxation of both responses implies that neuronal reuptake was still operative during and after the tetanus.

The mismatch between release, overflow and effector response suggests that the diffusion of released noradrenaline, away from the receptors or the electrode, to the reuptake sites or the effluent, was, in fact, restricted by nerve activity.

Finally, note the reasonably good agreement between the rapidly declining per pulse release of ATP[11] (Fig. 4.3*b*) and the transience of the small ATP-induced neurogenic contraction (Fig. 4.3*c*, trace 3). This was an expected effect: as released ATP is known to be rapidly degraded[5], the effector response to released ATP ought to be a somewhat delayed but reasonably good reflection of the per pulse release of ATP[2].

These findings raise two important questions. (i) How could the concentration of released noradrenaline at the carbon-fibre electrode continue to increase and that at the $\alpha$-adrenoceptors driving the contraction be maintained throughout the tetanus, even at a stage when the neural release of noradrenaline had declined to very low levels? (ii) How could both relax so rapidly upon cessation of nerve stimulation? The answers are not known, but it is tempting to speculate that clearance of released noradrenaline was actually slowed by the tetanus and returned to normal or even accelerated upon cessation of nerve stimulation. The cocaine effects show that neuronal reuptake was not abolished; the clearance depressed by the tetanus may, therefore, be washout of released noradrenaline. What is now needed is a search for a mechanism by which nerve activity may reduce the availability of released noradrenaline for reuptake transporters and washout but maintain its concentration at the muscle receptors driving the contraction (and at the electrode). It has been hypothesised that such 'trapping' of released noradrenaline may occur by reversible binding to an intra-junctional buffering site (S in Fig. 4.3*e*) whose noradrenaline affinity increased during nerve activity[16]. Whether this occurs remains to be established.

Meanwhile, the important lesson in the present context is that inferences concerning the per pulse release, based on the overflow of transmitter or on the contractile response, may be reasonably correct for some transmitters (in this case, ATP) but extremely misleading for others (in this case, noradrenaline).

## 2.7   Available methods measure release minus clearance: the fact and the consequences

In general, the problem of variable clearance affects the measurement of the release of different transmitters in different ways. As an example, Fig. 4.3d shows some features which complicate measurement of the release of a 'fast' ionotropic transmitter T, in this case acetylcholine at the neuromuscular endplate[1,10,15]. The principles probably apply as well to other ionotropic transmitters, e.g. ATP released as a sympathetic co-transmitter. The T molecules in the released quantum are under constant attack by T-ase, a low-affinity T-binding protein which is also a T-degrading enzyme. Degradation by T-ase, which resides in the basal lamina filling the narrow neuromuscular gap (width: < 50 nm), is normally the main reason for the rapid decline of the concentration of T, which initially is extremely high near the site of exocytosis (equal to that in the vesicle, i.e. up to 100 mM). Approximately one third of the T molecules in the quantum are lost during the passage of the small but dense packet through the basal lamina. At the effector membrane, T binds reversibly to the receptor R, opens its ion channel and generates, within a fraction of a millisecond, a brief postsynaptic current and potential (PSC and PSP). As T molecules dissociate from the receptors, most are destroyed by T-ase, within a few milliseconds. A membrane transporter takes up the metabolite (in this case, choline) into the nerve terminal. Only a small fraction of the T in the quantum escapes to the effluent. Block of T-ase does not change the amplitude of the PSC or PSP (suggesting

that a T quantum may normally saturate the receptor patch) but increases their duration and dramatically enhances the overflow of T into the effluent. The measured parameters PSC or PSP (or the overflow of T), thus, represent T release minus clearance. The rate of clearance is determined by properties of T-ase in the basal lamina. The amplitude of the PSC or PSP may represent the impact of 70% of the T molecules in a single quantum. However, in those synapses in which the T in single quanta saturates the local receptor patch, these responses do not distinguish between release of one quantum or several quanta from the same site.

A very different situation exists in the measurement of the release of a 'slow' metabotropic transmitter (T in Fig. 4.3e). In this case T could be noradrenaline released from the active zone of a sympathetic nerve varicosity junctionally related to a smooth muscle cell, for example in rat tail artery. The principles probably apply as well to other metabotropic, e.g. monoamine or amino acid, transmitters released from active zones of other neurones. The extremely high initial T concentration near the site of exocytosis (equal to that in the vesicle, in some cases up to 100 mM[15]) probably declines rapidly. In this case, the decline is not the result of enzymatic degradation of T but is thought to be caused in part by reversible binding to a local low-affinity buffering site S in the basal lamina that fills the narrow (< 100 nm) neuromuscular gap. A fraction of the T molecules in the quantum bind to the intrajunctional metabotropic receptor R. Free T is slowly eliminated from the junctional space by neuronal reuptake (extraneuronal uptake plays a role in other synapses but not in rat tail artery) and diffusion to the more numerous metabotropic receptors in the surrounding tissue, and then eventually into the effluent. As explained above (see Section 2.6), there are reasons to believe that the T affinity of the local buffering site S is increased by nerve activity[16]. The reuptake transporter of the releasing varicosity removes most of the T molecules in a single quantum but is saturated by rapidly repeated release from the same site; by contrast, neuronal uptake in the vicinity of active junctions remains fully operative[16]. Buffering and local saturation of reuptake may act in concert to maintain or amplify the T level at the receptors and thereby amplify and prolong the effector response to a given amount of T released during nerve stimulation[2]. Reversal of these mechanisms after cessation of nerve activity accelerates the removal of T and the relaxation of the effector response[2,16].

## 2.8   Conclusions

The overflow of ionotropic or metabotropic transmitters and the electrical or mechanical effector responses do not directly indicate the release of these transmitters, but rather reflect release minus clearance. This may explain why results using different methods in different tissues have led different researchers to hold quite different views about the composition of the transmitter cocktail released by nerve impulses, as well as about the prejunctional modulation of release[11,15,19].

# 3   Do current experimental methods resolve the probability of monoquantal release in individual sites?

The best spatial resolution of the secretory activity of individual active zones is obtained by extracellular recording of the PSC caused by release of ionotropic transmitters, especially when applied to preparations in which the active zones are widely separated. Measurement of the release of ATP from the 'string-like' sympathetic nerves in smooth muscle preparations is suitable for this purpose[5,16]. The concurrent use of an intravital dye and a small recording electrode (internal tip diameter ≤ 4 μm) has made it possible to visualise the varicose nerve terminals and characterise the pulse-by-pulse quantal release from individual varicosities along the strings[10]. In the future, examination of a large

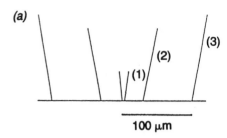

**100 μm**

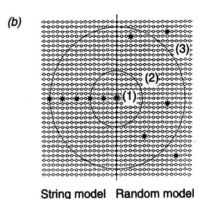

**String model   Random model**

Fig. 4.4.  When using extracellular recording to study the secretory activity in a varicosity population, more detail is paid for by less overview. (a) Recording electrodes (1–3) with internal tip diameters of 4, 40 or 200 μm 'see' a single varicosity, 50 varicosities or 1200 varicosities, respectively (if the density of junctional varicosities is 40 000/mm$^2$). (b) Two extreme possible models of the geometry of monoquantal transmitter release. In both a single pulse releases 10 quanta from 33 × 33 varicosities ($p$, the probability of monoquantal release in the average varicosity is 0.01; releasing varicosities are filled, silent varicosities open). In the string model, the release probability is non-uniform; all release occurs along one string in whose varicosities $0 < p < 1$; in all other strings $p$ is 0. In the random model, the release probability is uniform, $p$ is 0.01 in all varicosities. For further comments see text.

number of randomly chosen individual varicosities with this approach (Fig. 4.4) may give definitive answers to the currently debated crucial questions which follow (see Sections 3.1–3.5).

## 3.1   Are all sympathetic varicosities potentially secretory?

This is not known with certainty. The best evidence has been obtained using fluorescence light microscopy to study in whole-mount preparations of rat iris the effects of prolonged nerve stimulation at high frequency (20 Hz for 40 min) on the noradrenaline concentration in sympathetic nerve terminals in (i) the absence of drugs or in the presence of a noradrenaline-synthesis inhibitor, or (ii) in the presence of reserpine, a blocker of the catecholamine-uptake transporter of the transmitter vesicles. Nerve stimulation alone, in the absence of drugs, only slightly reduced the noradrenaline fluorescence of the varicosities. Nor did the presence of the drugs for 60 min in the absence of nerve stimulation markedly change the morphology of the terminals. However, when noradrenaline synthesis was inhibited, nerve stimulation caused a 'spotted' loss of fluorescence; some branches appeared to be depleted of noradrenaline while others remained unchanged. In addition, nerve stimulation in the presence of reserpine caused a uniform, profound loss of fluorescence in all varicosities. These findings indicate, first, that transmitter release during a tetanus is normally highly restricted (see Section 2.5), second, that release is normally non-uniform, and third, that all varicosities are likely to be potentially secretory[15].

## 3.2   Is release from individual sympathetic varicosities always monoquantal?

The present answer, based on studies of EJCs under optimal conditions, is probably yes, in the absence of drugs. But one cannot be absolutely certain, since the EJC amplitude does not distinguish between mono- and polyquantal release in junctions in which single quanta saturate the receptor patch[5,15]. However, calculations based on the fractional overflow of noradrenaline are compatible with monoquantal release[5,15]. This possibility

is also supported by the growing evidence that release from active zones may normally be monoquantal in most or all neurones (see Chapter 3).

## 3.3   What is the release probability in the average sympathetic varicosity?

The present answer is close to 0.01[5,15]. One reason is that the per pulse fractional overflow of noradrenaline in many tissues and species (approximately 1/50 000 of the tissue content) is consistent with the calculated release of the contents of a single vesicle from 1% of the varicosities. A second is the finding in several electrophysiological studies of the release of ATP as a sympathetic cotransmitter in a variety of rodent tissues (guinea-pig and mouse vas deferens, rat tail and femoral artery, guinea-pig mesenteric arteriole) that each nerve impulse appears to release a quantum (assumed to represent the contents of a single vesicle) from approximately 1% of the varicosities[5,15].

## 3.4   Is the release probability in individual sites constant or fluctuating?

The available evidence on this point is controversial. One approach to solving this problem is based on study of the 'discrete events' ($dV/dt$ of the rising phase of EJPs) or EJCs (using electrodes with internal diameters of $\geq 40$ $\mu$m) in guinea-pig or mouse vas deferens or rat tail or femoral artery. When recorded under conditions of high resolution, the discrete events fluctuated in amplitude and time course[5,15]. Some characteristic profiles occurred repeatedly during long trains at 0.5–1 Hz (with 1.3–1.8 mM $Ca^{2+}$ in the medium). Prominent responses which were closely similar ('identical') in amplitude and time course were used tentatively as 'fingerprints' of quantal release from individual sites. 'Identical' units appeared in pairs or triads, i.e. occurred at the most two or three times during several hundred impulses at 1 Hz, often within 10–15 s and occasionally even in response to two consecutive pulses. Based on these results, it was concluded that activity, at least in these individual sites, was periodic, i.e. that the release probability was mostly zero but transiently could reach unity, and that release of a quantum did not autoinhibit but rather transiently facilitated the releasing varicosity[5,15]. With the more direct approach described above, using a small extracellular electrode to examine release from individual visualised sympathetic varicosities in mouse vas deferens (during stimulation at 0.2 Hz, with 4 mM $Ca^{2+}$ in the external medium), the results were partly in agreement and partly at variance with these conclusions[10]. The release probability in varicosities on the examined strings was non-uniform, varied by up to 3-fold and in general was an order of magnitude higher $(p \geq 0.1)$ than reported in the studies described above. The activity in individual varicosities remained essentially constant for at least 30 min (see Chapter 3). The explanation for the variance between the two sets of experimental results is almost certainly that the methods sample the activity in different subpopulations of varicosities (Fig. 4.4b). Whether or not this is the case remains to be established.

### 3.5   Does release from individual varicosities obey a random or a string model?

The two alternatives are shown in Fig. 4.4b. In both, a single nerve impulse releases single quanta from 1% of the varicosities. In the random model, the release probability is uniform and low $(p = 0.01)$. The probability of monoquantal release in response to two consecutive pulses is therefore 0.0001, i.e. virtually zero: transmitter does not accumulate locally during a high-frequency train. In the string model, the release probability is highly non-uniform. In $< 5\%$ of the strings the probability in the average varicosity is high $(0 < p < 1)$, in $> 95\%$ of the strings it is zero. Short trains at high frequency release quanta repeatedly from a subpopulation of varicosities and cause released transmitter to accumulate locally in and around these active

junctions. A definitive choice between these models cannot be made at present, but the balance of the evidence seems to support a modified string model[16].

### 3.6   Conclusions

Present methods can resolve quantal release from some but not all individual sites. A drawback with some methods is that their resolution is too high (overview is lost), in others that it is too low (detail is lost). The available data by different methods are in apparent conflict and do not fit either the random or the string model, summarised in Fig. 4.4b. A new paradigm is needed in which the release probability of individual varicosities is high and stationary in some strings, high but non-stationary in other strings and, at any given time, virtually zero in the majority of strings. A working hypothesis which appears to meet these requirements is presented below (see Section 4.5).

## 4   'Local' or 'spreading' modulation of transmitter release?

Modulators of transmitter release, endogenous as well as exogenous, are currently assumed to act locally at targets (e.g. receptors to presynaptic agonists or ion channels) near the release sites. These fundamental assumptions have been challenged recently. Local agonist interaction with cell membrane receptors has been shown to generate spatially distributed, second messenger-mediated effects in other regions of the same cell. Such spreading effects may obviously be relevant, e.g. for neuronal function, by conveying signals over long distances along neurites[9]. Two concrete examples will be given. The first concerns 'local' and 'spreading' modulation of the probability of ATP release from sympathetic nerve terminals, the second 'spreading' long-term potentiation in synapses formed between a Schaffer collateral and different pyramidal cells[3].

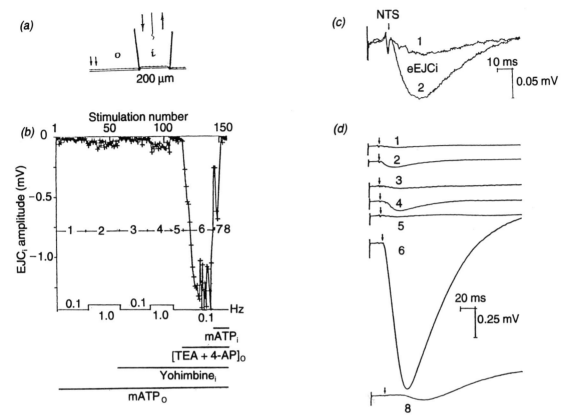

Fig. 4.5. 'Local' and 'spreading' control of ATP release from sympathetic nerve terminals. (*a*) The setup for extracellular recording: varicose nerve terminals on the surface of smooth muscle, stimulating electrode (vertical arrows) and the internally perfusable recording electrode; the medium can be changed independently outside (o) or inside (i) the electrode. The patch is probably innervated by approximately 1200 varicosities. Spontaneous tetrodotoxin-resistant EJCs (not shown) represent the release of single quanta but, even under control conditions, evoked EJCs are mostly caused by synchronous release of several ($p = 0.005$, an average of six) quanta. (*b–d*) A single representative experiment in mouse vas deferens, to show the effects of drugs added outside or inside the electrode on the nerve terminal spike (NTS) and EJC evoked by nerve stimulation at 0.1 or 1 Hz, as indicated. (*b*) Plot of peak amplitude of the EJCs versus the stimulus number. mATP, 10 μM α,β-mATP; yohimbine, 1 μM; TEA, 20 mM tetraethylammonium; 4-AP, 1 mM 4-aminopyridine. Each drug addition was followed by a 10 min stimulus-free interval (not shown). (*c*) Averaged original recordings from periods (1) and (2) in (*b*). Note that an increase in frequency from 0.1 Hz to 1 Hz had no marked effect on the NTS but greatly amplified the EJCs. (*d*) Averaged original recordings from periods 1–6, 8; note that the amplification was lower than in (*c*). For further comments see text.

## 4.1 Blockers of the K⁺ channel may enhance release by local and spreading effects

Potassium channels in nerve terminals play important roles in the control of the release probability and its presynaptic modulation. Here the sites and mechanisms involved in the enhancement of transmitter release induced by K⁺-channel blockade are considered.

### 4.1.1 Local action of K$^+$-channel blockers disrupts monoquantal release

Direct block of voltage-gated delayed rectifier and Ca$^{2+}$-activated K$^+$ channels in nerve terminals by drugs such as TEA and/or 4-AP has no effect on transmitter release evoked by depolarising concentrations of K$^+$. However, it does cause nerve stimulation with single nerve impulses to release transmitter from most or all vesicles at active zones, i.e. dramatically enhances nerve impulse-induced transmitter release[15]. The mechanisms which ensure that each nerve impulse normally releases maximally a single quantum from an active zone may, therefore, involve K$^+$ channels, or other actions of K$^+$ in the perineuronal space[15].

### 4.1.2 Local K$^+$-channel block may cause spreading enhancement of transmitter release

'Local' effects, action potential broadening and increased Ca$^{2+}$ influx in the releasing bouton are thought to be how TEA and 4-AP (see Section 4.1.1 above) enhance transmitter release[15]. The results in mouse vas deferens shown in Fig. 4.5 suggest that this may not be their only mode of action. This approach was employed to find out if modulation of the nerve impulse-induced EJCs, i.e. the quantal release of ATP from sites inside the electrode, is an exclusively 'local' or at least in part a 'spreading' effect. The assumption is that changes in the EJCs caused by adding agents to the medium internally perfusing the recording electrode are 'local' effects, while those caused by adding them to the bath are 'spreading' effects. It is important to note that the EJCs were unaffected by the presence of 10 μM α,β-mATP in the bath, added to desensitise P$_{2x}$ purinoceptors outside the electrode, but were profoundly depressed or complely blocked by further addition of this agent inside. This finding suggests, but does not conclusively prove, that leakage across the rim of the electrode was negligible, i.e. that agents added to the external medium indeed exerted their effects only on targets outside the electrode. Also important is that the procedures and agents employed in this approach have no marked effect on the frequency, amplitude or time course of spontaneous EJCs (not shown), i.e. they do not change quantal size or the rate of spontaneous release of quanta[15,17].

Consider first the enhancing effects on the EJCs, i.e. on the quantal per pulse release of ATP from sites inside the patch, caused by increasing the stimulation frequency (Fig. 4.5b–d). As shown particularly clearly in Fig. 4.5c, a rise in stimulation frequency (from 0.1 to 1 Hz) had no effect on the nerve terminal spike (NTS), i.e. the extracellularly recorded nerve terminal action potential, but caused a 4-fold increase in the EJC amplitude (i.e. the number of quanta released per pulse). This suggests that the increase in stimulation frequency had increased the probability of monoquantal release from the average release site in the patch from, approximately, 0.005 to 0.02.

Next, consider the effects on the EJCs caused by adding an α$_2$-adrenoceptor blocker inside the electrode ('local' block of α$_2$-adrenoceptor-mediated autoinhibition). As shown in Fig. 4.5b,d, addition of yohimbine to the medium superfusing the patch had no effect on the EJCs at 0.1 Hz, but at 1 Hz it further amplified the EJCs by 50%, i.e. it may have enhanced the release probability to approximately 0.03.

Then, consider the effects of adding TEA and 4-AP outside the electrode (a 'spreading' effect of K$^+$-channel block). As shown in Fig. 4.5b,d, this led (after a lag time of approximately 10 min) to a dramatic enhancement of the amplitude and duration of the EJCs. The presence of K$^+$-channel blockers some distance away from the release sites, thus, somehow caused each nerve impulse to induce massive release from sites inside the electrode[15,17].

Taken as a whole, these results suggest, first, that facilitation of release was not the result of a change in the nerve-terminal action potential but of improved depolarisation– secretion coupling. Second, they show that endogenous noradrenaline released at 1 Hz, but not at 0.1 Hz, tonically depressed release via presynaptic $\alpha_2$-adrenoceptors on nerve terminals inside the patch. Third, they show that TEA and 4-AP dramatically increased the nerve impulse-induced release, and they suggest that these drugs may do so even when they are not in direct contact with the releasing varicosities[15,17].

### 4.1.3 Structural and biochemical effects of K$^+$-channel block on transmitter release

Deduced from electron-microscopic data, the dramatic increase in the nerve impulse-induced release caused by K$^+$-channel blockers is not the result of increased mobilisation of transmitter vesicles from the reserve pool but of disruption of the mechanisms which normally cause active zones to release only single quanta. In the presence of the K$^+$-channel blockers, each nerve impulse may cause exocytosis from all vesicles docked at active zones[15]. The mechanisms by which TEA and 4-AP may exert this effect, when they are not in contact with the release site, are not known. Two 'unusual' effects, so far demonstrated only for 4-AP, may be involved[17]. The first is that this drug increases the number of large intramembrane particles at active zones, which may represent Ca$^{2+}$ channels or membrane proteins involved in vesicle docking and fusion. The second is that 4-AP increases the phosphorylation of B-50/GAP 43, a protein present on the cytosolic side of the plasma membrane of the entire axon as well as of the membrane of intra-axonal 'transport vesicles'. This protein binds calmodulin and is thought to act as a substrate for protein kinases and participate in transmembrane and intracellular signal transduction. Finally, it is tempting to speculate that K$^+$-channel blockers, even when applied at a distance, may ultimately promote 'activation' of docked vesicles by increasing the hydrolysis of GTP[8]; i.e. that this step may be normally restricted by K$^+$-channel activity (see Section 1.2).

### 4.1.4 Conclusions

The K$^+$-channel blockers TEA and 4-AP disrupt the mechanisms that normally cause each active zone to release maximally a single quantum per nerve impulse. In sympathetic nerves, they exert this effect even when applied some distance away, possibly without increasing the duration of the presynaptic action potential in the releasing varicosity. The mechanisms underlying this 'spreading' effect are not known. Whether they involve an increase in the number of Ca$^{2+}$ channels or docking proteins at the active zones, and/or phosphorylation of existing Ca$^{2+}$ channels, or of synaptic-vesicle proteins or proteins at the docking sites at the active zones, or occur by other mechanisms remains to be established[15,17].

## 4.2 Both 'local' and 'spreading' Ca$^{2+}$ effects may influence release probability

The important roles of Ca$^{2+}$ for transmitter release and its presynaptic modulation are described elsewhere (see Chapters 1, 3 and 10). Here the sites at which Ca$^{2+}$ may influence the release probability and the biochemical links involved in this control are considered. The Ca$^{2+}$ dependence of transmitter release is more complex than hitherto acknowledged. Specifically, at least in sympathetic nerves, nerve impulse-induced release seems to require Ca$^{2+}$ entry into the neurone through N-type Ca$^{2+}$ channels, both at the 'secretory' sites and at 'regulatory' sites some distance away[15-17].

### 4.2.1 'Local' actions of Ca$^{2+}$

Findings in squid giant synapse[1,8,20] indicate that the normal nerve terminal action potential opens only a small fraction (less than 10%) of the N-type Ca$^{2+}$ channels present near the active zone. The Ca$^{2+}$ influx increases, for a few tens of microseconds, the Ca$^{2+}$ level within tens of nanometres of the mouth of the open channels to extremely high levels ($\gg 100$ μM). It is probably this 'fast' and spatially restricted $Ca^{2+}$ signal which triggers transmitter release (see also Chapter 1). Agents that modulate the number and/or the duration of the open state of these channels are likely to strongly modulate the release from vesicles already docked at the active zones. However, there is also a 'slow', global $Ca^{2+}$ signal caused by influx through N-, L-, P- and 'leak' channels not necessarily concentrated near the active zone and activated by voltage, receptor, G-protein and second messenger changes. This $Ca^{2+}$ signal may be that which regulates the availability of vesicles for docking at active zones[7]. The channels which mediate this signal, therefore, could be targets of agents that lead to slow plastic changes in the release probability[7,8,20].

### 4.2.2 'Spreading' actions of $Ca^{2+}$?

Based on classical experiments in frog neuromuscular endplate, it is generally accepted that nerve impulses release transmitter even when $Ca^{2+}$ is not generally present in the medium but is restricted to the vicinity of the release sites[15]. However, this does not indicate that the perineuronal concentration of $Ca^{2+}$ in other regions is unimportant in events related to transmitter release. In presynaptic terminals of squid giant synapse, for example, the presence of $Ca^{2+}$ in the external medium is required for 'fast' axonal transport of synaptic vesicles towards the active zones[4,17]. In addition, as shown by extracellular recording (in experiments using the technique shown in Fig. 4.5), removal of $Ca^{2+}$ from the external medium or addition of N-type $Ca^{2+}$-channel blockers only outside the electrode blocks the nerve impulse-induced release of ATP from sympathetic varicosities in the patch inside the electrode[15-17]. Therefore, in order to induce release, nerve impulses may require the presence of $Ca^{2+}$ and also N-type $Ca^{2+}$ channels both locally and some distance away from the site of release. The 'spreading' $Ca^{2+}$-dependent effect has been found to be temperature sensitive, suggesting that it may involve active transport of

some regulatory factor, and was not demonstrable when the internal diameter of the recording electrode was $< 400$ μm[15,16]. The identity of the putative messenger remains to be established. Meanwhile, the results indicate that, at least in sympathetic nerve varicosities, active $Ca^{2+}$-dependent intra-axonal transport of an unknown permissive factor to the secretory sites may be required in order for the action potential to trigger transmitter release[15-17].

### 4.2.3 Intra-terminal biochemical links between $Ca^{2+}$ entry and transmitter release

Several recent studies show that the $Ca^{2+}$ current in nerve terminals and the concentration of $Ca^{2+}$ at the active zone do not directly determine the release probability. This does not contradict the findings in squid giant synapse under voltage-clamp conditions, which show that transmitter release is normally proportional to the strength of the presynaptic current pulses and the inward $Ca^{2+}$ current ($I_{Ca}$). These rules evidently apply only as long as the biochemical environment of vesicles remains unchanged. Microinjection of dephospho-synapsin I into the presynaptic terminal (to increase cross-linking of synaptic vesicles with actin filaments in the cytoskeleton) progressively depressed the evoked release. Conversely, injection of $Ca^{2+}$-calmodulin-dependent protein kinase II (to phosphorylate endogenous synapsin I and, thereby, free the vesicles and enable them to move to the active zone) progressively enhanced the evoked release. In both cases this occurred without altering $I_{Ca}$[7]. The ability of intra-terminal $Ca^{2+}$ to trigger release is, thus, ultimately biochemically controlled. This conclusion is supported by the aforementioned finding (see Sections 1.2 and 4.1.3), also in squid giant synapse, that prejunctional injection of GTPγS, a non-hydrolysable GTP analogue, blocked the action potential-induced exocytosis of vesicles docked at the active zone, without changing the $Ca^{2+}$ current[8] (see also Chapter 11). The functional state of a regulatory

G-protein-dependent mechanism may, therefore, decide whether or not the action potential-induced entry of $Ca^{2+}$ will trigger exocytosis from a docked vesicle.

### 4.3 Is modulation of release by prejunctional agonists a 'local' or a 'spreading' effect?

Presynaptic agonists that modulate release are generally believed to act only locally, via receptors near the active zone of the bouton or varicosity whose secretory activity they control[15]. However, the evidence on this point is ambiguous. As illustrated by the points below, it is unclear whether exogenous agonists modulate transmitter release only by an action on receptors at the releasing site ('local' effect), only by actions exerted some distance away ('spreading' effect), or both. Furthermore, it seems possible that the releasing site itself may be 'immune' to direct, local autoinhibition by transmitter in quanta it has just released.

#### 4.3.1 The machinery for 'local' control is present

The most direct evidence for 'local' regulation of release is that exogenous agonists modulate the $Ca^{2+}$-dependent secretion of transmitters from synaptosomes (torn-off nerve-terminal boutons or varicosities) induced by veratridine- or $K^+$-induced depolarisation. There can be no doubt, therefore, that boutons/varicosities possess the receptors and postreceptor mechanisms required to modulate depolarisation–secretion coupling[14,15,18]. This view is also supported by the finding by patch-clamp techniques that ion channels that control the release probability may be modulated locally. Presynaptically active agonists have been shown to depress $Ca^{2+}$ and enhance $K^+$ conductances, e.g. in sympathetic neurones, by receptors that are coupled via G-proteins directly to the ion channels and that, therefore, do not require a soluble second messenger. Two caveats should be kept in mind: first, that these observations were made in the cell soma, and, second, that the finding that ion channels which influence the release probability are locally modulated does not exclude the possibility that release itself is modulated by a mobile second messenger (see also Chapters 9 and 10).

#### 4.3.2 Autoinhibition may be 'lateral' rather than 'local'

In the experimental paradigm shown in Fig. 4.5, addition of exogenous $\alpha_2$-agonist to the medium perfusing the electrode dose-dependently depresses the EJCs[5]. Furthermore, addition of the sympathomimetic amine tyramine, inside the electrode, to increase the molecular leakage of noradrenaline from all regions of the terminals, profoundly depresses the EJCs[5,16]. The nerve impulse-induced release of transmitter from sites inside the patch is, thus, strongly inhibited by relatively low concentrations of diffusely applied endogenous or exogenous $\alpha_2$-adrenoceptor agonist. Nevertheless, as shown in Fig. 4.5b,d, addition of yohimbine inside the electrode to block the $\alpha_2$-adrenoceptors within the patch amplified the EJCs (at 1 Hz) by 'only' 50%. This effect may seem substantial, but it is 'small' when compared with the dramatic effect of $K^+$-channel blockers in the same experiment, showing that $K^+$-channel activity is much more important than $\alpha_2$-adrenoceptor-mediated autoinhibition for restricting release.

Surprisingly, therefore, 'active' varicosities seem to be not, or only weakly, inhibited by noradrenaline in quanta they have just released, even though the noradrenaline concentration in the junctional cleft would be extremely high (initial peak level: 70 mM[14]). In contrast, 'active' varicosities are strongly inhibited by endogenous or exogenous $\alpha_2$-adrenoceptor agonists, distributed diffusely, at much lower concentrations ($<< 1 \mu M$), in their surrounding environment. These observations have led to the hypothesis that noradrenaline in released quanta may be unable to inhibit the varicosity from which it was

76                                                L Stjärne

released but is capable of depressing release
from neighbouring varicosities ('lateral inhibition')[5,15]. A modification of this hypothesis
will be presented below (Section 5; see also
Chapter 5). Meanwhile, it is interesting to
note that this phenomenon may not be
unique to sympathetic varicosities: actively
releasing sites in other systems (neuromuscular synapses *in vitro*) have been reported to
be 'immune' to negative feedback (in that
case, by trans-synaptic signals)[6].

### 4.3.3 'Spreading' actions of presynaptic agonists

Suggestive evidence for 'spreading' modulation of release by prejunctional agonists has
been obtained in the experimental paradigm
shown in Fig. 4.5. Addition of $\alpha_2$-adrenocep-
tor agonists outside the electrode depressed
the nerve impulse-induced (but not the spontaneous) EJCs (i.e. evoked transmitter
release from sites within the patch) even
when the $\alpha_2$-adrenoceptors in the patch were
protected by the presence of an $\alpha_2$-adreno-
ceptor antagonist in the medium perfusing
the electrode[15].

### 4.4 Long-term potentiation may involve both 'local' and 'spreading' synaptic enhancement

The examples above of 'local' and 'spreading'
control of transmitter release are taken from
sympathetic nerves. The results in Fig. 4.6
show that both control mechanisms may be
involved in long-term potentiation (LTP) in
rat hippocampus[3]. Figure 4.6 shows that, as
predicted by Hebbian theory, simultaneous
stimulation of cell 1 and the afferent Schaffer
collateral fibre 'a' induced LTP in synapse A
but not in B. In apparent contradiction of
Hebbian theory, however, LTP was induced
in cell 2 as well. The mechanism which
strengthened synapse A, therefore, somehow
spread over a distance of up to 150 $\mu$m to
synapse C between fibre 'a' and cell 2. The
mechanism      underlying      this      intriguing

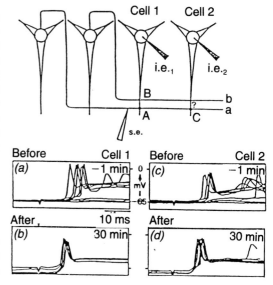

Fig. 4.6. 'Local' and 'spreading' long-term
potentiation (LTP) in rat hippocampus. *Upper panel.*
Four pyramidal cells are shown with two afferent
Schaffer collateral presynaptic fibres (a, b) which
form *en-passant* synaptic contact with the apical
dendrites of cell 1 and cell 2 (separated by up to
150 $\mu$m). s.e., stimulating electrode, i.e. intracellular
electrodes. *Lower panel.* A concrete example.
Simultaneous intracellular recordings from two
pyramidal cells in a hippocampal slice culture
(separation between cell 1 and cell 2: 30 $\mu$m),
showing responses to stimulation (at 0.25 Hz) of the
afferent Schaffer collateral fibre by which both cells
were innervated, before and 30 min after
simultaneous pre- and postsynaptic stimulation of cell
1. Contrary to Hebbian rule, this stimulation caused
the LTP in cell 1 to spread to cell 2 (note the many
failures in *a* and *c* and the non-intermittent response
in *b* and *d*). (From ref. 3, with permission.)

'spreading synaptic enhancement' is not yet
fully understood[3].

### 4.4.5    Conclusions

Suggestive evidence from different systems
indicates that modulators of transmitter
release may not exert their effects exclusively
via local targets (see Chapters 5 and 6) or only
by altering the intra-terminal concentration

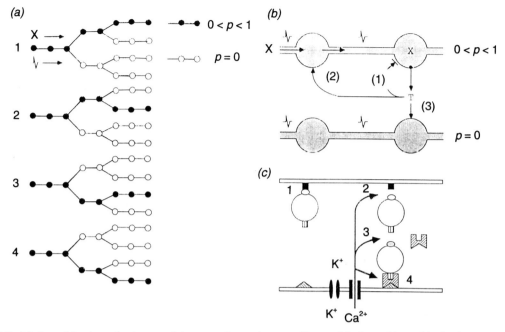

Fig. 4.7. (*a*) A working hypothesis to explain transmitter release and its modulation: a hierarchical string model of *p*, the probability of monoquantal release in individual varicosities. Filled circles: potentially active varicosities in strings in which X is present ($0 < p < 1$); open circles: 'silent' varicosities in strings lacking X ($p = 0$). For further comments, see the text. (*b*) Implications of the model at the microscopic level: 'lateral' autoregulation of the release probability? (1) The releasing varicosity is 'immune' to direct autoinhibition by T in the quantum it has just released. (2) Action of T on the T-autoreceptors of the next varicosity along the string inhibits the transport of X and silences the releasing varicosity ('lateral autoinhibition'). (3) T has no observable 'lateral' effects on the silent varicosities along the second string. For further comments, see text. (*c*) Implications of the model at submicroscopic and molecular levels: possible molecular levels of modulation of release. Top bar: actin filament; bottom bar: plasma membrane with a docking site at the active zone and (several) $K^+$ and $Ca^{2+}$ channels. (1) A synaptic vesicle in the reserve pool tethered to an actin filament by dephospho-synapsin I, associated with the vesicle via a subunit of $Ca^{2+}$-calmodulin protein kinase II on its surface. (2) A rise in $Ca^{2+}$ levels activates $Ca^{2+}$-calmodulin protein kinase II and releases the vesicle. (3) The vesicle is targeted to the docking protein at the active zone by its counterpart protein on the surface of the vesicle. (4) Fusion occurs only if a soluble factor is present. For further comments see text (see also Chapter 1).

of free $Ca^{2+}$ (see Chapters 1, 9, 10 and 11). They could exert their effects in part via 'biochemical' targets and may, in addition to their 'local' actions, influence release by 'spreading' mechanisms. In some cells, long-range actions are mediated by identified intracellular second messengers, such as Ins(1,4,5)$P_3$ and cAMP, or by intercellular messengers, such as nitric oxide[9]. The messengers mediating the 'spreading' actions in

sympathetic nerves described in Section 4.3 remain to be identified.

## 5 Sites and mechanisms of modulation of neurotransmitter release: models and hypotheses

Several of the results described above are difficult to explain in terms of existing models of transmitter release and its modulation. Figure 4.7 shows at the macroscopic, microscopic and submicroscopic levels a working hypothesis for control of nerve impulse-induced release in nerves with *boutons-en-passant* terminals that may explain the data.

## 5.1    A hierarchical string model

The view that the probability of nerve impulse-induced monoquantal transmitter release is determined exclusively by local factors cannot explain the puzzling geometry of transmitter release from sympathetic nerve terminals, i.e. that the release probability in varicosities appears to be high and stationary in some strings, high but non-stationary in others and in the majority, at any given moment, virtually zero. Nor can a local control model explain the observation that modulators influence release in sites with which they are apparently not in direct contact. These puzzling data are explainable in terms of a hypothetical hierarchical string model, the macroscopic aspects of which are shown in Fig. 4.7a (see ref. 16). Although based on data from sympathetic neurones, the model may be valid as well for other neurones with similar, repeatedly branching varicose terminals. In this model, each nerve impulse releases a quantum from 1% of the varicosities. The postulated reason for the low average-release probability is that the nerve impulse, although invading all varicosities, cannot release a transmitter quantum unless a soluble permissive factor is present. This factor, which has not been identified and hence is provisionally termed $X$[15-17], is carried towards the terminals by $Ca^{2+}$-dependent, fast intra-axonal transport. Because it is particle associated, it is forced to make binary 'choices' at each branch point. Varicosities in strings where $X$ is present have a finite release probability ($0 < p < 1$); in strings that at the moment lack $X$ the varicosities are 'silent' ($p = 0$). At low frequencies of nerve-impulse traffic, the release probability in parent string varicosities is relatively constant. The branches are activated in rotation; hence

activity in most individual branches is intermittent. The release probability in varicosities declines progressively in successive branch generation. As the majority of varicosities reside in distal branches, the release probability in the average varicosity within the total population will eventually become very low. With a sufficient number of branch generations, the nerve impulse will release a quantum from less than 1% of all varicosities. Note that, in this hypothesis, $X$ is a possible target of modulators of release[16].

## 5.2    'Lateral autoinhibition' of the releasing varicosity

Figure 4.7b shows some implications of the hierarchical string model, at the microscopic level[16]. All varicosities have receptors to transmitter T and the machinery by which exogenous T may depress their release mechanisms. The action potential releases quanta only from the varicosity in which $X$ is present at the moment. Furthermore the presence of $X$ makes the releasing varicosity 'immune' to direct autoinhibition by T in the quantum it has just released (1). During an impulse train, this varicosity therefore releases T quanta repeatedly, increasing the local T concentration and the diffusion of T to the surroundings. When the T concentration at the next varicosity on the same string becomes sufficiently high, T-induced activation of its autoreceptors (2) inhibits the transport of $X$ and thereby silences the releasing varicosity ('lateral autoinhibition'). In contrast, T has no observable 'lateral' effects on the silent varicosities along the second string (3).

In this hypothesis autoinhibition occurs under conditions when the repeated release of quanta from the same site has saturated the local receptor patch at and around the active junction. The physiological role of 'lateral autoinhibition' is to control the 'heat' in this 'hotspot' by restricting its diameter, i.e. to turn off release and thereby prevent a useless further increase in the local transmitter concentration.

## 5.3 Possible molecular mechanisms of release modulation

Figure 4.7c illustrates the part of the hypothesis that concerns events at the submicroscopic and molecular levels (but see also Chapter 1). The model presumes that $K^+$ efflux or a rise in periterminal $[K^+]$ are the main factors which cause each active zone normally to release maximally one quantum per nerve impulse[15-17], probably by modulating a G-protein-mediated mechanism required to make docked vesicles 'releasable'[8]. At the mouth of N-type channels at the active zones, $Ca^{2+}$ binds to low-affinity receptors and triggers exocytosis of a single vesicle (provided that an 'activated' vesicle[8] is present). The global $Ca^{2+}$ concentration influences a range of processes that affect the release probability. Synaptic vesicles in the reserve pool are tethered to actin filaments by dephospho-synapsin I, associated with the vesicle via a subunit of $Ca^{2+}$-calmodulin-dependent protein kinase II on their surface (Fig. 4.7c, 1)[7]. A rise in $Ca^{2+}$ activates $Ca^{2+}$-calmodulin-dependent protein kinase II, which phosphorylates synapsin I and releases the vesicle, allowing it to move to the active zone (Fig. 4.7c, 2). It is suggested that this step is restricted by autoreceptor activation, which possibly tonically depresses the global $Ca^{2+}$ concentration[7]. The 'free' vesicle is targeted to the docking protein(s) (t-SNARE[13]) at the active zone by its counterpart vesicle surface protein(s) (v-SNARE[13]). A soluble factor (NSF-SNAP-SNAP[13]) has to be present (Fig. 4.7c, 3) for fusion to occur (Fig. 4.7c, 4). The reason why the majority of vesicles docked at the active zone ignore the $Ca^{2+}$ signal could be either the presence of an unknown inhibitory component (a 'fusion clamp'[13]) or the lack of an unidentified permissive factor ($X$?)[15-17].

## 6 Summary

Technical difficulties complicate the analysis of neurotransmitter release and the sites at which it is modulated. Particularly problematical is the fact that methods available at present do not measure release *per se* but release minus clearance and that clearance of released transmitters is physiologically and pharmacologically variable. Data obtained using different approaches in different systems indicate that intrinsic mechanisms, as yet poorly understood, restrict the size of the releasable pool, set an upper limit to the release probability in individual potential-release sites and cause each active zone to release maximally one quantum per nerve impulse. The physiological role of these restrictive mechanisms is probably to prevent depletion of the transmitter store and maintain long-term transmission capability in the synapse.

Numerous modulatory factors influence the probability of monoquantal release: (i) the frequency and number of nerve impulses; (ii) agents released from the effector or from other neurones, or derived from the bloodstream, acting via prejunctional heteroreceptors; and, finally, (iii) the neurone's own transmitters acting via prejunctional autoreceptors. The role of heteroreceptor-mediated control is to fine tune neuro-effector transmission, whereas that of autoinhibition is to prevent excessive accumulation of transmitter in 'hotspots', i.e. the area around repeatedly releasing single sites.

The effects of local application of release modulators are not only local, on the release sites with which they are in contact, but may also spread longitudinally along nerve terminals, possibly by influencing an intra-axonally transported permissive factor whose presence may be necessary for the action potential to induce release.

An actively releasing bouton/varicosity is 'immune' to direct autoinhibition by the transmitter it has just released, but sensitive to 'lateral autoinhibition' via receptors on neighbouring boutons/varicosities along the same string.

It should be appreciated that these conclusions are tentative and concern the *possible* sites and mechanisms of prejunctional control of transmitter release. The current tremendous progress in this field made by molecular biologists promises that the molecular basis of many of these mechanisms will be clarified in the near future.

# References

1. Atwood HL and Wojtowicz (1986) Short-term and long-term plasticity and physiological differentiation of crustacean motor synapses. *International Review of Neurobiology* **28:** 275–361

2. Bao JX, Gonon F and Stjärne L (1993) Kinetics of ATP- and noradrenaline-mediated sympathetic neuromuscular transmission in rat tail artery. *Acta Physiologica Scandinavica* **149:** 503–519

3. Bonhoeffer T, Staiger V and Aertsen A (1989) Synaptic plasticity in rat hippocampal slice cultures: local 'Hebbian' conjunction of pre- and postsynaptic stimulation leads to distributed synaptic enhancement. *Proceedings of the National Academy of Sciences, USA* **86:** 8113–8117

4. Breuer AC, Bond M and Atkinson MB (1992) Fast axonal transport is modulated by altering trans-axolemmal calcium flux. *Cell Calcium* **13:** 249–262

5. Brock JA and Cunnane TC (1992) Electrophysiology of neuroeffector transmission in smooth muscle. In: Burnstock G and Hoyle CHV (eds) *Autonomic Neuroeffector Mechanisms*, pp 121–213, Harwood Academic, Reading

6. Dan Y and Poo M (1992) Hebbian depression of isolated neuromuscular synapses *in vitro*. *Science* **256:** 1570–1573

7. Greengard P, Valtorta F, Czernik AJ and Benfenati F (1993) Synaptic vesicle phosphoproteins and regulation of synaptic function. *Science* **259:** 780–785

8. Hess SD, Doroshenko PA and Augustine GJ (1993) A functional role for GTP-binding proteins in synaptic vesicle cycling. *Science* **259:** 1169–1172

9. Kasai H and Petersen OH (1994) Spatial dynamics of second messengers: $IP_3$ and cAMP as long-range and associative messengers. *Trends in Neurosciences* **17:** 95–101

10. Lavidis NA and Bennett MR (1992) Probabilistic secretion of quanta from visualised sympathetic nerve varicosities in mouse vas deferens. *Journal of Physiology* **454:** 9–26

11. Msghina M and Stjärne L (1993) Facilitation and depression of ATP and noradrenaline release during high frequency stimulation of sympathetic nerves. *Neuroscience Letters* **155:** 37–41

12. Müller CM (1992) A role for glial cells in activity-dependent central nervous plasticity? Review and hypothesis. *International Review of Neurobiology* **28:** 215–284

13. Söllner T, Whiteheart SW, Brunner M *et al.* (1993) SNAP receptors implicated in vesicle targeting and fusion. *Nature* **362:** 318–324

14. Starke K, Göthert M and Kilbinger H (1989) Modulation of neurotransmitter release by presynaptic autoreceptors. *Physiological Reviews* **69:** 864–989

15. Stjärne L (1989) Basic mechanisms and local modulation of nerve impulse-induced secretion of neurotransmitters from individual sympathetic nerve varicosities. *Reviews of Physiology, Biochemistry and Pharmacology* **112:** 1–138

16. Stjärne L, Bao JX, Gonon F, Msghina M and Stjärne E (1993) A two-compartment string model of sympathetic neuromuscular transmission. *News in Physiological Sciences* **8:** 253–260

17. Stjärne L, Stjärne E, Msghina M and Bao J-X (1991) $K^+$ and $Ca^{2+}$ channel blockers may enhance or depress sympathetic transmitter release via a $Ca^{2+}$-dependent mechanism 'upstream' of the release site. *Neuroscience* **44:** 673–692

18. Verhage M, McMahon HT, Ghijsen WEJM *et al.* (1992) Differential release of amino acids, neuropeptides and catecholamines from isolated nerve terminals. *Neuron* **6:** 517–524

19. von Kügelgen I and Starke K (1991) Noradrenaline- and ATP co-transmission in the sympathetic nervous system. *Trends in Pharmacological Sciences* **12:** 319–324

20. Zucker RS (1989) Short-term synaptic plasticity. *Annual Reviews of Neuroscience* **12:** 13–31

# 5 Modulation of neurotransmitter release by autoreceptors

James A. Brock

Modulation of neurotransmitter release was formally recognised in the late 1960s when it was reported that the amount of transmitter released from the neurone was inversely related to the magnitude of the postjunctional effector response. It was suggested that a substance liberated from the activated effector inhibited transmitter release. Subsequent experiments showed that the nerve terminals themselves possess receptors for the released transmitter and that their activation inhibits release. This assisted neurotransmitter economy at neuronal level: if there is already a high concentration of neurotransmitter in the synaptic cleft then from the perspective of the postjunctional effector there is perhaps less need to release more. This feedback inhibition has been demonstrated and is termed 'autoregulation' and the receptors are known as 'autoreceptors'. A common presumption is that it is autoreceptors located on a particular nerve terminal or varicosity which modulate the subsequent release from those particular sites. In this chapter, James Brock considers this and widens the definition of autoreceptors to accommodate the parallel concepts of co-transmission and modulation of neurotransmitter release from sites distant to those from which release has just occurred.

## 1 What are autoreceptors?

The term autoreceptor is applied to a receptor present on a neurone for a neurotransmitter released from that neurone. Autoreceptors have been described both at the soma-dendritic membrane and at the axonal membrane of neurones close to the sites of neurotransmitter release. The aim of this chapter is to consider the roles that autoreceptors located at the nerve terminal (presynaptic autoreceptors) play in the modulation of neurotransmitter release. Activation of presynaptic autoreceptors may either increase (facilitatory autoreceptors) or decrease (inhibitory autoreceptors) transmitter release evoked by nerve impulses. In addition they may alter the synthesis of the neurotransmitter, an effect that might indirectly modulate its release. Nerve terminals also possess transmitter release-modulating receptors responding to endogenous substances other than those released by that neurone (heteroreceptors). These heteroreceptors are the subject of the following chapter.

To date, the pharmacological evidence suggests that virtually all neuronal types, including adrenergic, noradrenergic, dopaminergic, histaminergic, serotonergic, cholinergic, GABAergic and glutamatergic neurones, possess presynaptic transmitter release-modulating autoreceptors. Indeed, single neurones have been found to possess presynaptic autoreceptors for more than one transmitter substance (i.e. for the

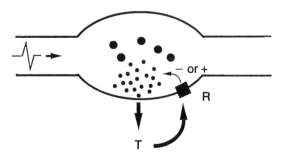

Fig. 5.1. Schematic representation of autoregulation of transmitter release. Transmitter (T) released from the nerve terminal by a nerve impulse feeds back locally at receptors (R) located on the same nerve terminal to facilitate or inhibit release evoked by subsequent nerve impulses.

co-transmitters released together with the main transmitter). The presence of auto-receptors on nerve terminals raises the possibility that these are sites at which the neurone's own transmitter acts to modulate (autoregulate) the amount of transmitter secreted; facilitatory and inhibitory autoreceptors being involved in a positive or a negative feedback regulation of transmitter release, respectively (Fig. 5.1). However, the functional role that presynaptic autoreceptors play in the regulation of transmitter release is a matter of considerable debate.

In this chapter, the types of evidence needed to establish the presence and a functional role for transmitter release-modulating presynaptic autoreceptors are briefly reviewed. The topic of presynaptic and, in particular, autoreceptor-mediated modulation of transmitter release has been extensively reviewed elsewhere[13,19,20,26–28,33] and the interested reader is referred to these articles for a more extensive discussion.

## 2    Evidence for the existence of presynaptic autoreceptors

Two basic observations suggest the existence of presynaptic transmitter release-modulating autoreceptors. First, application of the neurotransmitter or a related agonist modifies (increase or decrease) evoked transmitter release. Second, the presynaptic effects of the neurotransmitter or agonist is inhibited competitively by antagonists. However, such observations do not confirm the presynaptic location of the activated receptor. The possibility remains that the receptors activated are postsynaptic and a substance(s) released from the activated postsynaptic cell acts trans-synaptically to modulate neurotransmitter release. Furthermore, in tissues containing entire neurones (e.g. brain slices), the effects of the agonists and antagonists may be exerted either (i) at soma-dendritic receptors modifying the rate of action-potential generation in the cell body or (ii) at other synaptically connected neurones or even on other adjacent cells (e.g. glial cells).

Confirmation of the presynaptic (nerve terminal) location of the activated receptors has proved problematical. When preparations are free of neuronal cell bodies, it is possible in some cases to find agonists and/or antagonists that apparently act specifically on the nerve terminals and are without any discernible effects postsynaptically. In preparations containing cell bodies, the effects of the agonists and antagonists on transmitter release evoked by direct depolarisation of the nerve terminals (e.g. by raising the external $K^+$ concentration) in the presence of the $Na^+$ channel-blocking agent tetrodotoxin have been investigated. Tetrodotoxin prevents the generation of propagated nerve action potentials and, therefore, the effects of agonists and antagonists exerted at the cell body can be excluded. However, even then the possibility remains that the receptors activated are located postsynaptically or on other surrounding cells.

The cell bodies and dendrites of many neurones respond to application of their own neurotransmitters, demonstrating that they possess autoreceptors. Since responses can be obtained by focal application (e.g. ionophoresis) of the neurotransmitter or related agonists to the cell body, these receptors are most likely to be present in the soma-dendritic membrane. While *in situ* these soma-dendritic autoreceptors may play an important role in regulating neuronal function, their activation is unlikely to modulate transmitter release directly. However, pharmacologically, the soma-dendritic autoreceptors often appear to be identical to the transmitter release-modulating presynaptic autoreceptors, demonstrating expression of the gene encoding the receptor in the neurone. Since presynaptic autoreceptors synthesised in the cell body would have to be transported along the axon to reach the nerve terminals, demonstration of the axonal transport of such receptors would strongly support the nerve-terminal location of the autoreceptors.

If the receptors are located on the nerve terminals, then destruction of the nerve terminals should result in decreased receptor numbers in the innervated tissue. Changes in receptor numbers produced by nerve lesions have been quantified by radioligand-binding studies. However, the results of such studies are often equivocal and must be viewed with caution. For example, denervation may cause postsynaptic changes with resultant increases or decreases in receptor numbers. Furthermore, as the presynaptic receptors may only represent a small fraction of the total tissue population of receptors, any decrease caused by nerve lesioning might be undetectable by ligand-binding assays.

The only studies that appear to provide unequivocal evidence for the nerve-terminal location of autoreceptors are those where the effects of agonists and antagonists can be demonstrated in synaptosomes. Synaptosomes are pinched-off nerve terminals prepared by tissue homogenisation followed by their separation on density gradients. Transmitter release can be evoked from synaptosomes by raising the $K^+$ concentration of the bathing solution and modulation of this release by receptor activation can be determined. In this case, it is difficult to conceive that the effects of agonists and antagonists on transmitter release are being exerted at sites other than receptors on the nerve-terminal membrane.

## 3  Evidence for a functional role for autoreceptors

While much evidence supports the view that nerve terminals possess autoreceptors, the activation of which modulates neurotransmitter release, much debate has centred on the question of whether such receptors are involved functionally in the autoregulation of transmitter release. The primary criterion for proposing a functional role for presynaptic autoreceptors is the demonstration that an antagonist specific for a presynaptic autoreceptor alters evoked transmitter release in a manner consistent with these receptors being activated by the endogenous agonist (i.e. the released neurotransmitter). Conversely, failure of an antagonist to alter transmitter release implies that the autoreceptors are not operational, at least under the conditions of the experiment. This last point is of particular importance, since in many tissues it has been demonstrated that the extent to which presynaptic autoreceptors are activated depends on the experimental conditions.

It is predicted that as the concentration of the endogenous agonist at the presynaptic autoreceptors is increased the release-modulating action of exogenously applied agonists should decrease. Conversely, the effects of antagonists should increase. Therefore, the demonstration that the transmitter release-modulating action of an added agonist is decreased and of an antagonist is increased by procedures expected to raise the extracellular concentration of the endogenous agonist provides good evidence for a functional autoregulation.

In the following section, three specific examples of presynaptic transmitter release-modulating autoreceptors are described. In each case, the basic *in vitro* evidence for the existence and location of these autoreceptors is briefly reviewed. In addition, special attention is given to other information gained *in vitro* indicating a functional role for these receptors in the autoregulation of transmitter release. The role *in vivo* that some autoreceptors play in modulating transmitter release is dealt with elsewhere in this book (see Part 4).

## 4 Autoreceptors on noradrenergic nerves

### 4.1 Noradrenergic α-adrenoceptors

The increase in noradrenaline efflux (the noradrenaline diffusing from the tissue into the surrounding bathing medium) evoked by electrical stimulation of almost all tissues innervated by noradrenergic nerves (e.g. postganglionic sympathetic nerves) is inhibited by the application of α-adrenoceptor agonists (e.g. noradrenaline, clonidine), an effect reversed by α-adrenoceptor antagonists (e.g. yohimbine, idazoxan)[13,26,27]. Similarly, application of α-adrenoceptor antagonists alone generally causes an increase in evoked noradrenaline efflux[27]. Since the effects of the α-adrenoceptor agonists and antagonists cannot be explained by changes in the uptake and/or metabolism of released noradrenaline, it has been concluded that there is an alteration in the amount of noradrenaline released from the nerves. In support of this conclusion, α-adrenoceptor antagonists have been shown to increase the release of the vesicular protein dopamine β-hydroxylase from postganglionic sympathetic nerves, a protein for which there is no known mechanism of inactivation[9].

Early attempts to explain the transmitter release-facilitating action of α-adrenoceptor antagonists favoured a postsynaptic site, these agents being said to increase transmitter efflux by reducing the combination of released noradrenaline with its postsynaptic receptor. The key experiment that led to a change in interpretation was the finding that α-adrenoceptor antagonists increase noradrenaline release from cardiac tissues, where the effector response to sympathetic nerve stimulation is mediated through postsynaptic β-adrenoceptors[29]. In this case the action of α-adrenoceptor antagonists could not be

attributed to postsynaptic phenomena. Indeed, α-adrenoceptor antagonists were found to increase the response of cardiac tissues to sympathetic nerve stimulation, a finding consistent with their ability to increase transmitter release (see ref. 12). To explain this observation, Starke[24] proposed that noradrenergic nerve terminals possess α-adrenoceptors that, when activated by released noradrenaline, inhibit (autoregulate) transmitter release. The demonstration that exogenous noradrenaline inhibited the release of noradrenaline from cardiac tissue during nerve stimulation and that this action was antagonised by α-adrenoceptor antagonists supported this idea[25].

### 4.1.1 Which α-adrenoceptor subtype: $\alpha_1$ or $\alpha_2$?

On the basis of the differential sensitivity of pre- and postsynaptic α-adrenoceptors to the non-competitive adrenoceptor antagonist phenoxybenzamine, Langer[18] proposed a division of the α-adrenoceptor into $\alpha_1$ (postsynaptic) and $\alpha_2$ (presynaptic) subtypes. In support of this subclassification, the pre- and postsynaptic receptors in a number of different tissues have been shown to differ in their sensitivity to a range of α-adrenoceptor agonists and antagonists (see ref. 19). However, α-adrenoceptors with similar pharmacological characteristics to $\alpha_2$-adrenoceptors have been described at postsynaptic sites as well as on the noradrenergic nerve terminals (e.g. in vascular smooth muscle[32]) and there is evidence that supports the existence of transmitter release-inhibiting presynaptic $\alpha_1$-adrenoceptors (see ref. 28). Nevertheless, it is the effect of activating presynaptic $\alpha_2$-adrenoceptors that predominates, and it is these receptors that will be described further.

Besides inhibitory α-adrenoceptors, many noradrenergic nerves also possess transmitter release-facilitating $\beta_2$-adrenoceptors. However, these receptors are relatively insensitive to released noradrenaline and are not considered to play an autoregulatory role normally. It has been proposed that the presynaptic β-adrenoceptors may become functional 'autoreceptors' when circulating adrenaline released from the adrenal medulla is accumulated by postganglionic sympathetic nerves and released as a co-transmitter (see Chapters 14 and 17).

Evidence supporting the nerve-terminal location of transmitter release-modulating $\alpha_2$-adrenoceptors is as follows. (i) The $\alpha_2$-adrenoceptor agonists and antagonists modify transmitter release in a great range of tissues with differing perineuronal environments (blood vessels, heart, kidney, submandibular gland and cerebral cortex). The one common element in all these tissues is the noradrenergic nerve terminal. (ii) Noradrenergic neurones possess soma-dendritic $\alpha_2$-adrenoceptors, demonstrating that they express the gene encoding the $\alpha_2$-adrenoceptor[27]. (iii) In the submaxillary gland, $\alpha_2$-adrenoceptor-mediated modulation of transmitter release from the postganglionic sympathetic nerves innervating the secretory cells survives ligation of the collecting ducts, a procedure that causes atrophy of the (postsynaptic) secretory cells[12]. In this case, the effects of $\alpha$-adrenoceptor agonists and antagonists cannot be explained by an action at the effector cell. (iv) In various brain slice preparations, noradrenaline release evoked by raising the $K^+$ concentration (in the presence of tetrodotoxin) is inhibited by $\alpha_2$-adrenoceptor agonists (see ref. 27). This finding excludes a mechanism of action mediated through $\alpha_2$-adrenoceptors located at the soma or dendrites of the neurone or at other synaptically connected neurones. (v) Noradrenaline release from synaptosomes is inhibited by $\alpha_2$-adrenoceptor agonists (see ref. 27). This finding strongly supports the nerve-terminal location of the transmitter release-modulating $\alpha_2$-adrenoceptors.

Along with the above supportive evidence for the nerve-terminal location of the transmitter release-inhibiting $\alpha_2$-adrenoceptors, a number of studies have reported a decrease in binding of $\alpha_2$-adrenoceptor ligands in tissues following destruction of the noradrenergic nerve terminals (see ref. 27). However, in most nerve-lesioning experiments, no change in $\alpha_2$-adrenoceptor ligand binding has been detected.

### 4.1.2 The importance of the experimental conditions for demonstrating $\alpha$-adrenoceptor-mediated autoinhibition

To date, the *in vitro* experimental evidence indicates that $\alpha_2$-adrenoceptor-mediated autoregulation of transmitter release is a universal characteristic of noradrenergic neurones (see ref. 27). However, the extent of this modulatory influence depends on the experimental conditions. For example, in accordance with the view that autoreceptors on noradrenergic nerve terminals are activated by released noradrenaline, the transmitter release-inhibiting actions of $\alpha_2$-adrenoceptor agonists is decreased and the transmitter release-facilitating actions of $\alpha_2$-adrenoceptor antagonists is increased by procedures expected to raise the extraneuronal concentration of noradrenaline (see ref. 27). Failure to demonstrate this finding in all cases has been attributed to factors other than $\alpha$-adrenoceptor-mediated autoinhibition. In particular, the facilitatory effect of $\alpha$-adrenoceptor-antagonists often decreases with increasing frequencies of stimulation. It is suggested that this occurs because the intra-axonal $Ca^{2+}$ concentration rises during trains of high-frequency stimuli to saturation levels for transmitter release; i.e. transmitter release becomes maximally facilitated. In this regard, it is important to note that inhibition of transmitter release mediated by activation of $\alpha_2$-adrenoceptors is thought most likely to result from reduced $Ca^{2+}$ entry[5] (see Chapters 9 and 10).

The importance of the experimental conditions has been elegantly demonstrated by Story *et al.*[31]. In this study, they investigated the effects of stimulation train length and stimulation frequency on the ability of the non-specific $\alpha$-adrenoceptor antagonist phentolamine to increase tritium release from [$^3$H]-noradrenaline-labelled guinea-pig atria. They showed that the release of radioactivity evoked by a train of 4 pulses at

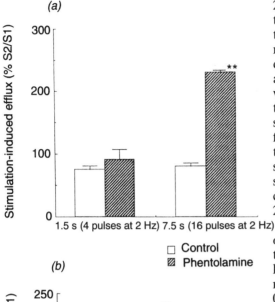

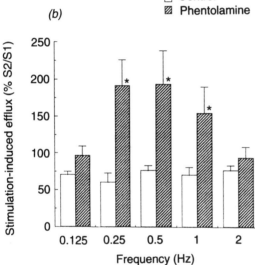

2 Hz was not significantly altered by the addition of phentolamine, while that evoked by a train of 16 pulses at 2 Hz was increased by more than 2.5-fold (Fig. 5.2$a$). These findings demonstrate that $\alpha$-adrenoceptor antagonists are unable to modify transmitter release when the concentration of noradrenaline at the autoreceptors is low, as it would be at the start of a train of stimuli. Furthermore, these findings indicate that there is a minimum time interval between the start of the train of stimuli and the time when the effect of presynaptic $\alpha_2$-adrenoceptor activation is discernible ($> 1.5$ s, the duration of 4 pulses at 2 Hz).

To investigate further the dependence of $\alpha_2$-adrenoceptor-mediated inhibition of transmitter release on the duration of stimulation, the effects of phentolamine on transmitter release evoked by trains of 4 pulses at 0.125, 0.25, 0.5, 1 and 2 Hz were compared (Fig. 5.2$b$). The release of radioactivity evoked at 0.125 and 2 Hz was not significantly altered, but that evoked at 0.25, 0.5 and 1 Hz was significantly enhanced by phentolamine. These findings suggest that there is a minimum time interval for the effects of $\alpha_2$-adrenoceptor activation to be manifested ($> 1.5$ s, the duration of 4 pulses at 2 Hz) and a limited period during which transmitter release evoked by one pulse can influence that evoked by subsequent pulses ($< 8$ s, the interval between two pulses at 0.125 Hz).

Fig. 5.2. Effect of the $\alpha$-adrenoceptor antagonist phentolamine (3 $\mu$M) on stimulation-evoked efflux of tritium from guinea-pig atria previously loaded with [$^3$H]-noradrenaline. Two periods of identical stimulation were given with an interval of 30 min between them. In test preparations, phentolamine was added 20 min before the second period of stimulation. In both histograms ($a$ and $b$) the radioactivity released by the second period of stimulation (S2) is expressed as a percentage of the radioactivity released by the first period of stimulation (S1). ($a$) The effects of stimulation with 4 or 16 pulses at 2 Hz in control (clear bars) and in phentolamine-treated (hatched bars) preparations. ($b$) The effects of stimulation with four pulses at 0.125, 0.25, 0.5, 1 and 2 Hz in control (clear bars) and phentolamine-treated (hatched bars) preparations. The results demonstrate that there is a minimum time interval for the effects of $\alpha_2$-adrenoceptor activation to be manifest ($> 1.5$ s) and a limited period during which transmitter release evoked by one pulse can influence that evoked by subsequent pulses ($< 8$ s). See text for further explanation. Significant differences: * ($p < 0.05$) ** ($p < 0.01$) from paired control. (Adapted from ref. 31, with permission.)

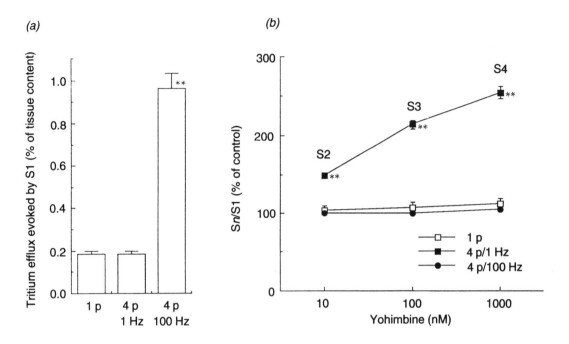

Fig. 5.3. Stimulation-evoked efflux of tritium from rabbit occipito-parietal slices previously loaded with [³H]-noradrenaline and effects of the $\alpha_2$-adrenoceptor antagonist yohimbine (10–1000 nM). After loading, the slices were superfused with medium containing the noradrenaline-uptake inhibitor desipramine (1 μM). The tissues were stimulated four times (S1 to S4) with 1 pulse (p) or 4 pulses at 1 or 100 Hz with an interval of 24 min between them. Solvent or increasing concentrations of yohimbine were added 12 min before S2, S3 and S4. (a) The efflux of tritium evoked by S1 as a percentage of the total tritium content of the tissue. (b) The ratios S$n$/S1 (S2/S1, S3/S1, S4/S1) obtained in the presence of yohimbine expressed as a percentage of the mean ratios obtained in control experiments without the drug. The results show a very pronounced autoinhibition of transmitter release following a single pulse of electrical stimulation and that a minimum time interval is required for the inhibitory effects of autoreceptor activation to be manifest: > 30 ms but < 1 s. See text for further details. Significant differences ** ($p < 0.01$) from release evoked by 1 pulse in (a) and from control in (b). (Adapted from ref. 23, with permission.)

A more striking demonstration of the impulse-by-impulse regulation of noradrenaline release has been described by Mayer *et al.*[23]. In this study, the release of radioactivity from [³H]-noradrenaline-labelled slices of rabbit cortex (occipito-parietal slices) in the presence of the monoamine-uptake inhibitor desipramine was investigated (Fig. 5.3). The release of tritium evoked by a single pulse was 0.19% of the total tritium content of the tissue (Fig. 5.3a). Stimulation with 4 pulses at 1 Hz released an amount of radioactivity similar to that released by a single pulse, while that released by 4 pulses at 100 Hz was 5.1-fold higher (Fig. 5.3a). In the presence of the $\alpha_2$-adrenoceptor antagonist yohimbine, the amount of tritium released by 4 pulses at 1 Hz was increased by up to 2.5-fold, but this treatment did not alter the release evoked by a single pulse or by 4 pulses at 100 Hz (Fig. 5.3b). This study demonstrates, as did that of Story *et al.*[31], that when the

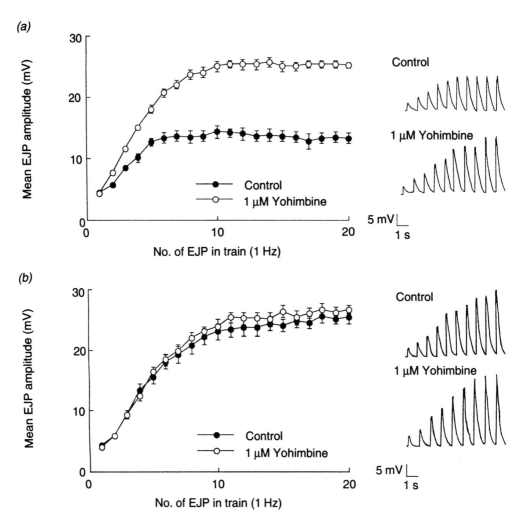

**Fig. 5.4.** Effect of the $\alpha_2$-adrenoceptor antagonist yohimbine (1 μM) on the EJP amplitude in control and reserpinised guinea-pig vasa deferentia. (*a*) In control tissues, EJPs increased in amplitude (facilitated) during the first five stimuli. (*b*) In reserpinised tissues, facilitation continues for 10–15 stimuli. Yohimbine markedly increased the amplitude of the fully facilitated EJPs in control tissues but had no effect on EJPs in reserpinised tissues. In control tissues, yohimbine also lengthened the period of facilitation, suggesting that activation of presynaptic α-adrenoceptors normally limits the magnitude of facilitation. Trains of 10 EJPs at 1 Hz after each procedure are shown to the right of each graph. See text for further details. (Adapted from refs. 5 and 6, with permission.)

extraneuronal concentration of noradrenaline is low (as it is when tissue is stimulated with only a single pulse) α-adrenoceptor antagonists are without effect. Further, a minimum time interval is required for the inhibitory effects of autoreceptor activation to be manifest: i.e. at least 30 ms (the duration of 4 pulses at 100 Hz) but less than 1 s (the interval between 2 pulses at 1 Hz). In addition, this study reveals a very pronounced autoinhibition of transmitter release following a single pulse of electrical stimulation ( 4 pulses at 1 Hz released little more tritium than did 1 pulse).

### 4.1.3   Presynaptic $\alpha_2$-adenoceptors also modulate the release of co-transmitters

The release of co-transmitters (e.g. ATP and neuropeptide Y) from noradrenergic nerves is also inhibited through activation of presynaptic $\alpha_2$-adrenoceptors by endogenous noradrenaline (see ref. 28). For example, in the rodent vas deferens and various vascular preparations, electrically evoked EJPs, which probably reflect the release of ATP (see Chapter 2), are altered by $\alpha_2$-adrenoceptor antagonists in a manner consistent with the autoinhibition hypothesis. Figure 5.4a shows the effects of the $\alpha_2$-adrenoceptor antagonist yohimbine on EJP amplitude in the guinea-pig vas deferens. In control tissues, EJPs increased in amplitude (i.e. were facilitated, see Chapter 3) during the first 5 pulses of a train of 20 stimuli at 1 Hz, after which a plateau level was maintained. Yohimbine increased the amplitude of all but the first EJP in the train; the plateau level EJPs are approximately double the size of control values. Yohimbine also lengthened the period of facilitation, suggesting that activation of presynaptic $\alpha_2$-adrenoceptor modifies the mechanism underlying the facilitation process.

### 4.1.4   Do $\alpha_2$-adrenoceptor antagonists enhance neurotransmitter release by mechanisms other than receptor blockade?

Although it is widely accepted that the potentiation of transmitter release by $\alpha$-adrenoceptor antagonists is the result of removal of $\alpha$-adrenoceptor-mediated autoinhibition, the possibility remains that the effects of such antagonists are not caused solely by blockade of $\alpha$-adrenoceptors located on the nerve terminals (see ref. 15). Instead, $\alpha$-adrenoceptor antagonists may

have a direct facilitatory action on the transmitter release mechanism. The demonstration that the release of co-transmitters from noradrenergic nerves is also inhibited through activation of presynaptic $\alpha_2$-adrenoceptors (see Section 4.1.3 above) has allowed this question to be addressed. Pretreatment of animals with reserpine selectively depletes the noradrenaline content of synaptic vesicles in postganglionic sympathetic nerves without, at least in the short term, any marked alteration in the storage of ATP[5] or neuropeptide Y[22]. In the guinea-pig vas deferens, the $\alpha$-adrenoceptor antagonist yohimbine had no effect on EJP amplitudes in reserpinised tissues[6] (Fig. 5.4b). Indeed, in these tissues, the EJPs behaved in a manner similar to the yohimbine-treated non-reserpinised control (Fig. 5.4a). Application of the $\alpha$-adrenoceptor agonist clonidine to these reserpinised tissues markedly reduced the amplitudes of EJPs, showing the presynaptic $\alpha$-adrenoceptors to be functionally intact. These findings support the view that yohimbine increases transmitter release by interrupting $\alpha$-adrenoceptor-mediated autoinhibition and not by some other mechanism, for example blockade of $K^+$ channels[15]. The release of neuropeptide Y from tissues pretreated with reserpine was also increased[22], suggesting that its release is normally inhibited through the presynaptic action of released noradrenaline.

## 4.2   Autoreceptors for co-transmitters on noradrenergic nerves

Present evidence indicates that noradrenergic nerve terminals possess transmitter release-modulating autoreceptors for the co-transmitters NPY, ATP, dopamine, somatostatin and opioid peptides[28]. However, it remains to be shown whether these receptors play a role in the autoregulation of noradrenaline and co-transmitter release. The postganglionic sympathetic nerves also possess presynaptic purinoceptors that, when activated by adenosine, inhibit transmitter release. While these purinoceptors are not strictly autoreceptors, they are considered to play a role in the feed-back modulation of transmitter release in some tissues (see ref. 28): the extracellular metabolism of released ATP by ecto-ATPases generating adenosine (see Chapter 6).

## 5   Autoreceptors on dopaminergic nerves

Dopamine-containing neurones are located mainly within the CNS. Major dopaminergic pathways (the nigrostriatal and mesolimbic pathways) originate in the substantia nigra and ventral tegmental areas and project pre-dominantly to the basal ganglia, limbic sys-tem and cerebral cortex. Another dopamin-ergic pathway (the tuberoinfundibular pathway) originates from the arcuate nucleus and projects mainly to the median eminence of the hypothalamus.

Inhibition of dopamine release, mediated by activation of dopamine receptors, has been detected in all regions of the CNS where it has been sought (see ref. 28). The principal central nervous tissue for studying dopamine release-modulating receptors *in vitro* has been the striatum (corpus striatum or neostriatum). Numerous studies have demonstrated that dopamine receptor antag-onists (e.g. chlorpromazine, haloperidol) applied to slices of striatum increase the efflux of radioactivity from tissues labelled with [$^3$H]-dopamine. Furthermore, applica-tion of dopamine and other dopamine recep-tor agonists (e.g. apomorphine, quinpirole) inhibits the release of radioactivity, an effect reduced by dopamine receptor antagonists. As the striatal slice contains the terminal axons of dopaminergic neurones, but not their cell bodies, an effect on the soma-den-dritic autoreceptors can be excluded.

The initial explanation for the effects of dopamine receptor agonists and antagonists on dopamine release involved postsynaptic receptors, some agent released from the post-synaptic cell acting trans-synaptically to inhibit transmitter release[10]. However, an action at presynaptic dopamine autorecep-tors located on the nerve terminal axons is now the preferred hypothesis[11,20] (see also Chapters 12 and 15).

### 5.1   Which dopamine receptor subtype: D$_1$ or D$_2$?

Pharmacologically, the receptors modulating dopamine release have the characteristics of D$_2$ receptors. D$_1$ receptor-selective agonists and antagonists are without effect on dopamine release (see ref. 20). However, all dopamine receptor agonists examined that are active at the D$_2$ receptor inhibit dopamine release, the effects of these agents being antagonised by sulpiride, an antagonist that is selective for the D$_2$ receptor[20]. Besides their presynaptic location, receptors with D$_2$-like characteristics are also located postsyn-aptically. The current available evidence sug-gests that D$_1$ receptors are only located postsynaptically.

Evidence supporting a nerve-terminal loca-tion for the D$_2$ receptors modulating transmit-ter release from dopaminergic neurones is similar to that for $\alpha_2$-adrenoceptors on nor-adrenergic nerve terminals (see ref. 28). (i) Soma-dendritic D$_2$ autoreceptors have been demonstrated electrophysiologically, establishing that dopaminergic neurones do express the gene encoding the D$_2$ receptor. (ii) Modulation of dopamine release has been shown in the presence of tetrodotoxin, which excludes the possible involvement of soma-dendritic receptors, or of other synaptically connected neurones. (iii) The transmitter release-modulating action of dopamine recep-tor agonists and antagonists has been demon-strated repeatedly in synaptosomes, providing strong supportive evidence for a nerve-termi-nal location of the release-modulating recep-tors. (iv) Loss of binding sites for dopamine receptor ligands has been observed following nerve lesion. However, since most ligand-binding studies have failed to show reductions in binding sites, it must be stated that loss of D$_2$-binding sites remains to be convincingly demonstrated.

## 5.2 Inhibition of dopamine synthesis

In addition to inhibition of transmitter release, activation of presynaptic dopamine autoreceptors has been reported to inhibit the synthesis of dopamine. This effect is probably exerted through an action on the enzyme tyrosine hydroxylase, which catalyses the hydroxylation of tyrosine to dihydroxyphenylalanine (dopa) and is the rate-limiting step in the synthesis of dopamine. Dopamine receptor agonists inhibit the synthesis of dopamine in various tissues including the striatum, an effect that is inhibited by dopamine receptor antagonists and is not dependent on transmitter release (see ref. 20). *In vivo*, following treatment with an inhibitor of dopa-decarboxylase, which converts dopa to dopamine, the dopamine receptor antagonist haloperidol increased dopa accumulation in the corpus striatum[16]. This finding suggests that synthesis of dopamine is autoinhibited through an action of released dopamine on presynaptic autoreceptors. In this *in vivo* study, the inhibitory action of the dopamine receptor agonist apomorphine on dopa accumulation survived section of the nigrostriatal axons, eliminating the possibility that a neuronal feedback input into dopaminergic cell bodies is involved.

The receptors modulating dopamine synthesis have a similar pharmacological profile to the transmitter release-modulating receptors ($D_2$ receptors) and it has been suggested that a single population of presynaptic dopamine receptors may be involved in the modulation of both dopamine release and dopamine synthesis[28]. However, the possibility that autoreceptor-mediated modulation of dopamine release is a consequence of modulation of dopamine synthesis is unlikely. The transmitter release-inhibiting effects of autoreceptor activation *in vitro* are apparent following a single pulse of electrical stimulation[21,23], while inhibition of dopamine synthesis is much slower in onset[34]. Furthermore, modulation of dopamine release has been demonstrated in tissues in which the *de novo* synthesis of dopamine has been blocked by pretreatment with α-methyl-*p*-tyrosine, a directly acting inhibitor of tyrosine hydroxylase[14].

## 5.3 Activation of presynaptic $D_2$ receptors by endogenous dopamine

In accordance with the idea that dopamine autoreceptors are activated by endogenous dopamine, the transmitter release-facilitating action of dopamine receptor antagonists has been shown to increase as the frequency of stimulation is raised. For example, in slices of rabbit caudate nucleus stimulated with 90 pulses at 0.3, 1, 3 and 10 Hz, the dopamine receptor antagonist haloperidol (30 nM) increased dopamine release by 10, 15, 50 and 110%, respectively[7]. Assuming that the extraneuronal concentration of dopamine is raised by increasing the frequency of stimulation, this finding strongly supports the view that released dopamine activates the transmitter release-modulating autoreceptors.

Further supporting evidence for an inhibitory autoreceptor activated by released dopamine is provided by the demonstration that inhibitors of dopamine uptake (e.g. nomifensin) reduce the transmitter release-inhibiting effects of dopamine receptor agonists but increase the transmitter release-facilitating action of dopamine receptor antagonists (see ref. 28). This presumably is caused by an enhanced autoinhibition resulting from an increase in the extraneuronal concentration of dopamine during periods of stimulation. Furthermore, the facilitatory action of dopamine receptor antagonists on transmitter release is markedly decreased in tissues taken from animals pretreated with reserpine to partially deplete the endogenous dopamine stores, a finding that presumably reflects a decrease in the extraneuronal concentration of dopamine (see ref. 20).

## 5.4 The importance of experimental conditions for demonstrating dopamine receptor-mediated autoinhibition

The importance of the stimulation conditions in determining the extent of activation of

(a)

(b)

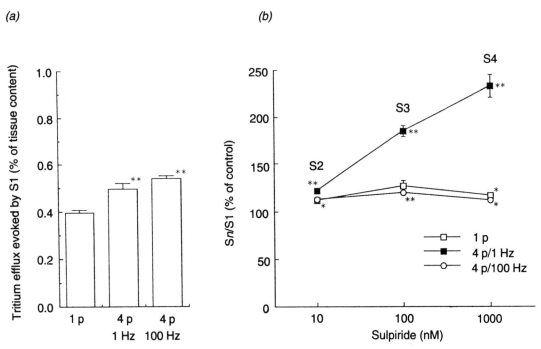

Fig. 5.5. Stimulation-evoked efflux of tritium from rabbit caudate nucleus slices previously loaded with [³H]-dopamine and effects of the $D_2$ receptor antagonist sulpiride (10–1000 nM). After loading, the slices were superfused with medium containing the dopamine-uptake inhibitor nomifensine (1 μM). The tissues were stimulated four times (S1 to S4) with 1 pulse (p) or 4 pulses at 1 or 100 Hz with an interval of 40 min between them. Solvent or increasing concentrations of yohimbine were added 20 min before S2, S3 and S4. (a) The efflux of tritium evoked by S1 as a percentage of the total tritium content of the tissue. (b) The ratios $Sn/S1$ (S2/S1, S3/S1, S4/S1) obtained in the presence of sulpiride expressed as a percentage of the mean ratios obtained in control experiments without the drug. The results show a very pronounced autoinhibition of transmitter release following a single pulse of electrical stimulation and that a minimum time interval is required for the inhibitory effects of autoreceptor activation to be manifest: > 30 ms but < 1 s. See text for further details. Significant differences: * ($p < 0.05$); ** ($p < 0.01$) from release evoked by 1 pulse in (a) and from control in (b). (Adapted from ref. 23, with permission.)

dopaminergic autoreceptors has recently been demonstrated using measures of both the efflux of radioactivity from [³H]-dopamine-labelled tissues[23] and the release of endogenous dopamine[21]. In the study of Mayer et al.[23], the release of radioactivity from labelled slices of rabbit caudate nucleus was assessed (Fig. 5.5). The experiments were performed in the presence of the dopamine-uptake inhibitor nomifensine to prevent reuptake of released dopamine. A single pulse of electrical stimulation released

0.39% of the total tritium content of the tissue. The release of radioactivity evoked by stimulation with 4 pulses at 1 Hz or 100 Hz was only 1.3-fold and 1.4-fold higher, respectively, than that evoked by a single pulse. Treatment with the dopamine receptor antagonist sulpiride increased up to 2.4-fold the release evoked by 4 pulses at 1 Hz but altered little the release evoked by 1 or 4 pulses at 100 Hz. These findings demonstrate, as did the experiments on α-adrenoceptor-mediated autoinhibition (see Section 4.1.2), that when the extraneuronal concentration of dopamine is low (1 pulse stimulation) the antagonist is without effect on transmitter release. The results also demonstrate that the presynaptic autoreceptors are powerfully activated by transmitter released by a single pulse of electrical stimulation and that a minimum time interval is required for the effect of their activation to be evident: >30 ms (which is the duration of 4 pulses at 100 Hz), but <1 s (the time interval between 2 pulses at 1 Hz). The reason why the amount of tritium released by 4 pulses at 100 Hz is only 1.4 times that evoked by 1 pulse remains to be explained. It clearly is not the result of activation of presynaptic dopamine receptors as the antagonist sulpiride did not increase the release of tritium evoked by 4 pulses at 100 Hz.

The findings of the study of Mayer et al.[23] have been confirmed and extended by Limberger et al.[21]. In this latter study, the release of endogenous dopamine from slices of rat neostriatum was measured, in the absence of an uptake inhibitor, using fast-cyclic voltammetry (Fig. 5.6). A single pulse of electrical stimulation evoked a transient increase in the extracellular concentration of dopamine. During a train of 4 pulses at 0.2 Hz, each pulse produced a peak, reflecting increased dopamine concentration, the second to fourth peak being considerably smaller than the first. Stimulation at 1 Hz (4 and 10 pulses) produced a shoulder on the declining phase of the peak caused by the first pulse, which reflected the release caused by subsequent pulses. Stimulation at 5 Hz (4 pulses) produced a monophasic response that was a little larger in amplitude than that evoked by a single pulse. Application of the dopamine receptor antagonist metoclopramide did not produce any significant changes in the release evoked either by a single pulse or by 4 pulses at 0.2 Hz. At 1 Hz (4 and 10 pulses) metoclopramide did not change the size of the initial peak but increased the height of the shoulder and at 5 Hz the peak amplitude was increased. These findings demonstrate, in the absence of

uptake inhibition, that the presynaptic autoreceptors are activated by dopamine released by a single pulse of electrical stimulation. In addition, the study revealed that there is a limited time interval during which transmitter release evoked by one pulse can modify that evoked by succeeding pulses: 5 s, which is the time interval between 2 pulses at 0.2 Hz. The results also indicate, as did those of Mayer et al.[23], that activation of dopamine autoreceptors is not the only factor contributing to the decline in transmitter release following a single pulse; at all frequencies of stimulation, both with and without the antagonist, the release of dopamine evoked by the first pulse was greater than that evoked by subsequent pulses. What this other factor is remains to be established.

## 5.5 Dopaminergic modulation of co-transmitter release

In various regions of the brain, dopaminergic neurones have been shown to contain a range of putative co-transmitter substances including GABA and the peptides cholecystokinin, neurotensin and galanin. Little evidence exists that supports a role for dopamine receptors in 'autoregulating' the release of these co-transmitters (see ref. 28). In addition, while all the above co-transmitters have been suggested to modify dopamine release, little evidence for an autoregulatory function exists (see ref. 28).

## 6 Nicotinic receptors on cholinergic nerves

Historically, the first proposal for transmitter release-modulating presynaptic autoreceptors was that acetylcholine released from somatic motor nerves and autonomic preganglionic cholinergic fibres acts back at nerve terminal nicotinic receptors to facilitate subsequent secretion[17]. At the somatic motor nerve terminal, this notion has been the cause of considerable controversy and only recently has evidence that directly supports

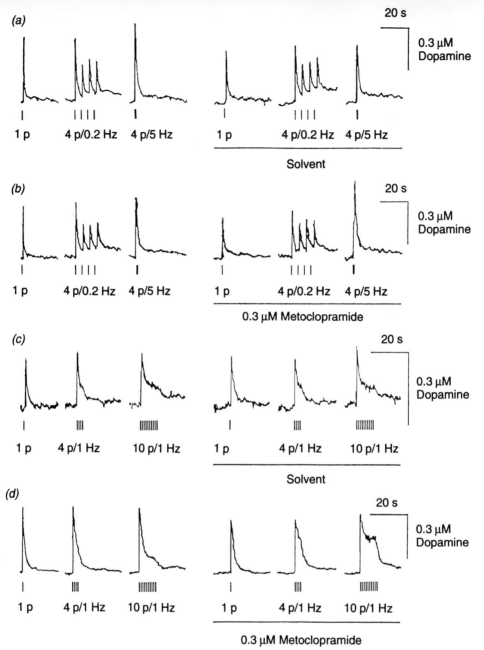

Fig. 5.6. Stimulation-induced increases in the extracellular dopamine concentration monitored by fast-cyclic voltammetry in slices of rat neostriatum and the effect of metoclopramide (0.3 μM). Recordings in (a), (b), (c) and (d) are from separate slice preparations. Tissues were stimulated at 5 min intervals: (a,b) a single pulse, 4 pulses at 0.2 Hz and 4 pulses at 5 Hz; (c,d) a single pulse, 4 pulses at 1 Hz and 10 pulses at 1 Hz. Solvent (a,c) or metoclopramide (b,d) was added to the superfusion medium after an initial cycle of nine stimulation periods (three times each of the three stimulation patterns). The cycle was then repeated twice. The traces show representative responses evoked by each of the stimulation patterns recorded during the first and third cycle. These findings demonstrate, in the absence of uptake inhibition, that the presynaptic autoreceptors are activated by dopamine released by a single pulse of electrical stimulation. In addition, the study revealed that there is a limited time interval (5 s) during which transmitter release evoked by one pulse can modify that evoked by succeeding pulses. See text for further details. (From ref. 21, with permission.)

the hypothesis been obtained. In these studies, endplate preparations of rat phrenic nerve were incubated with [³H]-choline, a procedure that produces an accumulation of [³H]-acetylcholine in the nerve terminals (see ref. 33). Released acetylcholine is normally rapidly broken down by cholinesterases to choline and acetate, choline being retrieved by the nerve terminals and reused for acetylcholine synthesis. Therefore, to ensure that the radioactivity measured is an accurate indicator of transmitter release, the choline-uptake blocker hemicholinium-3 was added to the tissues following the labelling period. Electrical stimulation of these labelled tissues produced an increase in the efflux of radioactivity that was inhibited by tetrodotoxin and had an absolute requirement for $Ca^{2+}$ in the bathing medium, indicating that it resulted from neurally released transmitter. Application of nicotine or dimethylphenylpiperazinium (a nicotinic receptor agonist) increased the stimulation-induced efflux of radioactivity, an effect reduced by the nicotinic receptor antagonist tubocurarine. Application of the nicotinic receptor antagonists tubocurarine (Fig. 5.7), pancuronium or hexamethonium alone decreased the stimulation-evoked increase in tritium efflux, a finding consistent with the idea that the transmitter release-facilitating presynaptic autoreceptors are activated by released acetylcholine.

An important feature of the above study is that an anticholinesterase, to prevent the extracellular breakdown of acetylcholine, was not required to allow the measurement of released acetylcholine. Indeed, when the experiments were undertaken in the presence of the anticholinesterase neostigmine, it was not possible to demonstrate the inhibitory effects of nicotinic receptor antagonists on acetylcholine release[33]. Previous attempts to detect the facilitatory nicotinic receptors in the presence of an anticholinesterase had also failed (see ref. 33). This failure to detect facilitatory nicotinic receptors in anticholinesterase-treated tissues can be explained by the assumption that these receptors are

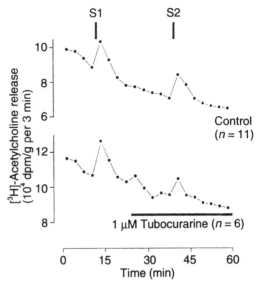

Fig. 5.7. Inhibition of the electrically stimulated release of [³H]-acetylcholine by tubocurarine (1 μM). The upper curve shows the basal tritium efflux and the stimulated tritium efflux evoked by two trains of 100 pulses at 5 Hz delivered 30 min apart under control conditions. The lower curve shows the effect of tubocurarine when added 15 min before S2. Tubocararine inhibited the release of tritium. (From ref. 33, with permission.)

readily desensitised in the continued presence of nicotinic receptor agonists (see ref. 33). Alternatively, it has been suggested that a second population of transmitter release-inhibiting nicotinic receptors exist on or near somatic motor nerve terminals that are not normally activated by released acetylcholine[3] (Fig. 5.8). In this scenario, following inhibition of acetylcholinesterase, released acetylcholine gains access to these receptors and inhibits transmitter release. In support of this suggestion, it has previously been reported that nicotinic receptor antagonists increase transmitter release in anticholinesterase-treated tissues (see ref. 3).

## 6.1  Nicotinic receptor subtypes

Nicotinic receptors have been divided into two types based on their pharmacological

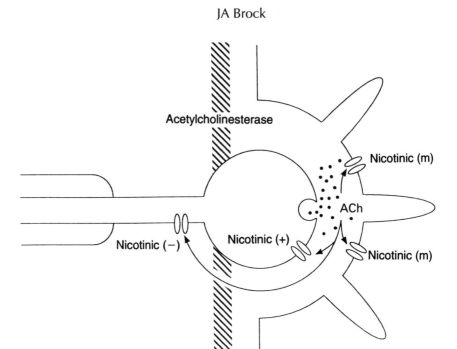

Fig. 5.8. Schematic representation of the sites at which neurally released acetylcholine (ACh) might act at the skeletal neuromuscular junction. Released acetylcholine activates postjunctional nicotinic receptors (Nicotinic (m)) and excites the muscle to contract. This acetylcholine may also access facilitatory prejunctional nicotinic autoreceptors (+), located close to the sites of transmitter release and, thereby, facilitate transmitter release. When the breakdown of acetylcholine is prevented by the addition of an anticholinesterase, the released acetylcholine may also diffuse to activate a more distant population of inhibitory nicotinic autoreceptors (−).

properties: the neuronal or ganglionic (those found on the postsynaptic neurones in autonomic ganglia) type, which is antagonised preferentially by hexamethonium, and the muscle type, which is antagonised preferentially by decamethonium. The receptors modulating acetylcholine release at the mammalian skeletal neuromuscular junction are similar to the neuronal type in that they show a greater sensitivity to hexamethonium than do the postsynaptic (muscle) receptors. In addition, the α-toxin antagonists of the muscle nicotinic receptor, erabutoxin-*b* and cobratoxin are without effects presynaptically[33]. However, another α-toxin, α-bungarotoxin, is effective at antagonising the transmitter release-modulating nicotinic receptor, a finding that distinguishes it from other neuronal nicotinic receptors of the ganglionic subtype[33]. It has been suggested that the transmitter release-modulating receptor is more sensitive to receptor desensitisation than the postsynaptic muscle nicotinic receptor (see ref. 33).

Direct evidence for the presynaptic location of transmitter release-modulating nicotinic receptors has been obtained by labelling somatic motor nerve terminals with α-bungarotoxin coupled to horseradish peroxidase (see ref. 33). However, it should be noted that others have failed to demonstrate α-bungarotoxin binding to motor nerve terminals (see ref. 33). Evidence suggesting the orthodromic axonal transport of α-bungarotoxin-binding sites in sciatic nerve has also been reported (see ref. 33). It may be that these binding sites are nicotinic receptors being transported along somatic motor nerves to their terminals.

## 6.2 Conditions under which presynaptic nicotinic receptors are operative

The radiolabelling technique for determining the release of acetylcholine has been used to investigate the conditions under which transmitter release-facilitating autoreceptors at the mammalian neuromuscular junction are activated (see ref. 33). Endplate preparations of rat phrenic nerve were stimulated with trains of 100 stimuli at 0.5, 1, 5, 25, 50 and 100 Hz, and the efflux of radioactivity measured. The nicotinic receptor antagonist tubocurarine did not significantly alter the tritium efflux evoked by 0.5 and 100 Hz but decreased that evoked by 1 Hz (30% reduction) and maximally inhibited efflux evoked by 5, 25 and 50 Hz (50–60% reduction). These findings indicate that the presynaptic nicotinic receptors are preferentially activated by frequencies of stimulation corresponding to the *in vivo* firing rates of motor neurones (up to 50 Hz) and support the suggestion of a physiological role for these receptors. Presumably at 0.5 Hz, the amount of acetylcholine accumulating at the presynaptic receptors is too low to activate them, while at 5, 25 and 50 Hz the concentration of acetylcholine at the receptors is sufficient to activate them maximally. The failure to detect an effect of tubocurarine at 100 Hz may be explained by the hypothesis that at this frequency the duration of stimulation (1 s) is too brief for the effect of autoreceptor activation to be observed. In support of this suggestion is the observation that when short trains of 15 stimuli at 5 or 25 Hz were given repeatedly application of tubocurarine did not significantly alter the efflux of radioactivity. This implies that the facilitatory nicotinic receptors are only substantially activated when the period of stimulation extends beyond a train of 15 pulses at these frequencies of stimulation. Prolonging the period of stimulation beyond 100 pulses (e.g. 300 pulses at 5 and 50 Hz) decreased the facilitatory effect of tubocurarine, an effect that is attributed to receptor desensitisation (see ref. 33).

## 6.3 Electrophysiological studies of nicotinic modulation of acetylcholine release

Electrophysiological techniques have been used to investigate the effects of nicotinic receptor antagonists on acetylcholine release at the mammalian skeletal muscle endplate (see ref. 3). For example EPPs or EPCs in rat diaphragm evoked by short trains of nerve impulses normally decline slightly in amplitude during the train, a phenomenon known as rundown. Nicotinic receptor antagonists (e.g. hexamethonium, tubocurarine, vecuronium) produce a marked pulse-by-pulse decrease in the amplitude of successive EPPs or EPCs, a finding that is consistent with these agents interrupting an autoreceptor-mediated facilitation of transmitter release (Fig. 5.9). These nicotinic receptor antagonists also reduce the amplitude of the EPPs or EPCs through blockade of postjunctional nicotinic receptors. However, the increased rate of rundown is not caused by an altered sensitivity of the postsynaptic membrane, as the amplitude of EPCs evoked by trains of pulses of acetylcholine applied ionophoretically in the presence of vecuronium did not decline (Fig. 5.9).

The effects of nicotinic receptor antagonists on rundown are already apparent by the time of arrival of the second pulse of a train of stimuli at 100 Hz (see ref. 33), whereas the biochemical measures of acetylcholine release reported above indicate that several stimuli (e.g. > 15 pulses at 5 or 25 Hz) are required before the transmitter release-facilitating nicotinic autoreceptors are activated. This discrepancy questions whether the radiolabelling technique for measuring acetylcholine release provides a good enough measure of transmitter release and its modulation during short trains of stimuli[2]. Perhaps

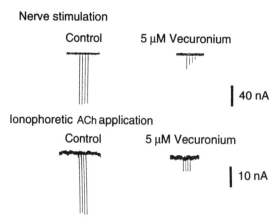

Nerve stimulation

Control        5 µM Vecuronium

                                      40 nA

Ionophoretic ACh application

Control        5 µM Vecuronium

                                      10 nA

Fig. 5.9. Effect of the nicotinic receptor antagonist vecuronium (5 µM) on the isolated phrenic nerve-hemidiaphragm preparation of rats. Endplate currents evoked by phrenic nerve stimulation (4 pulses at 2 Hz: a train of four stimuli) and by jets of acetylcholine applied ionophoretically (four jets at 2 Hz). Rundown, as distinct from depression of overall amplitude, was present only when the nerve was stimulated. (Adapted from ref. 3, with permission.)

the need (see above) to pretreat the radio-labelled preparations with hemicholinium-3 substantially alters presynaptic modulation of acetylcholine release. Alternatively, it has been suggested that the effects of tubocurarine on rundown are not the result of antagonism of facilitatory autoreceptors. Indeed, several alternate suggestions have been put forward to explain the electrophysiological findings (see ref. 33), but their discussion is beyond the scope of this chapter.

### 6.4    Role of nicotinic receptors in autoregulation of transmitter release from other cholinergic neurones

Studies of acetylcholine release from central cholinergic neurones suggest that transmitter release here may be influenced by presynaptic nicotinic autoreceptors in two distinct ways: nicotinic receptor agonists may both initiate the release of acetylcholine (directly evoking acetylcholine release from the nerve terminals in the absence of nerve impulses) and/or increase electrically evoked release (see ref. 28). However, little evidence exists which suggests that these receptors play a role in the autoregulation of transmitter release. Similarly, data supporting a role for presynaptic nicotinic autoreceptors in the autoregulation of transmitter release from peripheral autonomic cholinergic neurones are lacking (see ref. 28).

### 7    At what site does released transmitter act to modulate transmitter release?

The illustrative examples described above show that, *in vitro*, a pronounced impulse-to-impulse modulation of transmitter release, mediated through the activation of autoreceptors, occurs. The question remains as to the location on the nerve terminals of the receptors activated by released transmitter. It is commonly assumed that transmitter released from one release site acts locally to inhibit subsequent transmitter release from the same or a closely related release site (local inhibition: Fig. 5.1). However, recent studies of the transmitter release process at the sympathetic neuro-effector junction question whether such a local inhibition of transmitter release does operate in all cases.

At the sympathetic neuro-effector junction, the probabilities of quantal secretion determined electrophysiologically vary considerably from varicosity to varicosity (see Chapters 3 and 4), the majority having probabilities of secretion in the order of 0.01 (i.e. one quantum released per 100 applied stimuli). The observation that transmitter release at the level of the individual varicosity normally occurs with a very low probability means that transmitter is unlikely to accumulate locally near any one varicosity. Furthermore, it is difficult to envisage how

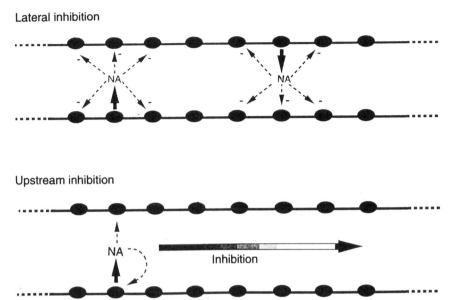

Fig. 5.10. Schematic diagram illustrating both the lateral regulation and the upstream regulation hypotheses for α-adrenoceptor-mediated autoregulation of transmitter release. The 'lateral inhibition' hypothesis proposes that noradrenaline (NA) released from one site diffuses to activate receptors located at release sites not yet activated. The 'upstream regulation' hypothesis proposes that noradrenaline released at a proximal site acts at presynaptic receptors close to its site of release. Activation of these receptors inhibits secretion from more distal sites, perhaps by the generation of a permissive factor which moves along the axon towards the nerve terminal (see also Chapter 4).

transmitter can feedback locally, on an impulse-by-impulse basis, if release from a particular varicosity is unlikely to occur again within the next 100 or so stimuli. Indecd electrophysiological studies of the occurrence of quantal release events from small populations of varicosities in the guinea-pig vas deferens, in the absence of α-adrenoceptor antagonists, have failed to demonstrate that endogenous transmitter regulates its own release locally[1,4,8].

How can this apparent lack of local inhibition be explained? It has been suggested that ATP, which is the transmitter that probably causes the electrical signals recorded postsynaptically, and noradrenaline are released differentially. If the release of noradrenaline from varicosities occurs with a much higher probability, then it could be suggested that it

is the released noradrenaline that acts locally to inhibit the secretion of both itself and ATP. However, estimates of the amount of noradrenaline released per nerve impulse from a varicosity suggest that on average about 1/100th of the transmitter content of a single transmitter storage vesicle is secreted[5]. If it is assumed that a varicosity normally secretes the entire transmitter content of a vesicle intermittently, then the probability of releasing single quanta of noradrenaline is similar to that of ATP (i.e. 0.01), supporting the view that they are co-secreted. Therefore, by extension, it can be concluded that noradrenaline released by nerve impulses is unlikely to inhibit subsequent release from its own site of release.

Another proposal is that the activated receptors are located at some strategic point in the nerve-terminal arbor, perhaps close to transmitter-release sites with a high probability of secretion, and that activation of these receptors inhibits secretion from varicosities located at some distance away (upstream regulation: Fig. 5.10*b*; see Chapter 4). Alternatively, it has been suggested that noradrenaline diffusing from its sites of release may produce a more global activation of presynaptic α-adrenoceptors (lateral inhibition: Fig. 5.10*a*).

These two hypotheses (upstream regulation and lateral inhibition) are not mutually exclusive, and there are studies that support both suggestions. These studies have used small diameter suction electrodes that are continuously perfused and allow the effects of local (within electrode) and of bath-applied drugs to be compared. Application of α-adrenoceptor antagonists to small populations of varicosities enclosed by the recording electrode increases their probability of quantal secretion, indicating that they are under the inhibitory influence of released noradrenaline[6]. This effect is apparent even when the probability of quantal secretion from the enclosed population of varicosities is low. This observation supports the idea of lateral inhibition, since it suggests that the extent of activation of autoreceptors located on, or near, a varicosity is not related to its secretory activity. Stjärne and his colleagues[30] have reported experiments in which, following perfusion of the electrode with the α-adrenoceptor antagonist yohimbine to protect the autoreceptors located within the electrode, bath application of the α-adrenoceptor agonist clonidine inhibited quantal secretion from the varicosities enclosed by the electrode, an effect that is reversed by bath application of yohimbine (see Chapter 4). This experiment demonstrates that it is possible to modulate secretion by activating α-adrenoceptors at some distance from the releasing varicosity. The question remains whether endogenous noradrenaline modulates secretion through these so called 'upstream' receptors. In the guinea-pig vas deferens, yohimbine applied through the recording electrode

maximally increased quantal secretion by approximately 2-fold. Under similar conditions, bath application of yohimbine also increased the amplitude of the intracellularly recorded EJP by about 2-fold (Fig. 5.4*a*). This finding suggests that it may be possible to account for all facilitatory effects of yohimbine on transmitter release by an action close to the secreting varicosities, an observation that would favour lateral inhibition. However, it is not possible at present to exclude a role for upstream receptors in the modulation of transmitter secretion.

The failure to detect local feedback inhibition of transmitter release at the level of the individual sympathetic nerve varicosity questions the role that presynaptic autoreceptors play in the regulation of transmitter release. Perhaps, since presynaptic α-adrenoceptors might respond to noradrenaline released from varicosities located on separate neurones, their function is to sense the general degree of nerve activation in the tissue. In this way, it would be possible to adjust the amount of noradrenaline secreted as the number of nerves activated is altered. In this manner, the presynaptic α-adrenoceptors could serve to limit the overall magnitude of transmitter release from the entire nerve terminal network. If noradrenaline released from one neurone inhibits secretion from other neurones, then autoinhibition should not be seen strictly as a negative feedback mechanism.

At the vertebrate somatic motor nerve terminal, it has been suggested that frequency-dependent facilitation of transmitter release involves the recruitment of release sites with previously low probabilities of quantal secretion (see Chapter 3). Perhaps activation of the presynaptic facilitatory nicotinic receptors also acts by recruiting sites with low probabilities of secretion. This implies that the facilitatory action of released acetylcholine would be at sites remote from its own site of release. At other nerve terminals, the situation is much less clear, since little is known about the way they release their transmitter on an impulse-by-impulse basis.

## 8   Summary

There is abundant pharmacological evidence that supports the existence of presynaptic transmitter release-modulating autoreceptors. There is also evidence that demonstrates, at least *in vitro*, that these receptors are activated by the endogenous transmitter and may play an important role in the regulation of transmitter release. However, it should be noted that in multiply innervated tissues, such as brain slices and smooth muscle, the demonstration of autoinhibition *in vitro* might give a false impression of its importance *in vivo*. This possibility arises because in the *in vitro* studies many nerves are activated synchronously, while *in vivo* only a small number of nerves may be activated at any particular time, and then asynchronously. Therefore, the *in vitro* situation might over-estimate the influence exerted by activation of autoreceptors on transmitter release.

In addition to the presynaptic autoreceptors for the 'classical' transmitters, the nerve endings of many neurones possess autoreceptors for their co-transmitters. To date, there is little convincing evidence to show that these receptors play a role in the autoregulation of transmitter release. However, in the case of the many peptides that are known to be co-transmitters, it has not been possible to determine their role in the autoregulation of transmitter release as, at present, antagonists for their presynaptic autoreceptors are generally unavailable.

Studies of transmitter release at the sympathetic neuro-effector junction have raised questions about the location of the autoreceptors activated by released noradrenaline. In particular, it appears that released noradrenaline does not act locally to inhibit subsequent transmitter release from its own site of release. Two alternate mechanisms have been suggested: lateral inhibition and upstream inhibition. However, the relative roles that these play in the regulation of noradrenaline release remains to be established.

The characteristic features of transmitter release from most other nerve terminals remain poorly understood. Therefore, in these cases it is not yet possible to state whether transmitter release is or is not regulated locally at its site of release.

Notwithstanding the above provisos, transmitter release-modulating autoreceptors may play an important role in maintaining the normal functioning of all synapses. Presynaptic autoreceptors are also potentially important sites of drug action. The possible roles that presynaptic autoreceptors play *in vivo* and, in particular, in the development and maintenance of various disease states are the subject of later chapters in this book.

## References

1. Blakeley AGH, Cunnane TC and Petersen SA (1982) Local regulation of transmitter release from rodent sympathetic nerve terminals? *Journal of Physiology* **325:** 93–109
2. Bowman WC (1989) Presynaptic nicotinic receptors. *Trends in Pharmacological Science* **10:** 136–137
3. Bowman WC, Prior C and Marshall IG (1990) Presynaptic receptors in the neuromuscular junction. *Annals of the New York Academy of Sciences* **604:** 69–81
4. Brock JA and Cunnane TC (1991) Local application of drugs to sympathetic nerve terminals: an electrophysiological analysis of the role of prejunctional $\alpha$-adrenoceptors in the guinea-pig vas deferens. *British Journal of Pharmacology* **102:** 595–600
5. Brock JA and Cunnane TC (1992) Electrophysiology of neuroeffector transmission in smooth muscle. In: Burnstock G and Hoyle CVH (eds) *Autonomic Neuroeffector Mechanisms*, pp 121–213, Horwood Academic, Reading
6. Brock JA, Cunnane TC, Starke K and Wardell CF (1990) $\alpha_2$-Adrenoceptor-mediated autoinhibition of sympathetic transmitter release in guinea-pig vas deferens studied by intracellular and focal extracellular recording of junction potentials and currents. *Naunyn-Schmiedeberg's Archives of Pharmacology* **342:** 45–52

7. Cubeddu LX and Hoffman IS (1982) Operational characteristics of the inhibitory feedback mechanism for regulation of dopamine release via presynaptic receptors. *Journal of Pharmacology and Experimental Therapeutics* **223:** 497–501

8. Cunnane TC and Stjärne L (1984) Transmitter secretion from individual varicosities of guinea-pig and mouse vas deferens: highly intermittent and monoquantal. *Neuroscience* **13:** 1–20

9. de Potter WP, Chubb IW, Put A and Schaepdryver AF (1971) Facilitation of the release of noradrenaline and dopamine β-hydroxylase at low stimulation frequencies by α-blocking agents. *Archives Internationales Pharmacodynamie et de Thérapie* **193:** 191–197

10. Farnebo LO and Hamberger B (1971) Drug induced changes in the release of $^3$H-monoamines from field stimulated rat brain slices *Acta Physiologica Scandinavica* Suppl. **371:** 35–44

11. Farnebo LO and Hamberger B (1973) Catecholamine release and receptors in brain slices. In: Usdin E and Snyder S (eds) *Frontiers in Catecholamine Research*, pp 589–593, Pergamon Press, Oxford

12. Filinger EJ, Langer SZ, Perec CJ and Stefano FJE (1978) Evidence for presynaptic location of alpha-adrenoceptors which regulate noradrenaline release in the rat submaxillary gland. *Naunyn-Schmiedeberg's Archives of Pharmacology* **304:** 21–26

13. Gillespie JS (1980) Presynaptic receptors in the autonomic nervous system. In: Sezekeres L (ed) *Handbook of Experimental Pharmacology*, vol 54: *Adrenergic Activators and Inactivators*, pp 352–425, Springer-Verlag, Berlin

14. Herdon H, Strupish J and Nahorski SR (1987) Endogenous dopamine release from rat striatal slices and its regulation by $D_2$-autoreceptors: effects of uptake inhibition and synthesis inhibition. *European Journal of Pharmacology* **138:** 69–76

15. Kalsner S and Quillan M (1984) A hypothesis to explain the presynaptic effects of adrenoceptor antagonists. *British Journal of Pharmacology* **82:** 515–522

16. Kehr W, Carlsson A and Lindqvist M (1972) Evidence for receptor-mediated feedback control of striatal tyrosine hydroxylase activity. *Journal of Pharmacy and Pharmacology* **24:** 744–747

17. Koelle GB (1961) A proposed dual neurohumoral role of acetylcholine: its functions at pre- and post-synaptic sites. *Nature* **190:** 208–211

18. Langer SZ (1974) Presynaptic regulation of catecholamine release. *Biochemical Pharmacology* **23:** 1793–1800

19. Langer SZ (1981) Presynaptic regulation of the release of catecholamines. *Pharmacological Reviews* **32:** 337–362

20. Langer SZ and Lehmann J (1988) Presynaptic receptors on catecholamine neurons. In: Trendelenberg U and Weiner N (eds) *Handbook of Experimental Pharmacology*, vol 90: *Catecholamines*, Part 1, pp 419–507, Springer-Verlag, Berlin

21. Limberger N, Trout SJ, Kruk ZL and Starke K (1991) 'Real time' measurement of endogenous dopamine released during trains of pulses in slices of rat neostriatum and nucleus accumbens: role of autoinhibition. *Naunyn-Schmiedeberg's Archives of Pharmacology* **344:** 623–629

22. Lundberg JM, Rudehill A, Sollevi A, Fried G and Wallin G (1989) Co-release of neuropeptide Y and noradrenaline from pig spleen *in vivo*: importance of subcellular storage, nerve impulse frequency and pattern, feedback regulation and resupply by axonal transport. *Neuroscience* **28:** 475–486

23. Mayer A, Limberger N and Starke K (1988) Transmitter release patterns of noradrenergic, dopaminergic and cholinergic axons in rabbit brain slices during short pulse trains and the operation of presynaptic autoreceptors. *Naunyn-Schmiedeberg's Archives of Pharmacology* **338:** 632–643

24. Starke K (1971) Influence of α-receptor stimulants on noradrenaline release. *Naturwissenshaften* **58:** 420

25. Starke K (1972) Influence of extracellular noradrenaline on the stimulation-evoked secretion of noradrenaline from sympathetic nerves: evidence for an α-receptor-mediated feed-back inhibition of noradrenaline release. *Naunyn-Schmiedeberg's Archives of Pharmacology* **275:** 11–23

26. Starke K (1977) Regulation of noradrenaline release by presynaptic receptors. *Reviews of Physiology, Biochemistry and Pharmacology* **77:** 1–124

27. Starke K (1987) Presynaptic α-adrenoceptors. *Reviews of Physiology, Biochemistry and Pharmacology* **107:** 73–146

28. Starke K, Göthert M and Kilbinger H (1989) Modulation of transmitter release by presynaptic autoreceptors. *Physiological Reviews* **69:** 864–989

29. Starke K, Montel H and Wagner J (1971) Influence of cocaine and phenoxybenzamine on noradrenaline uptake and release. *Naunyn-Schmiedeberg's Archives of Pharmacology* **270:** 210–214

30. Stjärne L, Bao J-X, Gonon FG, Msghina M and Stjärne E (1993) A nonstochastic string model of sympathetic neuromuscular transmission. *News in Physiological Sciences* **8:** 253–260

31. Story DF, McCulloch MW, Standford-Starr CA and Rand MJ (1981) Conditions required for the inhibition feedback loop in noradrenergic transmission. *Nature* **293:** 62–65

32. Timmermans PBMWM and Van Zwieten PA (1981) The postsynaptic $\alpha_2$-adrenoceptor. *Journal of Autonomic Pharmacology* **1:** 171–183

33. Wessler I (1992) Acetylcholine at motor nerves: storage, release and presynaptic modulation by autoreceptors. *International Review of Neurobiology* **34:** 283–384

34. Westfall TC, Besson MJ, Giorguieff MF and Glowinski J (1976) The role of presynaptic receptors in the release and synthesis of $^3$H-dopamine by slices of rat striatum. *Naunyn-Schmiedeberg's Archives of Pharmacology* **292:** 279–287

# 6 Modulation of neurotransmitter release by heteroreceptors

Bertil B. Fredholm

It has become clear that neurotransmitter release from an individual site is not only modulated by the specific transmitter released from that site or adjacent sites on that neurone, but by other substances, including transmitters of other classes of neurone, which are present at that time in the immediate extracellular space. The term 'heteroreceptor' was coined to express the concept that modulation can be mediated by receptors sensitive to substances other than that neurone's own transmitter. In this chapter, Bertil Fredholm considers what the term heteroreceptor has been commonly assumed to mean and discusses the role heteroreceptors might play in regulating neuro-effector transmission, particularly those sensitive to neurotransmitters released from adjacent nerves. The mutual adjustment of neuronal function that can be achieved by transmitters released from these adjacent neurones acting through heteroreceptors can result in a very precise balance of neurotransmitters in the neuro-effector junction, which will be reflected in a closely modulated postsynaptic response.

## 1    Introduction

In the periphery and particularly in the CNS, nerves using different neurotransmitters are located at close proximity. There is good evidence that monoamines and neuropeptides can diffuse over considerable distances from their sites of release. Even the amino acid neurotransmitters may act at sites removed from the synapse. Thus, a nerve will be exposed to an environment where there are many types of signal besides the ones that the nerve itself elaborates. Many of these can affect the release of transmitter from that nerve. To further complicate matters, each nerve may release many different types of transmitter (see Chapter 2) and there are hormones and local paracrine factors that have the ability to interact with neurotrans-

mitter release or synthesis. Thus, transmitter release can be regulated not only by autoreceptors, but also by heteroreceptors.

The term heteroreceptor is commonly used, even though it is not a very happy one. It is generally defined as the opposite of an autoreceptor: any receptor that is not an autoreceptor would qualify as a heteroreceptor. If the autoreceptor is defined as a receptor on a neurone to a transmitter released from that type of neurone, then the term is relatively unambiguous. The term autoreceptor is, however, often used in a stricter sense than this: a receptor that responds to that transmitter released from the *same* neurone. As pointed out by Kalsner[9], the word auto not only means 'self', but when applied to science it implies function, in this case autoregulation of transmitter release. If this strict, and

104

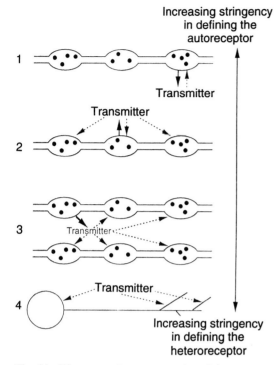

Increasing stringency
in defining the
autoreceptor

Transmitter

Transmitter

Increasing stringency
in defining the
heteroreceptor

Fig. 6.1. Diagrammatic representation of the different definitions of neurotransmitter release-modulating autoreceptors going from the most strict (1, uppermost) to the least strict (4, bottom). Since the term heteroreceptor is defined as the disjunctive of the term autoreceptor, its own definition is most strict for the least strict definition of the autoreceptor. A broken arrow defines the sites at which the transmitter can act to alter transmitter release. An unbroken arrow defines the site from which the transmitter is released. Note that the fourth case defines the autoreceptor very widely in that it may be a soma-dendritic as well as a terminal receptor. This use of the term is, in fact, quite common even though it is not the one advocated in this book. For further explanation see text.

probably original, definition is used, then a receptor might be an autoreceptor in one instance and a heteroreceptor in another, depending upon the origin of the agonist. For example, an $\alpha_2$-adrenoceptor on a noradrenergic neurone would be an autoreceptor if acted upon by noradrenaline released from the same neurone and a heteroreceptor if the noradrenaline molecule had been released by a neighbouring neurone. This is clearly confusing.

Finally, our conception of autoreceptors is often governed by pictures depicting a transmitter molecule released from a single varicosity acting on a receptor on the same varicosity limiting the release of further transmitter molecules from that same release site of the neurone. With this extremely restricted view of an autoreceptor, a transmitter molecule would be acting on a heteroreceptor if it regulates transmitter release at another varicosity than the one from which it had been released. These different definitions of the autoreceptor, and hence of the heteroreceptor, are illustrated in Fig. 6.1.

Neurotransmitter release is regulated not only by presynaptic receptors that alter the amount of release from the nerve terminal in response to a depolarising stimulus that passes along the terminal tree but also by the impulse flow. This in turn is controlled by soma-dendritic receptors, some of which respond to the neurone's own transmitter(s), and are, therefore, soma-dendritic autoreceptors. It is not uncommon that test models are unable to distinguish between presynaptic receptors and soma-dendritic receptors or whether the autoreceptor is an autoreceptor in any of the above-mentioned senses. Despite ambiguous data, interpretation may favour autoreceptors in the most strict sense. Referring to Fig. 6.1, there is sometimes a tendency to glide along the scale of strictness in the definition of autoreceptors.

For the purpose of the present chapter, a definition of low strictness will be used for the term autoreceptor. Consequently, a presynaptic heteroreceptor will be considered to mean a receptor, located in the terminal region of a nerve, for a substance that is not a transmitter in that nerve. There are numerous examples of such heteroreceptors. A partial list is given in Table 6.1. In the present chapter, only a few examples will be given and this selection is biased by personal interest. This is particularly evident in the treatment of adenosine receptors regulating transmitter release.

Table 6.1. *Examples of modulation of transmitter release via heteroreceptors.*

| Agent | Receptor type | Change (I, inhibition S, stimulation) | Transmitter affected |
|---|---|---|---|
| *Locally produced agents* | | | |
| Adenosine | $A_1$ | I | Noradrenaline, dopamine, acetylcholine, substance P, ATP, 5-HT, glutamate, dynorphin B, |
| | $A_2$ | S | Few absolutely clear examples |
| Prostaglandins | PGE | I | Noradrenaline, acetylcholine |
| | $TxA_2$ | S? | Noradrenaline |
| Hydroperoxy and hydroxy derivatives of arachidonic acid | ? | S | Glutamate |
| Nitric oxide | cGMP? | I | Noradrenaline |
| *Neurotransmitters* | | | |
| Acetylcholine | Nicotinic | S | Noradrenaline, acetylcholine |
| | $M_1$ | S | Noradrenaline, acetylcholine, dopamine |
| | $M_2$ ($M_4$) | I | Noradrenaline, acetylcholine, glutamate |
| Noradrenaline | $\alpha_2$ | I | Noradrenaline, acetylcholine, NANC transmitter (NO?), 5-HT, ATP |
| 5-HT (serotonin) | $5\text{-}HT_2$ | I | Noradrenaline |
| | $5\text{-}HT_{1D}$ | I | Acetylcholine |
| | $5\text{-}HT_3$ | I | GABA |
| Histamine | $H_3$ | I | Noradrenaline, 5-HT, acetylcholine, NANC (NO?, VIP?), histamine |
| Dopamine | $D_2$ | I | Acetylcholine |
| Glutamate | NMDA | S | Noradrenaline, acetylcholine, dopamine, 5-HT |
| | AMPA/kainate | S | Noradrenaline, acetylcholine, dopamine |
| GABA | $GABA_A$ | S | 5-HT, noradrenaline |
| | $GABA_B$ | I | Noradrenaline |
| Glycine | Ionotropic | S | Noradrenaline |
| *Neuropeptides* | | | |
| NPY | $Y_2$? | I | Noradrenaline, glutamate, SP/CGRP, 5-HT |
| CCK | ? | I | Dopamine |
| Enkephalins | $\delta$ | S | Dopamine |
| | $\delta$ | I | Noradrenaline, acetylcholine, substance P |
| | $\kappa$ | I | Dopamine, acetylcholine, noradrenaline, met-enkephalin |

NANC, non-adrenergic, non-cholinergic; NO, nitric oxide

## 2 Interaction between nerves releasing different transmitters

### 2.1 Noradrenaline–acetylcholine interactions in the autonomic nervous system

#### 2.1.1 Nicotinic modulation of noradrenaline release

It was realised quite early that nicotinic receptor stimulation in the heart may increase the release of noradrenaline. The exact nature of this phenomenon is controversial (see Löffelholz[10] and Chapters 5 and 16), even though it remains clear that the cardiostimulant effects of administered nicotine can be ascribed to the release of noradrenaline. Release of noradrenaline by nicotinic agonists has also been demonstrated in other tissues, such as the spleen and blood vessels. Interestingly, in the vas deferens, nicotinic receptors do not regulate release, even though muscarinic receptors can be demonstrated[10]. The presence of nicotinic receptors that regulate transmitter release is not limited to noradrenergic nerves but has also been clearly demonstrated in sensory nerves. Indeed, many of the effects of nicotine are the result of direct activation of sensory nerve endings.

The type of nicotinic receptor involved and the mechanism underlying the increased transmitter release remain unknown. The pharmacological evidence indicates that the receptors differ from those in skeletal muscle. However, as the ion channel is an integral part of the nicotinic receptor, it is reasonable to assume that either $Na^+$ or $Ca^{2+}$ are involved in the release modulation mechanism: $Na^+$ perhaps by inducing repetitive depolarisation, $Ca^{2+}$ potentially by acting at the release machinery. However, at none of the locations where presynaptic nicotinic receptors have been demonstrated is a physiological role clearly demonstrated. Indeed it is not even completely excluded that the effects are mediated by soma-dendritic receptors.

#### 2.1.2 Muscarinic modulation of noradrenaline release

Muscarinic receptors that modulate neurotransmitter release exist in several types of nerve terminal[16]. The muscarinic receptors that inhibit noradrenaline release appear to be of the $M_2$ subtype. There are also muscarinic receptors, apparently of the $M_1$ subtype, that increase the overflow of noradrenaline[13,17]. The relative importance of these inhibitory and stimulatory muscarinic receptors may vary in noradrenergic neurones from different locations.

The $M_1$ receptor is generally coupled via a pertussis toxin-insensitive G-protein (possibly $G_q$ or $G_{11}$) to the formation of inositol trisphosphate and diacylglycerol. The diffusible $Ca^{2+}$ message can give rise to numerous slow responses. The effectors involved include the L-type $Ca^{2+}$ channel and the M-type $K^+$ channel. An effect on the latter target explains the stimulatory effect in ganglia, but it is not certain that it adequately explains the actions in the terminal region. Here the $Ca^{2+}$ increase may act more directly, e.g. by mobilising more vesicles and causing their relocation to the release sites. The $M_2$ receptor (which may include both the $m_2$ and $m_4$ gene products) is coupled via a pertussis toxin-sensitive G-protein ($G_{i1-3}$ or $G_o$) rather directly to the N-type $Ca^{2+}$ channel[8], which it inhibits. This provides a fast, effective inhibition of transmitter release.

It is questionable whether the excitatory $M_1$ muscarinic receptors actually play a physiological role in most species. It is known that acetylcholine exerts a dual stimulatory effect in ganglia: an initial fast depolarisation (fEPSP) mediated by nicotinic receptors followed after a delay by a second, slow depolarisation (sEPSP) mediated via muscarinic ($M_1$) receptors. The major effect of these ganglionic stimulatory muscarinic receptors may be to facilitate nicotinic transmission rather than to initiate action potentials. Moreover it is possible that the presence of $M_1$ receptors in the terminal region is incidental to their presence on the cell soma and/or dendrites. Since the nerve cell has to synthesise the receptor for distribution to the soma and the dendrites, the $M_1$ receptor may be distributed fortuitously along the terminal network, unless the receptor molecule possesses a signal that acts as an address label. Indeed the situation may be similar for the nicotinic receptors.

By contrast, there is reasonably good evidence that the $M_2$ ($M_4$) inhibitory receptors on cholinergic and noradrenergic nerves are physiologically relevant. For example, inhibitory effects of muscarinic agonists on noradrenaline release are observed not only in isolated tissues in saline-perfused organs, but also in blood-perfused ones[10]. Several studies have shown that the stimulation of cholinergic postganglionic fibres decreases the release of noradrenaline during stimulation of postganglionic noradrenergic neurones. Likewise, acetylcholine release from postganglionic cholinergic terminals is inhibited by noradrenaline acting on presynaptic $\alpha_2$-adrenoceptors (see Section 2.1.4). At least in the periphery, these findings have important implications for the concept of reciprocal innervation of organs by the two divisions of the autonomic nervous system, which have opposing actions. Thus, the two divisions interact functionally not only at the effector cell level, but also at the level of transmitter release. This is schematically illustrated in Fig. 6.2.

### 2.1.3  Muscarinic receptors modulating dopamine and excitatory amino acid release

There is good evidence for muscarinic receptors in the brain modulating release of still other transmitters. In the striatum, there are muscarinic receptors that modulate dopamine release, in general by enhancing release. These receptors appear to be of the $M_1$ subtype. Since the effect of muscarinic agonists can be observed also in synaptosomes, the $M_1$ receptors are presumably located on the dopaminergic terminals[15]. Endogenous acetylcholine in a striatal slice may alter dopamine release, but this is seen only after blockade of acetylcholinesterase.

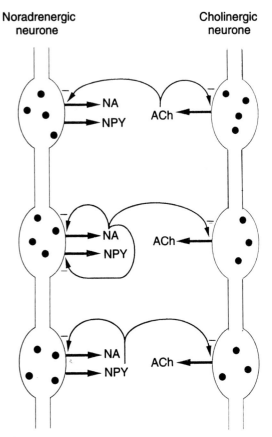

Fig. 6.2. Interactions between transmitters released by sympathetic and parasympathetic nerves. The left nerve profile represents a sympathetic nerve ending that releases noradrenaline (NA), neuropeptide Y (NPY) and possibly ATP (not illustrated). The right nerve profile represents a parasympathetic nerve ending that releases acetylcholine (ACh). The inhibitory actions of the released substance at presynaptic receptors are shown by arrows labelled $-$. Note that acetylcholine and noradrenaline act at both autoreceptors and heteroreceptors.

Interestingly, a lesion of the cell bodies in the striatum (removing the large cholinergic neurones) actually enhances the potency of $M_1$ receptor-stimulating agents to promote dopamine release. This could indicate that these receptors are tonically influenced by acetylcholine, leading to an agonist-induced down-regulation. When the tonic acetylcholine influence is removed, the receptors are then up-regulated. However, other explanations can also be found and the physiological significance of these $M_1$ receptors remains uncertain.

There is evidence that muscarinic receptors can modulate glutamate release in the hippocampus. Acetylcholine inhibits the $K^+$-evoked release of glutamate (and aspartate) from hippocampal synaptosomes. The effect is blocked by atropine, but not by pirenzepine. This indicates that, in contrast to the stimulatory effect on dopamine release, the effect on glutamate release is not mediated by $M_1$ receptors[15]. The physiological significance of the muscarinic receptors on glutamate neurones is unknown.

If both the above-mentioned mechanisms do in fact occur in the striatum, they might be functionally inter-related. Thus, acetylcholine would inhibit the major stimulatory input and stimulate a major inhibitory one. Since the glutamate and dopamine also (and predominantly) affect GABAergic neurones, the major effect of an increased amount of acetylcholine might be an altered GABAergic output (see Fig. 6.3).

### 2.1.4 Noradrenergic and dopaminergic modulation of acetylcholine release

It was shown quite early (by Paton and Vizi in 1969[14]) that noradrenaline can decrease the release of acetylcholine via an action on α-adrenoceptors. This has been shown to occur in several tissues. A careful examination of the pharmacology of the response revealed that the α-adrenoceptors involved are pharmacologically different from those on, for example, blood vessels and intestinal smooth muscle. This provided one of the first indications that there are distinct presynaptic α-adrenoceptors, later designated $\alpha_2$. As discussed in Section 2.1.2 above and shown in Fig. 6.2, this may provide one arm of a mechanism by which opposing divisions of the autonomic nervous system may antagonise each other's influence.

Another example of a catecholamine–

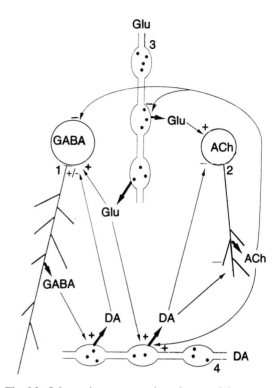

Fig. 6.3. Schematic representation of some of the interactions between neurones and nerve terminals in the striatum. In slices of rat striatum, there are two major types of neuronal cell body: (1) medium sized spiny neurones that are GABAergic and comprise more than 90% of all the neurones; and (2) large aspiny cholinergic interneurones. In addition, there are nerve endings from glutamatergic neurones (3) with their cell bodies in the cortex and thalamus, and dopamine (DA)-containing nerve endings (4) with their cell bodies located in the substantia nigra. Stimulatory actions are shown by (+) and inhibitory actions by (−). Note particularly that glutamate (Glu) has stimulatory effects at dopaminergic but apparently not at cholinergic nerve endings. Note also that acetylcholine has inhibitory effects on glutamatergic neurones and stimulatory effects on dopaminergic neurones. For further details see text.

acetylcholine interaction is the well-known inhibitory effect of dopamine on acetylcholine release. This effect is apparently mediated by dopamine $D_2$ receptors, which have been demonstrated in cholinergic interneurones. In this instance, however, it is

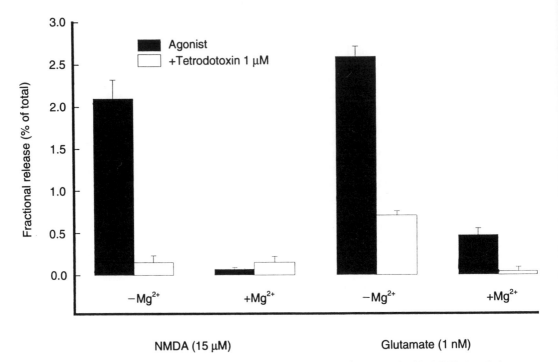

Fig. 6.4. Release of dopamine from dopaminergic nerve endings in striatum evoked by NMDA and glutamate. The effect of NMDA is completely blocked by $Mg^{2+}$; the effect of glutamate markedly reduced. This is consistent with the known $Mg^{2+}$-dependence of NMDA receptors. The incomplete blockade by $Mg^{2+}$ of the glutamate-induced dopamine release could be caused by glutamate actions at non-NMDA receptors. Note that tetrodotoxin blocks the effect of NMDA and glutamate on dopamine release despite the fact that there are no cell bodies in the preparation. For further details see text. (S. Jin and B. B. Fredholm, unpublished data).

not clear that presynaptic receptors are the most important. Instead soma-dendritic $D_2$ receptors that reduce the rate of firing of the cholinergic neurones may be more important (Fig. 6.3).

## 2.2 Excitatory and inhibitory amino acids in the CNS and their interaction with monoamines

Glutamate and GABA are quantitatively the most important neurotransmitters in the CNS. There is also some evidence that they may play a role in the periphery. Both transmitters have several types of receptor, which belong to two families: ion channels and G-protein coupled. In the case of GABA, there are $GABA_A$ receptors, which have integral $Cl^-$ channels, and $GABA_B$ receptors, which

are G-protein coupled. In the case of glutamate there are several classes of ion channel-associated receptors: $N$-methyl-D-aspartate (NMDA) receptors, α-amino-3-hydroxy-5-methyl-4-isoxazole proprionic acid (AMPA) receptors and kainate receptors. In addition, there are metabotropic receptors linked via a G-protein to the formation of inositol trisphosphate and diacylglycerol. It is commonly believed that all these receptor types are soma-dendritic and modulate neurotransmitter release mainly by affecting neuronal firing rate. However, there is increasing evidence that they may be present also presynaptically.

Activation of NMDA receptors has been shown to increase the release of several types of neurotransmitter in synaptosomes, provided that the $Mg^{2+}$ concentration is kept low and glycine is added. As expected, the effect of glutamate on NMDA receptors is increased if the preparation is somewhat depolarised, since such depolarisation leads to a removal of the $Mg^{2+}$ block of the NMDA receptor channel.

There is evidence from brain-slice experiments that there are presynaptic glutamate or GABA heteroreceptors. Two types of preparation have been useful in providing data. Cortical (and hippocampal) slices possess noradrenergic nerve endings that are functionally denervated, since the cell bodies are localised in the locus coeruleus, not included in the slice. Striatal slices similarly have dopaminergic nerve endings that are disconnected from their cell bodies (which are found in the substantia nigra).

One example of such experimental data is illustrated in Fig. 6.4. Here, release of dopamine from striatal slices was studied. There are clearcut effects of NMDA and of glutamate in causing this release. The interesting feature is that the release is clearly blocked by tetrodotoxin, despite the fact that there are no soma-dendritic receptors in this preparation. The implication is that tetrodotoxin blockade cannot be equated with actions at soma-dendritic receptors. Thus NMDA and glutamate can induce transmitter release that is dependent on $Na^+$-channel activation even in isolated nerve endings.

In all brain-slice preparations, there are glutamatergic and GABAergic neurones. However, these amino acids can be released in addition from non-neuronal elements in brain slices. Since glutamate and GABA themselves have been shown to increase the release of at least some other neurotransmitters, this is an important confounding factor in brain-slice experiments. When the entire slice is depolarised by field stimulation or, for example, by $K^+$, amino acids would be released, which in turn would cause, or modulate, the release of other transmitters under study. It is not known if this phenomenon has a physiological significance or is only an experimenter's nuisance. But, in this context,

a possible diffuse presynaptic receptor-mediated modulating role of amino acids in conditions such as ischaemia, where extracellular glutamate levels are much increased, would be an interesting topic for further study.

## 3   Co-transmitters and heteroreceptor-mediated modulation

It now appears to be the rule rather than the exception that nerves elaborate, store and release more than one type of transmitter (see Chapter 2). Often these co-transmitters belong to different classes of compound, for example peptides co-existing with amines or amino acids. One specific example is the 36 amino acid residue NPY, which is a known co-transmitter in peripheral noradrenergic neurones. It is known that NPY, acting on a putative $Y_2$ receptor, inhibits noradrenaline release. The presynaptic inhibitory effect of NPY appears to be dependent on a pertussis toxin-sensitive G-protein[1]. In sensory neurones, $G_o$ appears to be particularly important[1]. Furthermore, there is excellent evidence that the NPY receptor inhibits transmitter release by inhibiting $Ca^{2+}$ entry[1], in all probability via an action on N-type $Ca^{2+}$ channels. However, there is no good evidence that NPY released from a sympathetic nerve ending provides an important inhibitory influence on subsequent release of either NPY itself or its co-transmitters (e.g. Fig. 6.2). It is probable that the co-existing neuropeptide is predominantly released at high stimulation frequencies. By then, presynaptic $\alpha_2$-adrenoceptors would probably have been almost maximally activated. However, a final verdict on the physiological importance of presynaptic NPY (auto)receptors will have to await the development of selective antagonists.

NPY does, however, inhibit neurotransmitter release in several neurones where NPY is not a recognised neurotransmitter. For example, it inhibits neurotransmitter release in sensory neurones[1], and in cholinergic neurones as well as excitatory neurotransmitter release from the hippo-campus. It even inhibits the release of renin. A particularly interesting example is the release of NPY from noradrenergic nerves in the heart, which causes a decrease in the vagal release of acetylcholine (see Fig. 6.2).

On balance, it appears that the neuro-transmitter release-modulating effect of NPY is not related to it being a co-transmitter. In fact, it might be the case generally that actions at heteroreceptors are more impor-tant than actions at autoreceptors for all the peptide co-transmitters.

In sympathetic nerves, there appears to be three classes of compound that act like trans-mitters: the purine nucleotide ATP, the cate-cholamine noradrenaline and the peptide NPY. Of these, ATP is likely to be degraded most rapidly, NPY least rapidly. Therefore, of the three, NPY may be the one most likely to act at heteroreceptors and ATP the least likely.

# 4    Modulation of transmitter release by locally produced factors

There are several locally produced sub-stances that play little or no role as carriers of distinct signals but which act as local paracrine modulators of neurotransmitter release. These substances can be formed and released by a variety of cells, not only by local nerve endings, in response to signals from the environment. Three such locally produced factors are known to influence neurotransmitter release (and functions). (i) Prostaglandins (and other arachidonic acid metabolites) appear to be released from cells in response to stimuli that perturb the mem-brane structure and/or raise $Ca^{2+}$ levels in the proximity of the membrane to very high lev-els. (ii) Adenosine is released from cells whenever there is an imbalance between the rate of energy utilisation (ATP breakdown) and the rate of energy production (ATP syn-thesis). In addition, adenosine levels in the extracellular environment will increase as a consequence of local ATP release. (iii) Nitric

oxide can be released from several types of cell in response to a variety of stimuli. These local factors are generally released as a con-sequence of *de novo* synthesis and not from storage pools, as is the case for neurotrans-mitters or hormones. The first two will be dis-cussed here and nitric oxide in Chapter 7.

## 4.1    Prostaglandins and other eicosanoids

Arachidonic acid is the precursor of a variety of biologically active oxidation products. These are formed via a cyclooxygenase path-way, several lipoxygenase pathways and via a cytochrome P-450 epoxygenase pathway. Arachidonic acid is an abundant fatty acid found in the 2-position of many phospho-lipids. The major pathway to generate free arachidonic acid may be through the activa-tion of phospholipase $A_2$, but diacylglycerol formed by the activation of several forms of phospholipase C or via the activation of phospholipase D can also be a source (see also Chapter 9). These pathways are activat-ed by a variety of hormones and neurotrans-mitters that act on tyrosine kinase-coupled receptors, receptors with integral cation channels and, particularly, receptors coupled to the $G_i$ or the $G_q$ families of G-proteins. Thus, release of arachidonic acid metabolites is a general response to both neuronal and non-neuronal stimulation.

The neuromodulatory role of prostaglandins on noradrenaline release was discovered in the late 1960s (see ref. 7) and, therefore, actually predates the recognition that nor-adrenaline can regulate its own release. The effect is seen in several tissues and usually $PGE_2$ and $PGI_2$ (prostacyclin) are the most potent compounds. The receptor responsible may be similar to that which mediates inhibi-tion of lipolysis in fat cells. The mechanism underlying the inhibition of transmitter release is not entirely defined, as is the case for most other agents that act on receptors which have the capacity to couple with G-proteins. In some instances, inhibition of cAMP formation may play a role, but more often this is not the case. Instead a limitation of $Ca^{2+}$ entry or an effect on the $Ca^{2+}$-sensitive neurotransmitter-release machinery is likely to be most important. There is some evidence that thromboxanes and prostaglandin endoperoxides may enhance transmitter release.

Since prostaglandins may be formed as a consequence of α-adrenoceptor stimulation and then proceed to inhibit noradrenaline release, it has been suggested that prostaglandins may be part of the normal feedback loop (cf. refs. 7 and 11). In apparent support of this, there are several reports of a facilitatory effect of indomethacin (a prostaglandin-synthesis inhibitor) on noradrenaline release. This can be taken as evidence that prostaglandins are physiologically important regulators of noradrenaline release[7,11]. However, it is interesting to note that although such effects can be readily seen in smooth muscle strips *in vitro* or in organs perfused with a saline medium, they are not readily observed in more intact systems such as blood perfused tissues. It remains a possibility that, in those instances when endogenous prostaglandins do appear to play a role, the prostaglandins are formed as a consequence of tissue trauma during preparation rather than as a consequence of normal sympathetic tone. The more 'unphysiological' the preparation, the larger would be the stimulus for arachidonic acid release and consequent prostaglandin formation. In this context, it should be borne in mind that the overall rate of prostaglandin synthesis, as judged by the appearance of urinary metabolites, under physiological circumstances is quite low. It was reported[5] in 1975 that indomethacin may increase noradrenaline turnover in some, but not all, organs. This might be taken as evidence for a physiological role of prostaglandins in regulating the release of the sympathetic transmitter. However, indomethacin treatment causes gastrointestinal bleeding and hypoglycaemia. In short, the experimental animals would be severely stressed. Therefore, the increased turnover may have been the result of an increased impulse traffic in the sympathetic neurones rather than of a blockade of an endogenous brake on transmitter release.

Not only cyclooxygenase but also lipoxygenase products may influence transmitter release. In this context, 12-lipoxygenase metabolites of arachidonic acid have been suggested to mediate presynaptic inhibition in *Aplysia*. In the mammalian hippocampus, although LTP appears to be a postsynaptic phenomenon, fully established LTP appears to involve presynaptic elements also through increased neurotransmitter release. There is some evidence that an arachidonic acid metabolite, possibly a 12-lipoxygenase product, mediates the effect. It is hypothesised that NMDA receptor activation of the postsynaptic dendrite would lead to a $Ca^{2+}$-dependent enhancement of arachidonic acid metabolism. The lipoxygenase product would then diffuse back to the nerve terminal where it would enhance transmitter release.

Finally, and on a still more speculative note, arachidonic acid might by itself influence neurotransmitter release. This unsaturated fatty acid is known to act as a co-signal in the activation of protein kinase C. Activation of this enzyme has been repeatedly shown to enhance neurotransmitter release, for example by favouring a specific open state of nerve terminal $Ca^{2+}$ channels. Others have speculated that nitric oxide might fulfill the role of the retrograde signal. Yet others doubt that there is any retrograde signal at all.

Therefore, there is reason to consider the possibility that arachidonic acid, and many of its metabolites, could influence neurotransmitter release. They may not be very important under strictly physiological conditions, but many experimental preparations are far from physiological and are characterised by an increased arachidonic acid liberation. However, in several pathophysiological conditions, arachidonic acid metabolism is increased. In this context, it is perhaps of significance for neurotransmitter release and its modulation that non-steroidal anti-inflammatory drugs (NSAIDs) may alter the type of arachidonic acid product formed. Thus, the inducible form of cyclooxygenase normally generates prostaglandins, but after treatment with NSAIDs it generates lipoxygenase products.

## 4.2 Adenosine

### 4.2.1 Formation of adenosine

Adenosine is present in all body fluids even under basal physiological conditions. The concentration of adenosine in the extracellular space (usually between 50 and 500 nM) is in equilibrium with that in the cytosol of the surrounding cells. This equilibrium is maintained by a series of transporters. Some of these transporters are coupled to the $Na^+$ gradient and are, thus, directional, but the majority appear to be equilibrative; that is, the direction of transport depends on the direction of the adenosine concentration gradient. The relationship between the average intracellular and extracellular concentration of adenosine is complicated because in a given local environment some cells may be net producers and others net consumers of adenosine. When an inhibitor of adenosine transport is given, this usually leads to an increase in the intracellular adenosine concentration, but frequently there is also a clear-cut increase in extracellular adenosine. By comparison, extracellular inosine concentrations usually decrease following blockade of adenosine transport.

The intracellular concentration of adenosine is a function of several enzymatic processes (Fig. 6.5). The most important determinant is probably the intracellular level of AMP. AMP can be degraded either by AMP deaminase to IMP, or by 5'-nucleotidase to adenosine. The relative contribution of these two processes may vary between cells and organs. In brain slices, they appear to be roughly equal in magnitude. The intracellular adenosine is consumed by adenosine kinase forming AMP, and by adenosine deaminase, which degrades it to inosine, and, finally, by S-adenosyl-homocysteine hydrolase, which can, provided that the amount of homocysteine is high, convert the

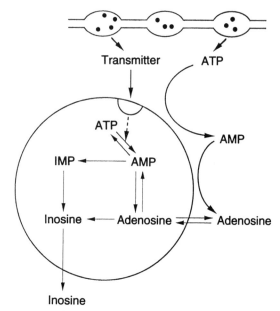

Fig. 6.5. Schematic representation of the mechanisms of adenosine formation. ATP can be released from nerve endings and from effector cells as part of, or as a consequence of, neurotransmission. The extracellular ATP is briskly degraded to adenosine. In addition, adenosine is formed intracellularly when the rate of ATP consumption locally exceeds the rate of ATP resynthesis. The adenosine formed intracellularly rapidly equilibrates with the extracellular space. For further details see the text.

adenosine to S-adenosyl-homocysteine. It appears that, in brain tissue, the adenosine kinase reaction is by far the most important mechanism to decrease intracellular adenosine.

When there is a discrepancy between the rate of ATP synthesis and ATP utilisation, the intracellular concentration of AMP increases. This then leads to an increased formation of intracellular adenosine. Because the ATP level can be somewhat decreased, the adenosine kinase reaction is also slowed down. The net result is a marked increase in intracellular adenosine and, consequently, in extracellular adenosine. Such an imbalance between ATP synthesis and ATP utilisation can result either from excessive nerve activity or from a decrease in energy supply.

Accordingly, there are numerous studies showing that nerve activity, particularly seizure activity, leads to an increase in adenosine production. Similarly, hypoxia, hypoglycaemia and ischaemia are potent stimuli for adenosine production.

In Fig. 6.5, which illustrates some of the metabolic pathways mentioned above, it is also shown that extracellular adenosine can be formed as a consequence of breakdown of extracellular adenine nucleotides. It is clear that the extracellular ATP content can increase as a result of increased nerve activity. ATP is co-stored and co-released by several peripheral, and probably also central, neurones. In addition, nerve activity can lead to ATP release from effector cells. Therefore, one might expect that there would be an increase in local adenosine concentration that matches the activity of an ATP-dependent neuronal pathway. So far, there is relatively little conclusive evidence to show that this is quantitatively important. This aspect is briefly discussed below.

The important conclusion to be drawn from the above is that nerve activity can lead to a local increase in adenosine level and that this in turn may affect the release of neurotransmitters.

### 4.2.2 Adenosine receptors and their mechanisms of action

There is now excellent evidence that adenosine and a variety of adenosine analogues can inhibit the release of many, if not all, neurotransmitters. There is evidence to suggest that the release of excitatory neurotransmitters may be inhibited to a greater extent than the release of inhibitory neurotransmitters, such as GABA. Since adenosine tends to limit its own formation, this can be understood if excitatory neurotransmission is a more powerful stimulus for adenosine production than inhibitory neurotransmission. The modulatory effects of adenosine and the adenosine analogues can be blocked by a variety of xanthine and non-xanthine adenosine receptor-blocking agents. It is thus clear

that the effect is mediated via adenosine receptors on the cell membrane.

The question of which particular receptor is responsible for the presynaptic effects of adenosine is more controversial. In the late 1970s, adenosine receptors were classified into two major groups, $A_1$ and $A_2$, based upon whether they decreased or increased, respectively, adenylyl cyclase activity. The classification was based both on the opposing actions on cAMP production and on the relative potency of a series of agonists. Clearly, these criteria are not suitable for detailed receptor subclassification. Relative agonist potency is a notoriously troublesome parameter to use in these circumstances and so is the mechanism of action of an agonist. Therefore, more recent attempts to classify the receptors have relied much more heavily on the use of selective inhibitors and on the identification of distinct gene products. There is now solid evidence for four types of adenosine receptor: $A_1$, $A_{2A}$, $A_{2B}$ and $A_3$, all of which have been cloned. The $A_1$ receptor is characterised by being potently inhibited by several xanthines including DPCPX (1,3-dipropyl-8-cyclopentyl xanthine). At the $A_2$ receptor, this xanthine is about three orders of magnitude less potent and at $A_3$ receptors it may be virtually inactive. Some characteristics of the adenosine receptors are summarised in Table 6.2.

There is essentially universal agreement that the $A_1$ (or perhaps an $A_1$-like) receptor mediates the inhibitory effect of adenosine on the release of neurotransmitters (see Fig. 6.6). The mechanism underlying the response is less clear-cut. As discussed by Fredholm and Dunwiddie[4], the reason for this could be that the adenosine $A_1$ receptor has the ability to inhibit neurotransmitter release, probably by four different mechanisms: (i) reduction in cAMP formation; (ii) stimulation of $K^+$ conductances; (iii) inhibition of N-type $Ca^{2+}$ channels; and (iv) effects, through so far poorly defined mechanisms, directly at the $Ca^{2+}$-responsive release machinery (see Chapters 1 and 11). There is also good reason to accept that these $A_1$

Table 6.2. *Some characteristics of adenosine receptors*

| | $A_1$ | $A_{2A}$ | $A_{2B}$ | $A_3$ |
|---|---|---|---|---|
| G-protein coupling | $G_{i(1-3)}$ $G_o$ | $G_s$ $(G_{olf})$ | $G_s$ | Yes, type unknown |
| Agonists | 2-Chloro-cyclopentyl-adenosine > cyclopentyl-adenosine > NECA > CGS 21680 | CGS 21680 > NECA (30 mM) > CV 1808 > R-PIA > CPA | NECA (1 mM) | APNEA (16 nM) > R-PIA = NECA > CGS 21680 |
| Antagonists | DPCPX, 8-cyclopentyl-theophylline | CP66713, KF17837 | No selective antagonist known | No tested xanthine acts as inhibitor |

APNEA, *N-p*-Aminophenethyladenosine; for other abbreviations refer to Fig. 6.6.

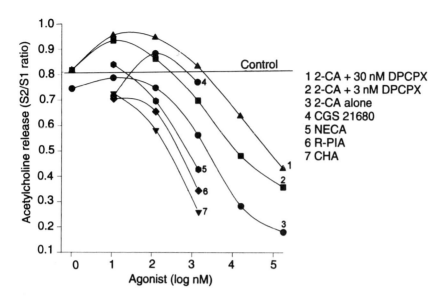

Fig. 6.6. Adenosine receptors and hippocampal acetylcholine release: the presence of stimulatory $A_{2A}$ and inhibitory $A_1$ adenosine receptors on cholinergic nerve endings in rat hippocampus. Acetylcholine release from rat hippocampal slices was evoked by two consecutive electrical field stimulation periods (S1 and S2, 0.5 Hz, 5 min). Drugs were administered 15 min before, during and 15 min after the second period (S2), as indicated in the figure. Inhibition of evoked acetylcholine release is shown by points below the control line, stimulation by points above. In the absence of any adenosine receptor antagonist, only inhibition could be detected. The potency order was: $N^6$-cyclohexyladenosine (CHA) $>$ $N^6$-($R$-phenylisopropyl)-adenosine (R-PIA) $>$ 5′-$N$-ethyl-carboxamidoadenosine (NECA) $>$ 2-chloroadenosine (2-CA) $>$ 2-[$p$-(2-carbonyl-ethyl)-phenylethylamino]-5′-$N$-ethylcarboxamidoadenosine (CGS 21680). When the highly selective $A_1$ receptor antagonist 1,3-dipropyl-8-cyclopentylxanthine (DPCPX) was administered, 2-CA caused a transient increase of transmitter release. For the sake of clarity, only mean values ($n = 4$–40) are given. The 95% confidence interval of the contents ranged from 0.87 to 0.77. The results are partly from ref. 2, with permission, and partly from unpublished experiments by S. Jin and B. B. Fredholm.

receptor effects are mediated by G-proteins. It is more controversial whether these G-proteins are pertussis toxin sensitive or not. In reconstitution studies, it has been found that the $A_1$ receptor is able to associate with $G_{i1}$, $G_{i2}$, $G_{i3}$ and $G_o$. All these G-proteins are pertussis toxin sensitive. At the same time, several carefully controlled studies have shown that the presynaptic inhibitory effect on neurotransmission mediated by $A_1$ receptors was not blocked by pertussis toxin, despite the fact that the toxin blocked several of the postsynaptic effects mediated by the same receptor (see ref. 6). The reason for this difference may not necessarily reside in the type of G-protein involved. Instead, factors such as the relative abundance of receptors and G-proteins at pre- and postsynaptic locations may be of greater importance.

Given that adenosine $A_1$ receptors have the potential to interact with neurotransmitter release in all the above-mentioned ways via the four known G-proteins, it is not surprising that evidence has accumulated in experimental systems in support of each of these possibilities.

The basic conclusion to be drawn is that there probably is no single mechanism that entirely explains the presynaptic inhibition of neurotransmitter release by stimulation of adenosine $A_1$ receptors. The rate-limiting step that is controlled by the presynaptic agonist seems to depend critically upon the experimental system used[4], for example on the mode of activation of neurotransmitter release. It may vary also between different types of nerve. It is probable that this basic conclusion applies to many presynaptic receptor systems.

There is some evidence to suggest that stimulation of adenosine $A_2$ receptors leads to an increased release of neurotransmitters. Such evidence has been obtained for the release of glutamate, acetylcholine, dopamine and noradrenaline. However it should be borne in mind that the effect of $A_2$ receptor stimulation is usually much smaller in magnitude than the $A_1$ receptor-mediated effect. Furthermore, the consensus amongst investigators is nowhere near as great as for the $A_1$ receptor-mediated effect. Different investigators using the same preparation either found or did not find evidence for $A_2$ receptor-mediated stimulation of transmitter release. Among those who found such an effect, some give evidence for high-affinity $A_{2A}$ receptors, others for low-affinity $A_{2B}$ receptors. The *only* clear example from our own studies (despite examining several systems) is shown in Fig. 6.6. An action at an $A_2$ receptor can be demonstrated if, and only if, the $A_1$ receptors are blocked. The stimulatory effect is exerted at low concentrations of the agonist, suggesting that an $A_{2A}$ receptor is involved. Further evidence for this is provided by data obtained with the use of selective antagonists (see Table 6.2).

### 4.2.3 Interactions between adenosine receptors and autoreceptors

In a number of instances, attempts have been made to study at the same time the influence of adenosine $A_1$ receptors and of autoreceptors on neurotransmitter release. It has often been the case that presynaptic receptor systems appear to interact. Therefore, the magnitude of the adenosine $A_1$ receptor-mediated inhibition of neurotransmitter release is invariably higher if the autoreceptors are blocked. There is also evidence from several laboratories that the magnitude of the autoreceptor control is higher if the adenosine $A_1$ receptors are blocked. One possible way to explain this is that the presynaptic receptor systems interact in a subtle way at the receptor or signal transduction level. Another possibility is that the two pathways interact functionally. Therefore, it is possible that both adenosine $A_1$-mediated control and autoreceptor control operate under basal experimental conditions. When one of these mechanisms is activated (or blocked), the consequence could well be that the other presynaptic regulatory system becomes less (or more) active, but that very little change is seen in net neurotransmitter overflow.

There are some indications that adenosine receptors and autoreceptors, even though they interact functionally, may use slightly different signal transduction mechanisms. In particular, there is evidence that blockade of some $K^+$ channels (probably an A- or D-type channel) by low doses of an aminopyridine preferentially antagonises the autoreceptor control of neurotransmitter release, leaving the effect of adenosine receptor-mediated inhibition of transmitter release virtually intact (but see Chapter 4). Such evidence has been obtained for both noradrenaline and acetylcholine release in the hippocampus and for dopamine release in the striatum. A typical finding is illustrated in Fig. 6.7. There are also findings which suggest that there may be differences in the degree of involvement of a protein kinase C-related mechanism between $\alpha_2$-autoreceptors and adenosine $A_1$ receptors in the control of noradrenaline release in the hippocampus.

### 4.2.4 Physiological role of adenosine heteroreceptors

The key question clearly is what is the physiological role of adenosine heteroreceptors? In the periphery, the evidence that adenosine plays a role in the regulation of noradrenaline (and acetylcholine) release under truly

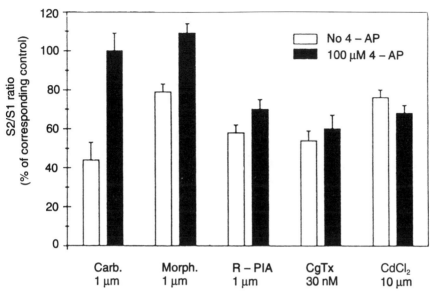

Fig. 6.7. Evidence that autoreceptors and heteroreceptors inhibit transmitter release via different mechanisms. Electrically evoked acetylcholine release from rat hippocampal slices was reduced by carbachol (Carb., 1 μM). The effect of this autoreceptor agonist was entirely blocked by blockade of $K^+$ channels with 4-aminopyridine (4-AP). The effect of morphine (Morph., 1 μM) was similarly antagonised. By contrast, the effect of the adenosine analogue R-PIA (1 μM) was unaffected by 4-AP, as was the effect of two agents, ω-conotoxin (CgTx, 30 nM) and cadmium chloride ($CdCl_2$, 10 μM), which block N-type $Ca^{2+}$ channels. (Reproduced from ref. 3, with permission.)

physiological conditions is poor. However, adenosine does seem to play a role both in tissues suffering from poor energy supply and in situations where the nerve activity is high and prolonged. These are also the situations when adenosine efflux from peripheral organs is elevated. During continuous nerve stimulation at frequencies between 3 and 5 Hz, it usually takes more than a minute before adenosine release is elevated and before it can be shown in experiments using blocking agents that adenosine modulates neurotransmitter release. This also tells us something about the source of adenosine that controls neurotransmission in the periphery. If the dominant source had been ATP released as a co-transmitter, it is expected that the adenosine control would be as rapid in onset as the autoreceptor control of neurotransmitter release. However, the observations are entirely compatible with a dominant

release of adenosine from the effector cells as a consequence of an imbalance between energy supply and energy demand.

In the CNS the situation seems to be somewhat different. In the brain, there is good evidence to show that low doses of adenosine receptor antagonists lead to an increased turnover of several central neurotransmitters, including noradrenaline, acetylcholine and serotonin (5-HT). Some studies have also suggested changes in dopamine turnover. Some years ago, it was shown that long-term treatment with theophylline leads to an augmented presynaptic adenosine receptor-mediated inhibition of neurotransmitter release. This finding is probably explained as an adaptation to a removal of a normal physiological inhibition. There is recent evidence from Dunwiddie and co-workers[12] that adenosine may be released from some effector neurones in response to only brief stimulations of the synaptic input. This could be caused by an increase in energy consumption in, for example, a dendrite. In such a structure, with a high surface area to volume ratio, the increased ATP utilisation cannot be rapidly met by increased ATP synthesis. Therefore, there are several mechanisms in the CNS that could indicate that adenosine is a physiologically important modulator of transmitter release.

The role of adenosine is likely to be much larger when there is a more global disruption of the energy supply or when a large number of neurones are firing at a high rate. Therefore, adenosine could be an important factor in hypoxia or ischaemia on the one hand, and in epilepsy on the other.

## 5  Summary

In the present chapter, a presynaptic heteroreceptor has been defined as a receptor that alters the release of a neurotransmitter that is *not* an agonist at the receptor. The agonists at such heteroreceptors can be neurotransmitters released from neighbouring nerves, local hormones and paracrine factors. The fact that neurotransmitters released from other neurones are able to influence not only the firing rate but also the release of a neurotransmitter at a nerve terminal is probably of very general significance. This provides a mechanism by which the activities of parallel neuronal pathways can be adapted to each other. In the periphery, this is nicely illustrated by the mutually antagonistic effects of noradrenergic and cholinergic nerves, not only at the effector level but also at the level of neurotransmitter release. The phenomenon is likely to occur also in the CNS where there is an extremely complex meshwork of neurones with different neurotransmitters. Heteroreceptor-mediated modulation of neurotransmitter release here can provide a patchy alteration of the activity in the basic neuronal networks. In particular, amines such as dopamine, noradrenaline and 5-HT might well exert their main actions by regulating nerve activity through combined presynaptic and soma-dendritic actions. In pathophysiological conditions, increased levels of amino acids and local paracrine factors could contribute to symptoms by exerting pronounced presynaptic actions. Therefore, in physiological, but particularly in pathophysiological conditions, drugs that affect presynaptic heteroreceptors may prove very important.

## References

1. Ewald DA, Sternweis PC and Miller RJ (1988) $G_o$ induced coupling of neuropeptide Y receptors to calcium channels in sensory neurons. *Proceedings of the National Academy of Sciences, USA* **85**: 3633–3637
2. Fredholm BB (1990) Adenosine $A_1$-receptor-mediated inhibition of evoked acetylcholine release in the rat hippocampus does not depend on protein kinase C. *Acta Physiologica Scandinavica* **140**: 245–255
3. Fredholm BB (1990) Differential sensitivity to blockade by 4-aminopyridine of presynaptic receptors regulating [$^3$H]-acetylcholine release from rat hippocampus. *Journal of Neurochemistry* **54**: 1386-1390
4. Fredholm BB and Dunwiddie TV (1988) How does adenosine inhibit transmitter release? *Trends in Pharmacological Sciences* **9**: 130–134
5. Fredholm BB and Hedqvist P (1975) Indomethacin-induced increase in noradrenaline turnover in some rat organs. *British Journal of Pharmacology* **54**: 295–300
6. Fredholm BB, Proctor W, van der Ploeg I and Dunwiddie TV (1989) *In vivo* pertussis toxin treatment attenuates some, but not all, adenosine $A_1$ effects in slices of the rat hippocampus. *European Journal of Pharmacology* **172**: 249–262
7. Hedqvist P (1977) Basic mechanisms of prostaglandin action on autonomic neurotransmission. *Annual Reviews of Pharmacology and Toxicology* **17**: 259–279
8. Hille B (1992) G protein-coupled mechanisms and nervous signaling. *Neuron* **9**: 187–195
9. Kalsner S (1990) Heteroreceptors, autoreceptors, and other terminal sites. *Annals of the New York Academy of Sciences* **604**: 1–6
10. Löffelholz K (1979) Release induced by nicotinic agonists. In: Paton DM (ed) *The*

*Release of Catecholamines from Adrenergic Neurons*, pp 275–301, Pergamon Press, Oxford

11. Malik KU and Sehic E (1990) Prostaglandins and the release of the adrenergic transmitter. *Annals of the New York Academy of Sciences* **604**: 222–236

12. Mitchell JB, Lupica CR and Dunwiddie TV (1993) Activity-dependent release of endogenous adenosine modulates synaptic responses in the rat hippocampus. *Journal of Neuroscience* **13**: 3439–3447

13. North RA, Slack BE and Surprenant A (1985) Muscarinic $M_1$ and $M_2$ receptors mediate depolarization and presynaptic inhibition in guinea-pig enteric nervous system. *Journal of Physiology* **368**: 435–452

14. Paton WDM and Vizi ES (1969) The inhibitory effect of noradrenaline and adrenaline on acetylcholine output by guinea-pig ileum longitudinal smooth muscle. *British Journal of Pharmacology* **25**: 10–28

15. Raiteri M, Marchi M and Paudice P (1990) Presynaptic muscarinic receptors in the central nervous system. *Annals of the New York Academy of Sciences* **604**: 113–129

16. Starke K (1981) Presynaptic receptors. *Annual Reviews of Pharmacology and Toxicology* **21**: 7–30

17. Starke K, Göthert M and Kilbinger H (1989) Modulation of neurotransmitter release by presynaptic autoreceptors. *Physiological Reviews* **69**: 864–989

# 7 Modulation of neurotransmitter release by hormones and local tissue factors

Julianne J. Reid, Zeinab Khalil and Philip D. Marley

The previous chapter introduced the concept that neurotransmitter release from a particular class of neurone may be modulated by neurotransmitters released by other classes of neurone, acting through heteroreceptors. In this chapter, Julianne Reid, Zeinab Khalil and Philip Marley extend this discussion to show that, besides neurotransmitters, other substances which are normally present in the body can also act through heteroreceptors to modulate neurotransmitter release. Such substances include hormones secreted at locations remote from the nerve terminals and locally derived factors that are produced in the vicinity of the nerve terminals. Implicit here is the concept that modulation of transmitter release may occur over a more extended time scale than that which would normally prevail with neurotransmitter-induced modulation. This chapter gives an account not only of the situation that prevails at the terminals of autonomic efferent neurones (from which most information on this subject has been derived experimentally), but also the situation in primary (sensory) afferent fibres and at the neuromuscular junction. The account clearly illustrates the ubiquity of modulatory control of, and the variety of potential modulators involved with, neuro-effector transmission.

## 1    Introduction

Neurotransmission at synapses operates over both short and long time frames. The duration of postsynaptic events depends on the nature of the transmitter, the type of receptor and the effector system to which it is coupled. Postsynaptic responses may last only a few milliseconds or endure for tens of minutes. The mechanism and consequences of presynaptic modulation of neurotransmission must, therefore, be considered in light of the temporal aspects of the postsynaptic response.

In addition to autoreceptors for transmitters and their co-transmitters, and heteroreceptors for transmitters released from adjacent nerves, many synapses are influenced physiologically by the presynaptic action of non-neuronally derived factors. These factors include those generated within the tissue that is innervated and circulating hormones that are released from endocrine cells distant from the affected nerve terminals. The release of these local tissue factors and hormones is usually controlled quite independently of the activity of the nerves they modulate. Furthermore, some have actions that are prolonged, since the agents concerned may have long half-lives, their receptors may have high affinity or the intracellular mechanisms they act through can be persistent.

Studying the actions of such factors on neurotransmitter release is complicated for a number of reasons. They may be generated by an endocrine organ some distance away from the nerves they modulate and this endocrine organ may not be part of an isolated tissue preparation containing the nerves being studied. Alternatively, the release of these agents may not be under nervous control but under the control of yet other local tissue events or of systemic factors. Furthermore, the time course of effects of many endocrine factors may be too slow to be detectable over the duration of normal *in vitro* experiments. Despite these, and other technical considerations, a large amount of information is now available on the presynaptic modulation of neurotransmitter release by non-neuronally derived factors.

It should be noted that a hormone is normally defined as a substance released by ductless glands and carried to a distant site of action by the blood. In contrast, local tissue factors are released by cells that do not form glands (e.g. mast cells, vascular endothelial cells) and reach their site of action directly through the interstitial fluid. In addition, a number of regulatory substances are known to be generated within the bloodstream from circulating precursors or by cells that do not form glands, yet are carried by the blood to a distant site of action. The systemic (cardiovascular) effects of histamine released from mast cells during anaphylactic shock are one example.

In recent years, the distinction between hormones and local tissue factors has become less clear. Many substances have now been found to have multiple regulatory roles: they may act as a hormone (because they are carried to their site of action by the bloodstream), but may also act as a local tissue factor (in that they can also be generated within a tissue in which they produce effects). Because the same substance may act in different ways, it is inappropriate to label *the substance* as a hormone or a local tissue factor, since it can be both; it is better to describe *the actions* of these substances as being endocrine or local in nature. In this chapter, a number of specific substances that act on nerve terminals are considered and in each case their actions are described as being endocrine or local in nature, as appropriate.

The main aim of this chapter is to consider the influence of certain hormones and local tissue factors on neurotransmitter release. In each case, the source of the substance is described and the physiological conditions under which it acts, followed by consideration of its endocrine and local actions on nerves.

One special group of non-neuronal substances that act on nerve terminals is produced by the postsynaptic effector cells responding to the neurotransmitter. These are called trans-junctional modulators and are best typified by adenosine and prostaglandins. Both compounds are liberated during the activation of effector cells and act trans-junctionally to inhibit the stimulation-induced release of noradrenaline from sympathetic varicosities, for example. The functional significance of trans-junctional modulation may be to place a restraint on excessive activation of effector cells.

Note that hormones and local tissue factors ('autacoids') may not only influence transmitter release from nerve terminals but may also modulate the postsynaptic effects of the transmitter, or themselves have direct effects on the innervated tissue. Some of these postsynaptic effects will be commented on in passing, to highlight the multiple sites of action of hormones and local factors. The examples chosen are ones for which there is good evidence that their prejunctional modulatory actions are of physiological significance, rather than an experimental curiosity.

Three types of peripheral nerve terminal only will be dealt with here: the terminals of postganglionic efferent autonomic nerves, the peripheral (sensory) terminals of primary afferent sensory nerves and the terminals of somatic motor nerves at the skeletal neuromuscular junction.

## 2 Modulation of autonomic neurotransmission by hormones and local tissue factors

### 2.1 Angiotensin II

The renin–angiotensin system functions as a centralised system, consisting of the enzyme renin (synthesised and released by the juxta-glomerular cells of the kidney), the $\alpha_2$-globu-lin precursor angiotensinogen (a plasma pro-tein synthesised by the liver) and angiotensin converting enzyme (localised mainly on the surface of pulmonary vascular endothelial cells). Renin cleaves the substrate angiotensinogen in plasma to generate angiotensin I, which is then converted to angiotensin II by angiotensin converting enzyme (Fig. 7.1). Angiotensin II is carried to many target tissues by the blood. More recent-ly, it has been demonstrated that there are also complete renin–angiotensin systems located in many tissues, including the heart and blood vessels, that can produce angiotensin II locally. Therefore, angiotensin II may act both as a hormone and as a local tissue factor.

The actions of angiotensin II are manifold and include direct vasoconstrictor and car-diac-stimulant actions in the cardiovascular system, an enhancement of both the synthesis and the release of aldosterone by the adrenal cortex and a number of interactions with the sympathetic nervous system to modulate its function. The interactions with the sympa-thetic nervous system include stimulation of central sympathetic outflow, activation of sympathetic ganglion cells, stimulation of adrenal chromaffin cells to release cate-cholamines and enhancement of noradrener-gic transmission through both pre- and postjunctional mechanisms. As depicted in Fig. 7.2, angiotensin II enhances tissue responses to noradrenergic nerve stimulation (and other vasoconstrictor agents) by a num-ber of mechanisms: an increase in the rate of synthesis of noradrenaline, enhancement of the stimulation-induced release of noradren-aline, inhibition of neuronal uptake (uptake$_1$, the amine-transport mechanism primarily responsible for terminating the action of noradrenaline at the neuro-effector junction) and enhancement of the responsiveness of effector cells to noradrenaline and other exci-tatory agents[13]. Angiotensin II also activates the synthesis and release of prostaglandins (mainly of the E type) in cardiovascular tis-sues, which act to oppose the prejunctional

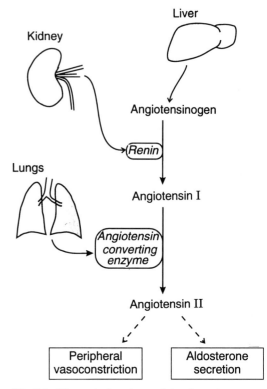

Fig. 7.1. The central renin–angiotensin system, showing the formation of angiotensin I and angiotensin II and the main physiological effects of angiotensin II. Note that local renin–angiotensin systems also exist in peripheral tissues, such as the heart and blood vessels.

enhancing effects of angiotensin II on neuro-effector transmission (see Fig. 7.2).

The effects of angiotensin II are mediated through the activation of specific membrane-bound receptors, which have recently been subdivided into two distinct receptor sub-types, designated AT$_1$ and AT$_2$. There is pre-liminary evidence that the AT$_1$ receptor sub-type is that subserving not only the direct vasoconstrictor action of angiotensin II, but also the actions of angiotensin II to increase neurotransmitter release from sympathetic nerve terminals and to facilitate postjunction-al responses to noradrenaline.

In addition to these direct interactions with noradrenergic neurotransmission,

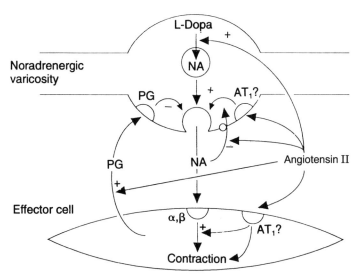

Fig. 7.2. The interaction of angiotensin II with noradrenergic neurotransmission. Angiotensin II acts directly on smooth muscle to produce contraction, thought to be mediated by $AT_1$ receptors. It also enhances noradrenergic neurotransmission by (i) activation of prejunctional receptors (possibly $AT_1$) on sympathetic nerve terminals to augment noradrenaline (NA) release; (ii) inhibition of the neuronal uptake of noradrenaline (uptake$_1$); (iii) stimulation of noradrenaline synthesis from L-dopa; and (iv) increasing effector cell responsiveness to noradrenaline, again possibly through $AT_1$ receptor activation. The augmentation by angiotensin II of neurotransmitter release may be opposed by a prejunctional inhibitory action of prostaglandins (PG), whose release from effector cells is stimulated by angiotensin II.

locally generated angiotensin II may also modify or mediate indirectly the effects of other substances. This appears to be the case for β-adrenoceptor-mediated enhancement of noradrenergic neuro-effector transmission: the enhancement of noradrenaline release induced by β-adrenoceptor agonists in some vascular and non-vascular tissues is inhibited not only by β-adrenoceptor antagonists but also by angiotensin converting enzyme inhibitors and angiotensin receptor antagonists[13]. However, this possible link between β-adrenoceptors and local renin–angiotensin systems does not exclude the existence of direct-acting facilitatory prejunctional β-adrenoceptors (see Chapters 9 and 14). Indeed, in some tissues, inhibition of the renin–angiotensin system has no effect on the enhancement of transmitter release caused by β-adrenoceptor activation.

The relative importance of each of the actions of angiotensin II to its overall action on the cardiovascular system has not yet been fully resolved. It is known that the postjunctional enhancing action of angiotensin II on effector cell responsiveness to noradrenaline is manifested at concentrations well below those that produce direct stimulatory actions on effector cells. Likewise the prejunctional action of angiotensin II to increase transmitter release occurs at lower concentrations than those required to elicit the postjunctional enhancing action. Therefore, under most conditions, modulation of noradrenaline release would appear to be the predominant influence of angiotensin II on neurotransmission.

It is probable that the enhancing effect of angiotensin II on noradrenergic function has a physiological role in cardiovascular regulation. Inhibitors of the renin–angiotensin system, such as inhibitors of angiotensin converting enzyme and antagonists at angiotensin receptors, have been shown in whole animal studies to reduce pressor responses to sympathetic stimulation, suggesting that there is, normally, facilitation of vascular noradrenergic transmission by endogenous angiotensin II.

The effectiveness of orally active angiotensin converting enzyme inhibitors to lower blood pressure in human hypertension has provided considerable stimulus to the study of renin–angiotensin systems and their role in cardiovascular regulation. The available evidence indicates that the antihypertensive effect of angiotensin converting enzyme inhibitors is dependent on inhibition of angiotensin II production, mainly by local renin–angiotensin systems. Certainly, there is evidence for enhanced facilitation by angiotensin II of noradrenaline release in cardiovascular tissues in animal models of hypertension. For example, the prejunctional effect of angiotensin II to increase transmitter release is more marked in (genetically) spontaneously hypertensive rats than in normotensive rats (see also Chapter 14).

### 2.2   Adrenaline

Adrenaline is synthesised in chromaffin cells of the adrenal medulla and is released by splanchnic nerve activity into the circulation, both tonically and during stress to prepare the body for increased physical demands typified by a fear, fight or flight reaction. Adrenaline increases blood glucose, decreases blood coagulation time, increases heart rate and force and increases blood perfusion of skeletal muscles (see also Chapters 13 and 14). In addition to these postjunctional effects, experimental results from both animal and human studies suggest that adrenaline released from the adrenal medulla can activate presynaptic $\beta_2$-adrenoceptors to facilitate noradrenaline release[9] (Fig. 7.3). This has been demonstrated in many isolated tissues (including human tissues) at adrenaline concentrations that are within the range occurring physiologically in the circulation (0.5–10 nM; see also Chapter 14). Adrenaline may also reduce noradrenaline release

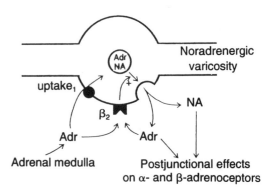

**Fig. 7.3.** Modulation of noradrenaline (NA) release by adrenaline. Adrenaline (Adr) secreted by the adrenal medulla can activate prejunctional $\beta_2$-adrenoceptors on noradrenergic nerve terminals to increase evoked noradrenaline release. Adrenaline can also be taken up into terminals by uptake$_1$ and stored with noradrenaline in storage vesicles, from which it can be released subsequently as a co-transmitter. The released adrenaline can act on prejunctional $\beta_2$-adrenoceptors to increase subsequent transmitter release, thus forming a positive feedback loop.

through activation of inhibitory $\alpha_2$-adrenoceptors, but concentrations in excess of 30 nM are required for this action. Therefore, it is likely that the only physiological effect of circulating adrenaline at sympathetic nerve terminals is on prejunctional $\beta_2$-adrenoceptors.

Sympathetic nerve endings can accumulate adrenaline from the circulation by the neuronal transport system for catecholamines (uptake$_1$), resulting in the storage of small amounts of adrenaline with noradrenaline in noradrenergic neurones[9] (Fig. 7.3). Adrenaline that has been taken up into sympathetic nerve terminals can subsequently be released as a co-transmitter along with noradrenaline (see Chapter 2). The participation of adrenaline as a co-transmitter has a number of potentially significant consequences. First, the nerves can concentrate the relatively low levels of adrenaline in the plasma. Second, it is likely that the adrenaline subsequently released into the synapse will be close to the prejunctional $\beta_2$-adrenoceptors. Third, since adrenaline taken up into noradrenergic nerves has a half-life of several hours, occasional bursts of adrenaline secretion from the adrenal medulla can accumulate in nerves and have a prolonged effect on sympathetic neurotransmission. Therefore, co-transmission involving adrenaline would allow a more intense and prolonged facilitation of noradrenaline release than would otherwise occur with circulating adrenaline alone. Indeed, it has been shown that adrenaline released from the adrenal medulla in humans causes a rise in plasma noradrenaline levels that continues well after plasma adrenaline levels have returned to normal. This further supports the suggestion that adrenaline has been taken up into sympathetic nerve terminals from the plasma and released as a co-transmitter to produce a persistent facilitation of noradrenaline release. The importance of adrenaline as a co-transmitter probably depends on the amount released from the adrenal medulla, so that factors such as prolonged stress may play a critical role. Consequent activation of prejunctional $\beta_2$-adrenoceptors by adrenaline has been implicated in the development of hypertension and there is considerable evidence for such a role for adrenaline in both animal models and humans[9]. In particular, studies suggest a direct involvement of adrenaline where environmental stressors appear to be involved in the development of hypertension (see also Chapter 14).

## 2.3 Histamine

Histamine is predominantly synthesised and stored in mast cells, which are present in connective tissue throughout the body. It is, therefore, found in high amounts in tissues that contain large numbers of mast cells such as skin, bronchial mucosa and intestinal mucosa. In plasma, histamine is stored in basophil leucocytes and, under normal conditions, circulating plasma concentrations of free histamine are generally very low, approximately 10 nM. There is also evidence

that histamine is present in histaminergic nerves in the CNS and in peripheral sympathetic nerves in tissues such as the heart and blood vessels.

The physiological postjunctional effects of histamine include contraction of gastrointestinal smooth muscle, increased gastric acid secretion and vasodilatation caused by subsequent release of nitric oxide and prostacyclin from the vascular endothelium. These effects are mediated through specific histamine receptors of which there are at least three distinct classes, discriminated pharmacologically and designated $H_1$, $H_2$ and $H_3$. Prejunctional receptors of the $H_3$ subtype have been described on histaminergic (histamine-containing) nerve terminals in the brain, where they regulate the synthesis, and modulate release of, histamine through an autoreceptor-mediated negative feedback mechanism. Release-inhibiting $H_3$ receptors have been demonstrated on central serotonergic neurones, on peripheral noradrenergic nerves and on parasympathetic cholinergic nerves of the intestine, airways, heart and blood vessels[5].

It is still not clear whether the $H_3$ receptor-mediated effects on sympathetic and parasympathetic transmission observed in *in vitro* pharmacological models indicate that histamine mediates a tonic influence either in normal or in pathophysiological conditions. At present, there is no evidence to show that endogenous histamine modulates autonomic neurotransmission under physiological conditions.

The ability of histamine, released from mast cells, to affect transmitter release from peripheral terminals of sensory nerves through the activation of $H_1$ receptors, is discussed in Section 3.2.1 below.

## 2.4 5-Hydroxytryptamine

5-Hydroxytryptamine (5-HT, serotonin) is principally synthesised and stored in enterochromaffin cells in the gastrointestinal tract. These cells, which may be innervated by preganglionic parasympathetic nerves, have a basal secretion of 5-HT that is augmented by mechanical stimulation, hypertonicity of the gut lumen contents, noradrenaline and vagal stimulation. On release from enterochromaffin cells, much of the 5-HT is taken up by platelets. It is also present in some noradrenergic nerve terminals in the periphery and is the chemical transmitter of serotonergic nerves within the CNS. Thus, the modulation of autonomic neuro-effector transmission by 5-HT can arise by virtue of its release as either a transmitter, a co-transmitter or a local hormone.

5-HT has varied and complex prejunctional and postjunctional actions in the cardiovascular, gastrointestinal and respiratory systems, as well as in the CNS. The specific receptors for 5-HT are divided on the basis of their pharmacology into four main types: $5\text{-}HT_1$, $5\text{-}HT_2$, $5\text{-}HT_3$ and $5\text{-}HT_4$, with further subdivision of the $5\text{-}HT_1$ and $5\text{-}HT_2$ groups, although the classification is still in a state of flux.

Receptors of the $5\text{-}HT_1$ subtype are located on the terminals of some noradrenergic and cholinergic autonomic nerves and mediate inhibition of noradrenaline and acetylcholine release, respectively. Autoinhibitory prejunctional $5\text{-}HT_1$ receptors are also located on central serotonergic nerve terminals. The $5\text{-}HT_2$ receptor subtype appears to be located mainly postjunctionally and subserves contraction of gastrointestinal, respiratory and vascular smooth muscle, as well as platelet aggregation and depolarisation of neurones in the CNS. Receptors of the $5\text{-}HT_3$ subtype are also postjunctional and occur on autonomic and enteric nerves and also on peripheral sensory neurones. The activation of these $5\text{-}HT_3$ receptors causes depolarisation and is associated with the ability of 5-HT to cause pain and itching, as well as pulmonary and cardiovascular reflexes (see Section 3 below). The most recent addition to the 5-HT receptor family, $5\text{-}HT_4$ receptors, have been located (postjunctionally) in the heart (on myocardial cells and the sino-atrial node), the CNS and in the gastrointestinal tract (on both neurones and smooth muscle); their function is still being defined.

Circulating 5-HT in the plasma is rarely observed, and the physiologically relevant responses of 5-HT as a mediator appear to be those produced locally in the vascular system by its release from platelets. A striking example of the modulation of neurovascular transmission by hormonal 5-HT comes from observations on dog isolated coronary artery segments[3]. In this tissue, 5-HT (along with adenosine-containing compounds) released from platelets can diffuse through the medial layer of the artery in sufficient amounts to inhibit stimulation-evoked noradrenaline release from the axons at the medial-advential border and thereby inhibit the vasoconstrictor response to noradrenergic nerve stimulation.

## 2.5 Adrenocorticotrophic hormone (ACTH)

ACTH (also termed corticotrophin) is secreted by the anterior lobe of the pituitary and controls the synthesis and release of the glucocorticoid steroid hormones of the adrenal cortex and, to a much lesser extent, aldosterone. The release of ACTH is controlled physiologically by a balance between stimulatory factors (mainly corticotrophin-releasing factor from the hypothalamus) and inhibitory factors (mainly glucocorticoids from the adrenal cortex) (Fig. 7.4; see also Chapters 8 and 13).

Besides regulating the release of adrenal steroids, ACTH and active fragments of ACTH, principally $ACTH_{1-24}$, are known to enhance stimulation-induced noradrenaline release from sympathetic postganglionic nerves in cardiovascular tissues of the rabbit through the activation of prejunctional ACTH receptors. There is some evidence that these receptors may have physiological significance. For example, 0.1 nM $ACTH_{1-24}$ (which is within the physiological range achieved in human plasma under conditions in which ACTH release is strongly stimulated) enhances noradrenaline release by sympathetic nerve stimulation in the rabbit isolated heart[14]. Therefore, ACTH may have a

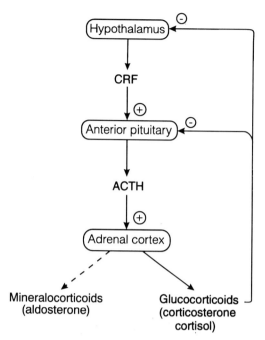

Fig. 7.4. Regulation of the secretion of ACTH from the anterior pituitary. ACTH release is stimulated (+) by corticotrophin-releasing factor (CRF) from the hypothalamus and inhibited (−) by circulating glucocorticoids acting directly on the anterior pituitary secreting cells and on the hypothalamic cells that secrete CRF. ACTH has only a small effect on mineralocorticoid secretion (indicated by a dotted line).

role to play in the modulation of noradrenaline release (at least in the rabbit), especially when ACTH levels are raised by stressful situations.

Although prejunctional facilitatory ACTH receptors have been demonstrated on the terminals of both cardiac and vascular sympathetic nerves in the rabbit, they have not been found in cardiovascular tissues from other species, such as rat and guinea-pig. It has been proposed though that activation of other prejunctional receptors, such as $\alpha_2$-adrenoceptors, normally masks the response of activation of prejunctional ACTH receptors, because the magnitude of their effect is considerably larger than that of ACTH receptors.

## 2.6   Nitric oxide

The importance of nitric oxide in intercellular communication, cardiovascular regulation and cytotoxicity has only been recognised since the late 1980s. It was initially identified as an endothelium-derived vasodilator but has since been shown to be released from many cell types in addition to endothelial cells, such as neurones, platelets, macrophages, neutrophils and smooth muscle cells. Nitric oxide is synthesised by the conversion of the amino acid L-arginine to L-citrulline, the reaction requiring molecular oxygen and a number of co-factors including NADPH. It is catalysed by the enzyme nitric oxide synthase (Fig. 7.5).

Nitric oxide can act directly to produce relaxation of vascular and non-vascular smooth muscle through activation of the cytosolic enzyme soluble guanylyl cyclase, which causes an elevation of cyclic GMP (cGMP) levels and a decrease in intracellular free $Ca^{2+}$ (Fig. 7.5).

Recently, it has been suggested that endothelium-derived nitric oxide may have a functional role in (postjunctional) modulation of vascular noradrenergic transmission and smooth muscle reactivity[15]. Inhibition of nitric oxide synthase causes a marked enhancement of the vasoconstrictor responses to sympathetic nerve stimulation and noradrenaline, as well as to other endogenous vasoconstrictor agents such as 5-HT. The enhancement is dependent on the presence of vascular endothelial cells. It has, therefore, been postulated that nitric oxide is released from the endothelium during vasoconstriction to cause relaxation of the vascular smooth muscle, to oppose the vasoconstrictor response and to act as a physiological brake, possibly to limit damage to blood vessels during the contractile response[15].

There are conflicting findings concerning a possible prejunctional action of nitric oxide on noradrenaline release from sympathetic nerves. Nitric oxide donors such as the antianginal agents glyceryl trinitrate and sodium nitroprusside have been shown either to

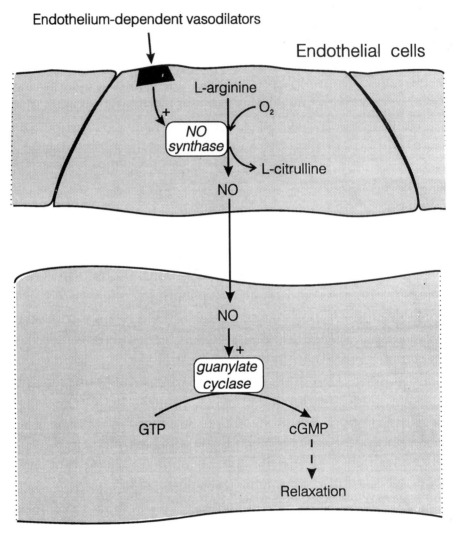

Fig. 7.5. Synthesis and mechanism of action of endothelium-derived nitric oxide (NO). NO release occurs basally from vascular endothelial cells or is stimulated by endothelium-dependent vasodilator agents (such as acetylcholine and bradykinin). NO is synthesised on demand by the conversion of L-arginine to L-citrulline, which is catalysed by the enzyme NO synthase. The released NO activates soluble guanylyl cyclase in smooth muscle cells, which in turn increases the production of cGMP from GTP, which causes vascular relaxation.

increase, decrease or have no effect on stimulation-induced noradrenaline release from sympathetic nerve terminals in blood vessels. The prejunctional action of nitric oxide apparently depends on the tissue and the species. Inhibition of endogenous nitric oxide synthesis using inhibitors of the synthase enzyme appears not to affect noradrenaline release[15], suggesting that endogenous nitric oxide does not exert a tonic influence to modulate basal noradrenaline release.

### 2.7 Endothelins

The endothelins are a group of peptides each containing approximately 21 amino acid residues and are found in at least three distinct isoforms (which differ by two to six residues). These have been termed endothelin-1, endothelin-2 and endothelin-3. Endothelin-1 was identified in 1988 as a potent vasoconstrictor agent released from vascular endothelial cells, but the endothelins are now known to be produced also by non-vascular cells within the brain, kidney, lung, intestine and elsewhere. In addition to vasoconstriction, the endothelins have been found to exert a wide variety of effects on both vascular and non-vascular tissues through the activation of specific endothelin receptors.

Endothelin-1 has been found to modulate neuro-effector transmission by both pre- and postjunctional mechanisms. The prejunctional actions of endothelin-1 are dependent on the tissue and species, with reports either of an increase, a decrease or no effect on the stimulation-induced release of noradrenaline from both vascular and non-vascular smooth muscle preparations. The physiological importance of the prejunctional effect of endothelin-1 is not clear, but it is possible that endothelin-1 released locally may reach sufficiently high tissue concentrations to modulate neurotransmitter release.

The most consistent effect of endothelin-1 on neuro-effector transmission is a postjunctional enhancement of the contractile response in vascular smooth muscle and in non-vascular smooth muscle from the intestinal and urogenital tracts. This enhancing effect of endothelin-1 may have physiological relevance, since it has been shown recently that sub-vasoconstrictor concentrations of endothelin-1, at or close to circulating plasma endothelin-1 levels (approximately 1 pM), can facilitate contractile responses in some vascular beds[10].

## 3 Regulation of transmitter release from peripheral terminals of sensory nerves

### 3.1 Neurotransmitter release at peripheral terminals of sensory nerves

Peripheral sensory (primary afferent) nerves are responsible for detecting changes in the external or internal environment and transmitting this information to the CNS. Sensory nerves have two sets of terminals. One is at the periphery and detects sensory stimuli and transduces them to nerve impulses. These are conducted along the sensory fibres to the second set of terminals in the CNS. The latter terminals synapse on to other central neurones (secondary afferents) that project to higher centres where the sensory information is processed.

Some primary afferent (sensory) nerves not only conduct action potentials towards the CNS (i.e. in the 'orthodromic' direction as above) in response to specific peripheral stimuli but also convey nerve impulses back to the periphery along collateral branches of the sensory nerve trunk to blood vessels near the site of stimulation. These are called 'antidromic' impulses, since they run in the opposite direction to their normal conduction direction. This recurrent pathway is called an axon reflex (Fig. 7.6). Axon reflexes are activated particularly when impulses are generated in small unmyelinated sensory fibres (C fibres) in response to noxious stimuli at the skin surface. Stimulation of the axon reflex results in the release of a number of neuropeptides from the *peripheral* terminals of the sensory nerves. Consequently, sensory nerves may be considered to have a dual function: to send nerve impulses to the CNS and release neurotransmitters from their central nerve terminals, and to send impulses along their peripheral collateral branches and release neurotransmitters from these peripheral terminals.

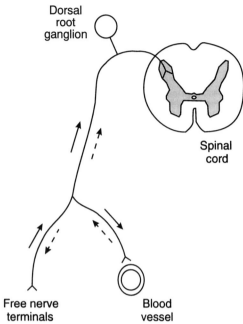

Fig. 7.6. Release of neurotransmitters from the *peripheral* terminals of primary afferent sensory nerves by the axon reflex. Sensory stimuli are detected by free nerve terminals of sensory fibres and produce action potentials in these nerves. The action potentials propagate along the fibre (solid arrows) past the dorsal root ganglia to the CNS thereby conveying sensory information to higher centres. The action potentials may also invade nearby peripheral branches of the sensory nerve and be conducted peripherally (antidromically) to their terminals around blood vessels. The antidromic impulses may, thus, lead to release of sensory neurotransmitters from these terminals around blood vessels. It is also possible that the blood vessel sensory terminals are activated by sensory stimuli (e.g. blood-borne factors, products of tissue injury) and send nerve impulses along the sensory nerve to the CNS (dotted arrow). In addition, these impulses may invade the other peripheral branches of the sensory nerve, such as those containing the free nerve endings, in the antidromic direction and cause neurotransmitter release from these terminals. A variety of local tissue factors and circulating hormones can, thus, affect the function and activity of these peripheral terminals of sensory nerves, either by modulating evoked transmitter release from the terminal or by sensitising them to sensory stimuli (see Figs. 7.7 and 7.8).

### 3.1.1 Neuropeptides released from sensory nerve terminals

Sensory primary afferent nerves contain several neuropeptides, including substance P and other tachykinins (neurokinin A, neuropeptide K, neurokinin A(3–10), neuropeptide γ), CGRP, VIP, cholecystokinin, angiotensin II, somatostatin, galanin and dynorphin. It is not yet clear which combinations of these peptides are present in the same sensory nerves and which, therefore, may be released together. The neurotoxin capsaicin, an extract of hot red peppers, can selectively destroy unmyelinated primary afferent sensory nerves that generate axon reflexes in peripheral tissues. Capsaicin subsequently produces a long-lasting reduction in neuropeptide release from peripheral terminals of sensory nerves and hence a reduction in the peripheral actions of these nerves during axon reflexes. Neonatal capsaicin treatment of experimental animals has been used as a method for studying the function and regulation of peripheral terminals of sensory nerves in a variety of tissues.

Neuropeptides are released predominantly from sensory nerve collaterals that terminate around nearby blood vessels, but they may also be released from collaterals that form free endings in the adjacent tissues. It is possible that stimulation of the sensory terminals around blood vessels may generate an axon reflex to other nearby blood vessels or to other free nerve endings on the collateral branches of the nerve (see Fig. 7.6). The release of the peptides and their subsequent actions are modulated by endogenous tissue factors released at the site of tissue injury, by circulating hormones and by neurotransmitters released by efferent autonomic nerves that innervate the tissue.

It should be noted that release of neurotransmitter from the central terminals of sensory neurones in the spinal cord is also subject to presynaptic modulation by neurotransmitters (e.g. opioid peptides) released by central neurones.

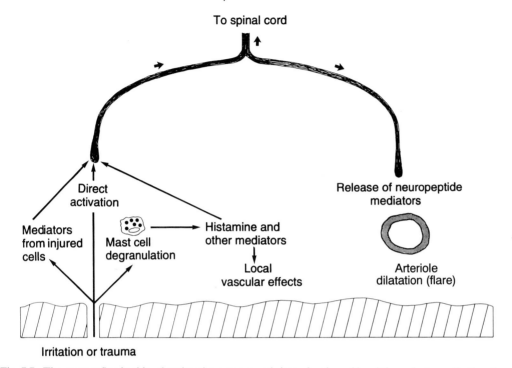

**To spinal cord**

Direct
activation

Release of neuropeptide
mediators

Mediators
from injured
cells

Mast cell
degranulation

Histamine and
other mediators

Local
vascular effects

Arteriole
dilatation (flare)

Irritation or trauma

Fig. 7.7. The axon reflex in skin, showing the sources and sites of action of local tissue factors affecting the peripheral terminals of sensory nerves. Separate peripheral branches of individual sensory fibres end as free nerve terminals in the skin and around cutaneous blood vessels. Irritation, noxious stimuli or trauma to the skin results in activation of the sensory nerves, which conveys the information to the spinal cord and also transmits antidromic impulses along other branches of the sensory nerve to local blood vessels. Sensory neuropeptides are released at the blood vessels that cause vasodilatation and plasma extravasation in the areas adjacent to the site of injury. A large number of locally produced tissue factors from injured cells, immune cells and mast cells, as well as circulating hormones, can influence the sensitivity of the axon reflex and affect the release of the sensory neuropeptides. Similar processes occur in the respiratory epithelium (see Fig. 7.8). (Reprinted from ref. 6, with kind permission from P. Holzer and Pergamon Press Ltd.)

### 3.1.2   The role of released neuropeptides

The neuropeptides from sensory nerves mediate local effects in the peripheral tissues, mainly serving to integrate the functioning of the microvasculature[4,6]. The role of sensory nerves as triggers of protective responses to noxious stimuli is well established: peripheral release of neuropeptides from primary afferents leads to a cascade of events which mediate inflammation, pain sensation and wound healing. Two of the most commonly investigated actions associated with peripheral sensory nerve endings involved in axon reflexes are arteriolar vasodilatation and an increase in venular permeability ('neurogenic inflammation', see Fig. 7.7). The released neuropeptides function physiologically to accelerate the wound healing process by promoting hyperaemia, chemotaxis of immune cells and plasma extravasation. Although this serves to protect the tissue from extensive damage, these same actions may also contribute to tissue damage during pathological conditions. For example, neurogenic inflammation has been shown to contribute to many disease states, including asthma, gastric ulcer, headache, arthritis, and in the pathogenesis

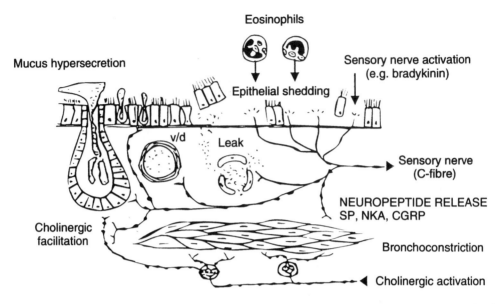

Fig. 7.8. The axon reflex mechanism in asthma. Damage to the respiratory epithelium causes activation of sensory nerves. These send impulses not only to the CNS, but also antidromically along local branches of the sensory nerves that end in proximity to blood vessels and epithelial glands. The sensory nerve terminals release neuropeptides, which cause mucus hypersecretion, vasodilatation (v/d), plasma extravasation (leak), contraction of airway smooth muscle (bronchoconstriction) and attract infiltrating eosinophils. Many local tissue factors as well as activation of cholinergic nerves can amplify this local reflex, augmenting the release of sensory neuropeptides and exacerbating the mucosal inflammation. SP, substance P; NKA, neurokinin A; CGRP, calcitonin gene-related peptide. (Reprinted from ref. 1, with kind permission from P. Barnes and Marcel Dekker Inc.)

of skin ulcers in patients with diabetes mellitus. Current evidence suggests that, of the neuropeptides released from peripheral terminals of sensory nerves, substance P is the most likely mediator of the neurogenic inflammatory response.

In the respiratory tract, the 'axon reflex hypothesis' for the deleterious role of sensory nerves in asthma[1] was proposed in 1986. It was suggested that epithelial desquamation stimulates sensory nerves and subsequent antidromic conduction leads to the local release of tachykinins in the airways (see Fig. 7.8). Furthermore, substance P-immunoreactive nerves proliferate in asthmatic airways, particularly in the submucosa. Axon reflexes could then amplify the inflammatory response and would spread inflammatory changes in the airway mucosa from patchy areas of epithelial damage.

## 3.2 Modulation of neuropeptide release from peripheral terminals of sensory nerves

Several endogenous tissue factors appear to modulate the release of neuropeptides from the peripheral terminals of sensory nerves. These factors are produced during the inflammatory process following tissue injury and act on receptors located on the primary afferent terminals. Antagonists directed at these neuronal receptors could be potentially useful compounds to alleviate pain in injured tissue and even reduce the extent of tissue injury. The inflammatory mediators include histamine, prostaglandins, leukotrienes,

5-HT, ATP, bradykinin and endothelium-derived mediators.

It should be noted that the *central* terminals of sensory nerves could also be a target for modulation of release of their neurotransmitters. Presynaptic modulation is known to occur on the central terminals of the unmyelinated C fibre sensory nerves that generate axon reflexes in the periphery and convey information about noxious stimuli to the CNS (e.g. the inhibitory effects of opioid peptide transmitters released at axoaxonic synapses in the dorsal horn of the spinal cord). Furthermore, the release of neurotransmitter from the other class of sensory nerves (large diameter, myelinated sensory afferents) is modulated presynaptically in the spinal cord at axoaxonic synapses by amino acid neurotransmitters released from other nerve terminals. However, the presynaptic modulation of neurotransmitter release from sensory nerve terminals in the CNS will not be discussed further here.

### 3.2.1  Modulators that enhance neuropeptide release

**Histamine.**  Histamine is released from mast cells at the site of tissue injury and has been implicated as a mediator in many inflammatory diseases. A considerable part of the histamine effect has been found to be indirect, acting through activation of capsaicin-sensitive sensory nerves. Histamine receptors have been localised on the peripheral terminals of these nerves and the effects of histamine are significantly reduced in animals pretreated as neonates with capsaicin. There is evidence suggesting involvement of $H_1$ receptors in causing vasodilatation and increasing plasma extravasation to substance P in the skin[7]. In the airways, histamine has multiple effects, which are mediated by at least three histamine receptor subtypes. The $H_3$ subtype is involved in the inhibition of neurogenic vascular leakage through presynaptic inhibition of neuropeptide release from airway sensory neurones[1]. However, $H_1$ receptors mediate bronchoconstriction,

vasodilatation and microvascular leakage by enhancing neuropeptide release from sensory nerve terminals. The $H_2$ subtype appears to be important in mediating bronchial vasodilatation and mucus secretion, probably by direct (postsynaptic) effects not involving the sensory nerves.

**The kinins.**  The kinins, bradykinin and kallidin, are other local tissue factors released as a consequence of tissue damage and are potent arterial vasodilators and venoconstrictors that cause increased vascular permeability and pain. They are generated from kininogens by a group of proteases called kallikreins, either in plasma (where bradykinin is generated) or in glandular tissues, such as the pancreas, and salivary and sweat glands. The kallikreins are generally kept in an inactive state and are activated to produce the kinins during inflammatory conditions, such as those caused by trauma, burns and allergy. They are also activated during circulatory shock. Kinins exert their effects through at least two different receptors, which have been named bradykinin $B_1$ and $B_2$. Many of their effects are mediated through the release of other endogenous agents, such as catecholamines released from sympathetic nerves and the adrenal medulla and vascular endothelium-derived nitric oxide and prostaglandins.

Bradykinin-induced venoconstriction and prostaglandin release could contribute to the plasma extravasation response. There is evidence for bradykinin sensitisation of nociceptive sensory nerve terminals, and high-affinity (presynaptic) bradykinin ($B_2$) receptors have been found on sensory nerve fibres. In the skin, a significant part of the response to bradykinin is mediated through an excitatory action on peripheral nociceptive C fibres. These fibres release sensory neurotransmitters (see below) that induce vasodilatation and plasma extravasation by releasing nitric oxide from vascular endothelial cells[8]. In the airways, bradykinin selectively activates nociceptive C fibre sensory nerve endings causing increased release of neuropeptides such as substance P, neurokinin A and CGRP from local collateral branches of sensory nerves. This results in bronchoconstriction (particularly caused by neurokinin A), exaggerated cholinergic reflexes (neurokinin A), mucus hypersecretion (substance P), hyperaemia (CGRP) and microvascular leakage (substance P) leading to oedema of the airway and extravasation of plasma into the lumen[1]. The bronchoconstriction and bronchial oedema result in dyspnoea. Whether the bradykinin acts at the primary afferent terminal to evoke neuropeptide release or to modulate the release evoked by antidromic impulses is not known.

**Eicosanoids.** Eicosanoids are the family of molecules derived from arachidonic acid. Among them are cyclooxygenase products, including prostaglandins and 5-lipoxygenase products, including leukotrienes. The role of prostaglandins in inflammation has been studied since the early 1960s. Most cells are able to generate prostaglandins, including macrophages, vascular endothelial cells, mast cells and airway smooth muscle cells. The finding that exogenous prostaglandins potentiate plasma exudation in the skin and bronchial oedema produced by other mediators such as histamine, leukotrienes and bradykinin suggests that modulation of plasma extravasation may be the primary role of prostaglandins in inflammation. One mechanism by which they achieve this is by enhancing neuropeptide release from the peripheral terminals of sensory nerves.

Studies have shown that prostaglandins enhance substance P release in skin blisters caused by antidromic sensory nerve stimulation. They also enhance substance P-induced plasma extravasation in the skin and capsaicin-induced protein extravasation in the respiratory tract. The ability of prostaglandins to cause these effects is explained by their ability to sensitise primary afferents. Sensitisation is characterised by a decreased threshold and increased excitability of nociceptors, that is by making them responsive to lower levels of noxious stimuli and thereby preconditioning them for the actions of other mediators that normally would be ineffective at exciting the sensory nerves. Most recently, prostaglandins have been shown to induce release of substance P from injured peripheral endings of sensory nerves in rat saphenous nerve neuroma (a mass of regenerating nerve fibres at the end of a cut nerve). These actions of prostaglandins on primary afferent neurones are thought to be mediated via receptors coupled intracellularly to stimulatory G-proteins, which in turn modulate the cAMP second messenger system.

**Leukotrienes.** Leukotrienes are slow-reacting substances of anaphylaxis generated by neutrophils, eosinophils, basophils, mast cells and macrophages. They increase microvascular leakiness and produce oedema in the skin. They are also potent stimulants of mucus secretion in human airways. It has been suggested that some of the effects of leukotrienes could result from enhancement of neuropeptide release from primary afferents, but this has not yet been proved.

**5-Hydroxytryptamine.** 5-HT is a potent pain-producing substance and a major mediator of inflammation. A number of studies have shown that 5-HT can increase the responsiveness of sensory receptors linked to nerve fibres of small diameter (C, possibly some Aδ) located in the skin and ankle joint tissues of normal and arthritic rats. It has been suggested that endogenous 5-HT could increase the responsiveness of sensory mechanoreceptors in chronically inflamed tissue. In addition, endogenous 5-HT contributes to ongoing neural afferent activity seen in inflamed joints. It is possible that endogenous 5-HT, released from platelets or nerve fibres, is responsible for sensitisation of sensory nerves during the acute inflammatory response. In most cases, the pharmacological identity of the 5-HT receptor associated with sensory endings has not been established, but it may be a $5-HT_3$ receptor.

**Platelet-activating factor.** Platelet-activating factor (PAF) is produced by several types of cell that participate in the inflammatory response, including macrophages, eosinophils and neutrophils. In the skin, PAF causes vasodilatation and increases vascular permeability, and an enhanced release of neuropeptides from sensory nerves has been suggested to be the mechanism involved. In addition, PAF induces bronchial hyper-responsiveness by triggering a series of inflammatory responses including activation of sensory nerves. The effects of PAF could also be mediated more indirectly by the release of 5-HT from platelets, since 5-HT is known to activate sensory nerves that release sensory peptides (see above). The receptor involved in the activation of sensory nerves by PAF has not yet been characterised.

### 3.2.2 Modulators that inhibit neuropeptide release

**Adenosine.** Several different cell types have now been shown to have the capacity to release adenosine, a compound that appears to act as a local modulatory factor of neurotransmitter release. In the present context, adenosine has been found to inhibit neuropeptide release from sensory nerve terminals in guinea-pig trachea and in guinea-pig isolated bronchi. Adenosine inhibits tachykinin release evoked by field stimulation of the sensory nerve terminals, but it has no effect on the tissue response to exogenous substance P. A prejunctional inhibition mediated by $A_1$ receptors has been proposed. In guinea-pig atria, endogenous adenosine inhibits neurotransmitter release from capsaicin-sensitive sensory nerves via a prejunctional $A_1$ adenosine receptor. In the airways, adenosine has an indirect bronchoconstrictor action that involves the release of histamine from mast cells. It is possible, therefore, that adenosine could affect primary afferents indirectly via released histamine.

It has been suggested that adenosine may also have a facilitatory action on sensory nerve terminals, mediated by direct activation of $A_2$ receptors. The two adenosine receptor subtypes and their spectrum of effects are similar to those on somatic nerve terminals at the skeletal neuromuscular junction (see below).

**Opioids.** Presynaptic inhibition of sensory transmitter release from primary afferent C fibres by opioid peptides in the CNS is well documented. Immunoreactive opioid receptors have also been demonstrated on peripheral terminals of sensory neurones, and increased amounts of opioid peptides have been localised in immune cells infiltrating inflamed tissue in the rat hindpaw. Therefore, endogenous opioids could produce localised effects in inflamed tissue. Activation of μ-opioid receptors located on peripheral terminals of sensory afferents has been shown to inhibit neuropeptide release and, as a consequence, to reduce neurogenic vasodilatation, plasma extravasation and also heat-induced oedema. In chronically inflamed tissue, there is an over-expression of μ- and δ-opioid receptors on the sensory fibres, which may play an anti-inflammatory role and mediate an analgesic effect via inhibition of neurotransmitter release.

Capsaicin-sensitive primary afferent sensory nerves in the guinea-pig atrium are endowed with μ-opioid receptors, which inhibit transmitter release from these terminals. The opioid peptides that affect these cardiac sensory nerve terminals may originate from nearby terminals of efferent autonomic fibres or be released from adrenal medullary chromaffin cells (along with adrenaline) to act as hormones. The suggestion has been made that prejunctional μ-opioid receptors on sensory nerves may play a role in modulating activity of the cardiovascular system.

Opioid peptides are effective inhibitors of the release of substance P from primary afferent collaterals in the airways. This action inhibits bronchoconstriction, reduces neurogenic microvascular leakage in guinea-pig airways and inhibits capsaicin-induced mucus secretion in human airways via an action on μ- and δ-opioid receptors located on local sensory nerve terminals.

**Catecholamines.** As with opioids and adenosine, catecholamines can inhibit transmitter release from sensory afferents. An $\alpha_2$-adrenoceptor-mediated inhibitory modulation of sensory C fibre function in the skin has been demonstrated *in vivo* in the allergen-induced wheal and flare reaction.

# 4 Presynaptic modulation of skeletal neuromuscular transmission

Although the molecular events of neurotransmission are probably better understood at the skeletal neuromuscular junction than at any other class of synapse, our knowledge of presynaptic receptors at the neuromuscular junction is not extensive. This is, in part, because skeletal muscle is sparsely innervated compared with many other tissues, and because methods for studying directly the release of acetylcholine from such sparsely innervated tissues have only been available relatively recently (see Chapters 3 and 4). Most information on presynaptic control and modulation of neuromuscular transmitter release has been obtained using sensitive and sophisticated electrophysiological techniques, which have been used to analyse the frequency of spontaneous miniature endplate potentials (MEPPs), caused by the release of single packets of transmitter, and the quantal content of the muscle EPP. The technique of labelling the presynaptic transmitter pool of acetylcholine with [3H]-choline and following the subsequent release of isotopically labelled transmitter has only recently been employed at this synapse (Section 6).

So far there is evidence for presynaptic modulation of transmitter release at the neuromuscular junction by adrenaline acting as a hormone and by adenosine acting as a local tissue-derived factor. There is also evidence that presynaptic nicotinic and muscarinic autoreceptors regulate transmission at the skeletal neuromuscular junction. However,

there are as yet very few data for modulation by other factors, such as angiotensin II, 5-HT, histamine or prostaglandins, which are effective at other peripheral nerve terminals (see above).

## 4.1 Adrenoceptors and the actions of circulating catecholamines

In common with a large number of other central and peripheral nerve terminals (see Chapters 5 and 6, for example), neurotransmitter release from neuromuscular nerve terminals is modulated by adrenoceptors. It has been known since the early 1960s that adrenaline, released into the bloodstream by adrenal medullary chromaffin cells, can partially overcome neuromuscular blockade induced *in vivo* by the nicotinic receptor antagonist curare. Detailed studies identified two actions of adrenaline: an initial effect mediated by α-adrenoceptors to overcome curare block, and a secondary effect mediated by β-adrenoceptors to potentiate the effects of curare.

The facilitatory effects of α-adrenoceptor agonists on skeletal neuromuscular transmission have been demonstrated *in vitro* using preparations of mammalian, amphibian, fish and earthworm neuromuscular junctions, suggesting this action has been well preserved during evolution. Noradrenaline and other α-adrenoceptor agonists increase the frequency of MEPPs, without changing their amplitude. By comparison, noradrenaline does not affect the postsynaptic potential resulting from iontophoretic application of acetylcholine to the muscle. These data, therefore, indicate a presynaptic site of action of the α-adrenoceptor agonists to increase acetylcholine release. In contrast, similar studies found that β-adrenoceptor agonists increased the frequency of MEPPs (a presynaptic action) and increased the amplitude of MEPPs and of acetylcholine-induced potentials (postsynaptic effects). Following 3H-labelling of the acetylcholine pools in phrenic nerve terminals of the rat isolated diaphragm preparation, both α- and β-adrenoceptor agonists were found to increase [³H]-acetylcholine release during stimulation of the nerves[16,17]. This confirmed that both types of adrenoceptor are present presynaptically and when stimulated evoke acetylcholine release at the neuromuscular junction.

Structure–activity studies of the presynaptic facilitatory α-adrenoceptors on cat sciatic nerve and rat phrenic nerve indicate that they are similar pharmacologically to vascular postjunctional $\alpha_1$-adrenoceptors. They are quite distinct from the inhibitory prejunctional α-adrenoceptors on sympathetic and sensory nerve terminals, which are predominantly of the $\alpha_2$-subtype (see Chapter 5, for example).

The facilitatory presynaptic β-adrenoceptors on rat phrenic nerve terminals are also unusual for prejunctional β-adrenoceptors since they are of the $\beta_1$-subtype[16]. In contrast, the postsynaptic β-receptors, known to be present on skeletal muscle (see below), have the pharmacology of $\beta_2$-adrenoceptors, similar to the facilitatory prejunctional $\beta_2$-adrenoceptors on sympathetic nerve terminals.

The ability of $\alpha_1$-adrenoceptor agonists to enhance [³H]-acetylcholine release at the skeletal neuromuscular junction was recently found to be prevented by the N-type $Ca^{2+}$-channel blocker ω-conotoxin GVIA but not by the L-type $Ca^{2+}$-channel blocker nifedipine, suggesting that the $\alpha_1$-adrenoceptors modulate N-type $Ca^{2+}$ channels. The $\beta_1$-adrenoceptor-mediated effect was blocked by nifedipine but not by ω-conotoxin GVIA, suggesting that the $\beta_1$-adrenoceptors modulate L-type $Ca^{2+}$ channels (see Chapters 9 and 10, for example).

It is unclear whether circulating catecholamines released from nearby sympathetic nerves or the adrenal medulla enhance neuromuscular transmission under physiological circumstances. In humans experiencing fright, tremor is a common symptom and is clearly caused by the action of circulating catecholamines on skeletal muscle. However, this effect is likely to be the result of a postsynaptic action. The concentrations of adrenaline and noradrenaline needed, *in vitro*, to enhance neuromuscular transmission by presynaptic actions are in the 0.1–1 μM range, more than ten times the concentrations needed to enhance autonomic transmission via prejunctional $\beta_2$-adrenoceptors (see above), and 10–100 times the plasma levels of these catecholamines experienced even during hypoglycaemia, myocardial infarction or with phaeochromocytoma. It is possible that other co-transmitters, local tissue-derived factors or hormones could sensitise somatic nerve terminals to circulating catecholamines and reveal a physiological facilitatory effect on neuromuscular transmission.

**Adenosine.** In the mid 1970s, using electrophysiological techniques, adenosine-containing compounds were shown to inhibit transmitter release at the mammalian and amphibian neuromuscular junction[12]. Although ATP has long been known to be stored in synaptic vesicles in somatic nerve terminals and to be released along with acetylcholine during skeletal nerve activation, it is now clear that the primary agent which inhibits acetylcholine release is not ATP but the nucleoside adenosine. It appears that the adenosine is not released as such from the nerve terminal at the neuromuscular junction, but is generated locally by extracellular hydrolysis of released ATP by the sequential action of ecto-ATPases and ecto-5'-nucleotidases[11] (see Fig. 7.9 and also Chapter 6). Early studies had shown that ATP, ADP, AMP and adenosine were of similar potency in inhibiting acetylcholine release at the neuromuscular junction. However, the necessity for extracellular degradation of adenine nucleotides to produce the active agent was shown by the lack of effect of non-hydrolysable ATP analogues on neuromuscular transmission: α,β-mATP had no influence on the frequency of MEPPs or on the quantal content of evoked EPPs[11]. Furthermore, inosine (the metabolic product from the deamination of adenosine by adenosine deaminase) (see Fig. 7.9) was inactive. The source of the ATP that generates

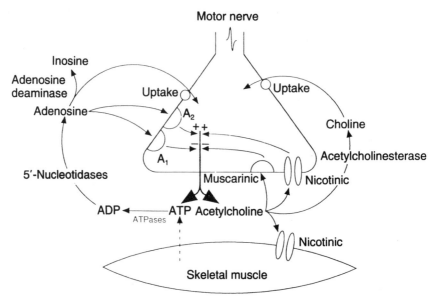

Fig. 7.9. The local production and presynaptic actions of adenosine at the neuromuscular junction. Motor nerves, and to a lesser extent the skeletal muscle, release ATP, which is hydrolysed by ecto-ATPases to ADP and then by ecto-5′-nucleotidases to adenosine. Adenosine may act on presynaptic $A_1$ receptors to inhibit cholinergic transmission to the muscle, or on presynaptic $A_2$ receptors to facilitate transmission. The action of adenosine is terminated by reuptake into the motor nerve terminal, rather than by deamination to inosine.

adenosine at the neuromuscular junction is mostly the somatic nerve terminals; however, some of the ATP may be released by the skeletal muscle. Consequently, in this action, adenosine may be considered to be a local tissue-derived factor generated extracellularly in the interstitial fluid.

Although local extracellular generation of adenosine from released ATP appears a rather indirect way of generating adenosine to act as a presynaptic modulator, this is clearly a mechanism of physiological significance[11]. During stimulation of the motor nerves to the frog sartorius muscle, it can be shown that adenosine is produced extracellularly and inhibits transmission via presynaptic adenosine receptors. The amplitude of evoked EPPs was increased by addition of exogenous adenosine deaminase (to degrade any adenosine that might be produced) or by the addition of adenosine receptor antagonists such as 8-phenyltheophylline or theophylline. Neurotransmission was reduced in

the presence of dipyridamole, an adenosine-uptake blocker (see Fig. 7.9) that potentiates the action of adenosine, but not in the presence of 2-chloroadenosine, which is not a substrate for the uptake transporter. In addition, the 5′-nucleotidase inhibitor $\alpha,\beta$-mADP, at a concentration that inhibited the action of exogenous ATP (which needs to be hydrolysed by ATPases and 5′-nucleotidases to produce adenosine), increased the size of evoked EPPs but did not affect the inhibitory action of exogenous adenosine. The effect of $\alpha,\beta$-mADP was overcome by adding exogenous purified ecto-5′-nucleotidase. These observations indicate clearly that endogenous ATP is released during nerve stimulation, is broken down to adenosine and that it is the adenosine that acts presynaptically to inhibit acetylcholine release from the somatic nerve terminals. Subsequently, the adenosine is inactivated by a dipyridamole-sensitive uptake system and not by degradation by adenosine deaminase (Fig. 7.9). This is quite a different mechanism from that which operates presynaptically to inhibit neurotransmission in frog sympathetic ganglia or in guinea-pig ileum, where ATP is the active agent (acting on $P_2$ purinoceptors) and adenosine is inactive.

Similar results have been obtained by studying acetylcholine release after loading the transmitter pool with [³H]-choline. In these experiments, exogenous adenosine inhibited nerve stimulation-induced [³H]-acetylcholine release, theophylline (an adenosine receptor antagonist) enhanced it and theophylline blocked the effect of exogenous adenosine.

Pharmacological studies indicate that adenosine may act at two receptors to produce opposite effects and, furthermore, that both effects can be seen at a single endplate (Fig. 7.9). The predominant effect is mediated by an $A_1$ receptor. This causes a reduction in spontaneous MEPP frequency and in quantal content of evoked EPPs and produces an inhibition of stimulation-induced [³H]-acetylcholine release. In the presence of $A_1$ receptor antagonists, the effects of $A_2$ receptors are revealed. These *increase* MEPP frequency and EPP quantal content and *enhance* [³H]-acetylcholine release. These actions are not blocked by theophylline, which is a selective $A_1$ receptor antagonist.

Adenosine generated locally outside the somatic nerve terminal clearly plays a physiological role in modulating cholinergic transmission by a presynaptic action. Adenosine reduces the amplitude of the EPP, particularly at junctions that release low amounts of acetylcholine, and is more effective at morphologically smaller terminals. Furthermore, when trains of stimuli are applied to the presynaptic nerve, it appears that adenosine does not affect successive impulses at a single site but rather reduces acetylcholine release from nearby sites[2] (see also Chapter 4). The physiological significance of this modulation of transmission at smaller terminals and from adjacent sites is not yet clear.

## 4.2  Seasonal changes in neuromuscular transmitter release

There have been several reports concerning seasonal modification of presynaptic modulation of transmitter release at neuromuscular junctions. It seems likely that humoral factors, including substances released from the skeletal muscle and circulating hormones, act on the somatic nerve terminals to contribute to long-term seasonal adaptation of the 'safety factor' for neuromuscular transmission, this being the likelihood that an action potential will result in release of sufficient transmitter to activate the skeletal muscle.

## 5  Summary

The presynaptic effects of a number of locally generated factors and circulating hormones on neurotransmitter release from peripheral autonomic, somatic and sensory neurones have been described. Local tissue factors and hormones clearly play a major role in presynaptic modulation of transmitter release from peripheral nerve terminals. The examples given in this chapter show the extensive effects these agents have in modulating neurotransmission. It is noteworthy that the agents considered have analogous actions to neurotransmitters, which act either as feedback modulators of their own release (see Chapter 5) or as heterologous modulators of release from adjacent nerves (see Chapter 6). Indeed with respect to their modulatory role, there are few functional distinctions between transmitters, local tissue factors and hormones. Each may act over short periods of time, affecting pulse-to-pulse release of transmitter, or have a very extended duration of action, affecting transmitter release for hours. Hormones may act at substantial distances from their site of release, while autacoids may act very locally. Both temporally and spatially, however, these two categories of compounds are functionally indistinguishable and, therefore, should be considered together as a single category of extracellular regulators that have powerful influences over neurotransmitter release.

It has been noted here that many of the local tissue factors and hormones that affect neuro-transmission presynaptically also have post-synaptic actions. These may be either direct effects of the agents or indirect, by the agent modifying the postsynaptic effects of the neuro-transmitters released at that synapse. It is clear that local tissue factors and hormones can play a significant role in modulating the total func-tion of the synapse. A number of agents may act both locally and systemically: for example, angiotension II may be generated as a local tis-sue factor and act to affect local transmitter release at a discrete locus but may also be gen-erated in the circulation and have widespread effects on transmitter release at many loci.

In some cases, more than one receptor sub-type for a particular local tissue factor or hor-mone may be present on a given nerve terminal (e.g. adenosine and acetylcholine receptors on nerve terminals at the skeletal neuromuscular junction; see Fig. 7.9). In these cases, the differ-ent receptor subtypes may mediate opposing effects that appear to cancel out. However, often because of different receptor sensitivities, it is usual for one action to dominate so that there is a net effect. Alternatively, long-term adaptive changes may affect the relative repre-sentation of a receptor subtype and hence alter the effect of the modulator at the synapse.

# References

1. Barnes PJ (1992) Neurogenic inflammation and asthma. *Journal of Asthma* **29:** 165–180
2. Bennett MR, Karunanithi S and Lavidis NA (1991) Probabilistic secretion of quanta from nerve terminals in toad (*Bufo marinus*) muscle modulated by adenosine. *Journal of Physiology* **433:** 421–434
3. Cohen RA (1986) Adenine nucleotides and 5-hydroxytryptamine released by aggregating platelets inhibit adrenergic neurotransmission in canine coronary artery. *Journal of Clinical Investigation* **77:** 369–375
4. Donnerer J and Amann R (1991) Sensory pharmacology. *Pharmacological Toxicology* **69:** 228–232
5. Hill SJ (1990) Distribution, properties, and functional characteristics of three classes of histamine receptor. *Pharmacological Reviews* **42:** 45–83
6. Holzer P (1988) Local effector functions of capsaicin-sensitive sensory nerve endings: involvement of tachykinins, calcitonin gene-related peptide and other neuropeptides. *Neuroscience* **24:** 739–768
7. Khalil Z and Helme RD (1989) Sequence of events in substance P mediated plasma extravasation in rat skin. *Brain Research* **500:** 256–262
8. Khalil Z and Helme RD (1992) The quantitative contribution of nitric oxide and sensory nerves to bradykinin-induced inflammation in rat skin microvasculature. *Brain Research* **589:** 102–108
9. Majewski H and Rand MJ (1986) A possible role of epinephrine in the development of hypertension. *Medical Research Reviews* **6:** 467–486
10. Reid JJ (1993) Endothelin-1 may be a physiological modulator of vasoconstriction in rat kidney. *Journal of Cardiovascular Pharmacology* **22:** S267–S270
11. Ribeiro JA and Sebastiao AM (1987) On the role, inactivation and origin of endogenous adenosine at the frog neuromuscular junction. *Journal of Physiology* **384:** 571–585
12. Silinsky EM, Hunt JM, Solsona CS and Hirsh JK (1990) Prejunctional adenosine and ATP receptors. *Annals of the New York Academy of Sciences* **603:** 324–333
13. Story DF and Ziogas J (1987) Interaction of angiotensin with noradrenergic neuroeffector transmission. *Trends in Pharmacological Sciences* **8:** 269–271
14. Szabo B, Hedler L, Schurr C and Starke K (1988) ACTH increases noradrenaline release in the rabbit heart. *Naunyn-Schmiedeberg's Archives of Pharmacology* **338:** 368–372
15. Vo PA, Reid JJ and Rand MJ (1992) Attenuation of vasoconstriction by endogenous nitric oxide in rat caudal artery. *British Journal of Pharmacology* **107:** 1121–1128
16. Wessler I and Anschütz S (1988) β-Adrenoceptor stimulation enhances transmitter output from rat phrenic nerve. *British Journal of Pharmacology* **94:** 669–674
17. Wessler I, Ladwein E and Szrama E (1989) Stimulation of $\alpha_1$-adrenoceptors increases electrically evoked [$^3$H]-acetylcholine release from rat phrenic nerve. *European Journal of Pharmacology* **174:** 77–83

# 8 Modulation of neurotransmitter release by corticosteroid hormones

Marian Joëls and E. Ronald de Kloet

It has commonly been assumed that steroid hormones affect cellular function principally by regulating the expression of the genome, which they do from within the cell after passing through the plasma membrane to interact with cytosolic receptors. This allows the possibility that steroid hormones can modulate neurotransmitter release at a point well before the exocytotic event. It has recently been shown, however, that steroid hormones can act also at neuronal cell surface receptors. There is, therefore, the additional possibility that steroid hormones may modulate neurotransmitter release in a manner similar to that described in the earlier chapters. In this chapter Marian Joëls and Ronald de Kloet evaluate these possibilities in general and describe specifically instances where steroid modulation may occur physiologically. They briefly consider also the neurosteroids: a class of compound chemically related to the adrenal steroids but produced by certain neurones in the CNS and which could be involved in modulating neuronal function.

## 1    Corticosteroids and the nervous system

Stress activates the hypothalamo–pituitary–adrenal axis. Noxious agents, trauma, pain and environmental changes, but also uncertainty, fear and lack of control, are conditions that stimulate hypothalamo–pituitary–adrenal activity. These trigger a cascade of humoral events, initiated by the release of hypothalamic corticotrophin-releasing hormone (CRH) and vasopressin into the portal vasculature that supplies the anterior pituitary (see also Chapter 13). Vasopressin potentiates the action of CRH on the anterior pituitary cells, leading to increased synthesis and release of pituitary pro-opiomelanocortin products, e.g. the endorphins and ACTH. The stress-induced ACTH surge stimulates secretion of corticosterone from the adrenal cortex (in man cortisol; see Fig. 8.1), which reaches maximal circulating levels after 15–30 min. It is emphasised in this chapter that corticosterone not only circulates in the blood but also enters the brain where it affects neuronal activity (for reviews see refs. 3, 4 and 17).

The hypothalamo–pituitary–adrenal axis displays a circadian variation[3]. In the rat, levels of corticosterone peak at about 750 nM at the beginning of the active period, while trough levels at the beginning of the inactive period are below 25 nM. Circulating corticosterone is bound to corticosteroid-binding globulin with a rather high affinity. Accordingly, at the trough of the circadian cycle, less than 10% of the steroid circulates in the free (unbound) form that is available for binding to the receptor. Imposed upon this circadian variation, stress causes a rise in

143

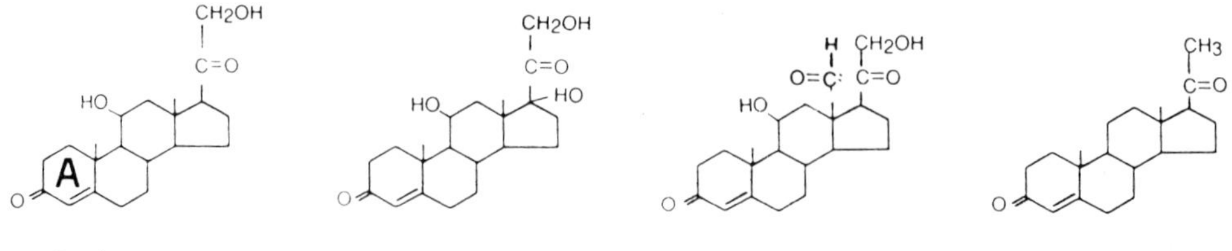

Fig. 8.1. Chemical structure of corticosteroid hormones and the related neurosteroids. Note that in all of the neurosteroids the A-ring is reduced.

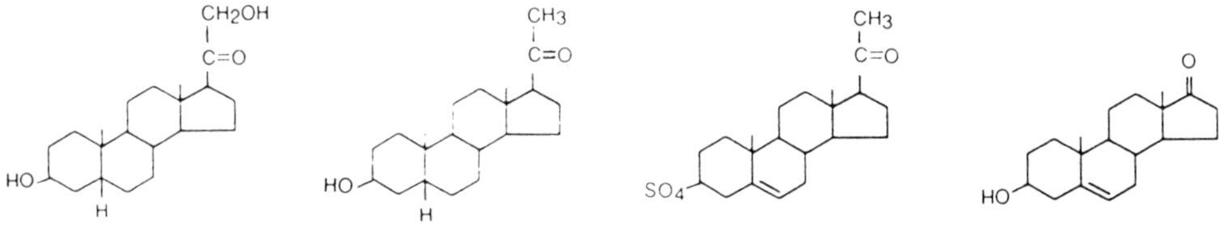

plasma corticosterone concentration, up maybe to 1000 nM, which exceeds the saturation of the binding to corticosteroid-binding globulin and results in an exponential rise in the level of free, circulating steroid.

Corticosterone (or cortisol in humans) has long been known to be connected with stress and adaptation, but the way in which the steroid contributes to the regulation of the stress response is not precisely known. One hypothesis emphasises the role of the steroids in the promotion of energy metabolism. High concentrations of corticosterone or doses of synthetic glucocorticoid analogues, such as dexamethasone, modify the conversion of metabolic energy from lipids and protein to carbohydrates to provide a readily available energy resource for the brain and heart during stress. In Tausk's[24] and Munck's[19] hypotheses, glucocorticoids are thought to prevent over-reaction of defence mechanisms to stress: defensive inflammatory and immune responses, as well as cardiovascular and central nervous responses, to stress may become damaging if not controlled, for example by glucocorticoids.

An important aspect of the action of (adrenal) corticosteroid hormones is their action on the brain and pituitary through which they modulate the neuroendocrine stress response[3]. While the feedback action of high corticosteroid concentrations at the pituitary and hypothalamic level was well-documented even in the early 1960s, the putative effects of corticosteroids in higher brain centres were only first appreciated later that decade when Bruce McEwen and his colleagues showed that circulating corticosteroid hormones enter the brain and are retained by specific intracellular receptors in neuronal tissue, particularly in the hippocampus[18]. Later it became clear that there are at least two structurally different types of this receptor in the brain to which corticosteroid hormones can bind[4,22]. Local factors, such as steroid-metabolising enzymes, may add to the phenotypical diversity of brain corticosteroid receptors.

Upon activation, the intracellular steroid receptor complexes bind to specific DNA-responsive elements and modulate gene transcription (Fig. 8.2). In neurones, gene-mediated steroid effects include transcriptional control of proteins involved in neuronal

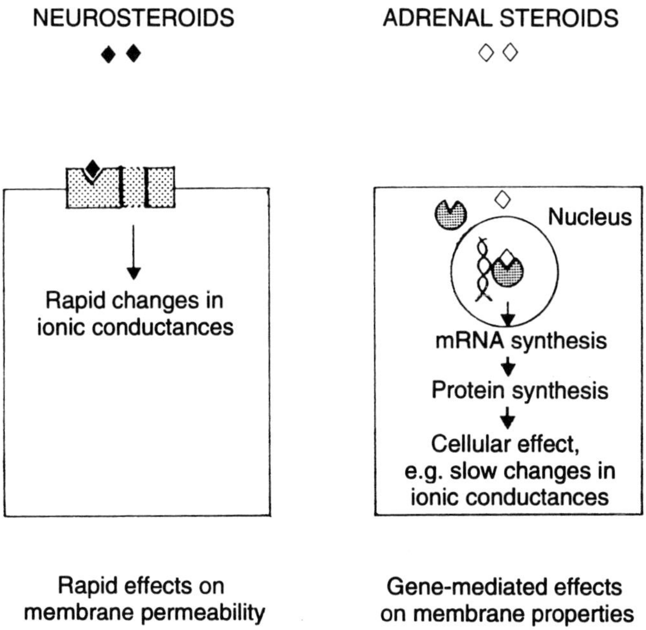

NEUROSTEROIDS              ADRENAL STEROIDS
◆ ◆                        ◇ ◇

Rapid effects on          Gene-mediated effects
membrane permeability     on membrane properties

Fig. 8.2. Adrenal steroids generally bind to intracellular receptors acting as transcription factors on the genome (right). As a result, any effects on membrane properties will be slow. Neurosteroids can induce rapid effects on membrane conductance through direct changes in ligand-gated ionic conductances (left).

structure, as well as in the regulation of cell metabolism and neuronal communication. In turn, the latter includes control of the synthesis of neuropeptide precursors, transmitter-synthesising enzymes, receptors, enzymes for signal transduction and, putatively, proteins regulating the activity of ionic channels. The process of changing gene expression and subsequent intracellular events, such as axonal transport of the gene products, is responsible for the slow onset and long duration of steroid effects on cell metabolism and neuronal communication. The long-lasting nature of these effects would allow the hormones to modulate transmission over a timespan that differs from most other compounds active in the brain.

The corticosteroid hormones described so far are produced in the adrenal gland and, as a result of their lipophilic nature, readily pass the blood–brain barrier. Once within the brain there is a diffuse distribution. However, there is also a class of structurally related steroids that are generated within the brain

and are termed the neurosteroids (Fig. 8.1). Neurosteroids have a reduced A ring (3α-hydroxy-5α-dihydro substituents) and derive either from conversion of precursor adrenal steroids entering the brain or are synthesised locally in glial cells. The neurosteroid-mediated effects that have been documented so far are rather fast in onset but short lasting in contrast with the corticosteroid effects mediated by the 'classical' intracellular receptors described above. It is conceivable, therefore, that neurosteroid effects are mediated by membrane receptors and do not directly involve gene transcription (Fig. 8.2). In the 1990s, extensive evidence has accumulated on neurosteroid modulation of the GABA$_A$ receptor complex. For further reading there are some excellent reviews concerning cellular actions of neurosteroids[1,2,15,16].

The following sections deal with the characteristics of corticosteroid hormone receptors associated with nervous tissue, followed by a review of the cellular actions mediated by these receptors. Next is a discussion of the significance of the cellular steroid actions for the process of neurotransmitter release. Attention is focused on actions mediated by corticosteroid hormones, but there are brief allusions to the effects induced by other steroid hormones when appropriate.

## 2   Neuronal corticosteroid receptors

In the brain, corticosteroid actions appear to be mediated by two distinct intracellular receptors, currently referred to as the mineralocorticoid receptors (MRs or type 1) and the glucocorticoid receptors (GRs or type 2)[22]. The MR and GR genes have been cloned and their primary structure is known[7].

The receptor structure of MR and GR is closely related to that of receptors for thyroid hormone, oestrogens, androgens, progestagens, retinoic acid and to receptors for certain oncogene products. Rat MR and GR contain 981 and 777 amino acid residues, respectively[7]. Proteolytic digestion and mutation analysis have revealed a clearcut domain structure: (i) an N-terminal immunogenic region of about 400 amino acid residues that displays potent transactivational activity and which is highly variable among species; (ii) a highly conserved DNA-binding domain of 70 amino acid residues containing two zinc fingers; (iii) the C-terminal steroid-binding domain. The last region binds also to a 90 kDa heat-shock protein dimer, which is dissociated from the receptor upon steroid binding and allows increased binding affinity of the receptor complex to glucocorticoid-responsive elements.

Rat MR and GR have a 76% sequence homology in the DNA-binding domain, and a 59% homology in the steroid-binding domain (94% and 57%, respectively, for human MR and GR)[7]. There are species differences: between rat and man, for example, the DNA-binding domain is 90% homologous. The similarity between the MR and GR DNA-binding domains has been taken as evidence that both receptors potentially interact with the same, or closely related, hormone-

responsive elements on particular genes[7]. This was actually demonstrated in cultured kidney CV-1 cells in which MR and GR were expressed. It appeared that not only GRs but also MRs were able to activate a typical GR-responsive promotor of the mouse mammary tumour virus. In brain tissue, there is only indirect evidence for an interaction of MRs and GRs at the level of the DNA; these data are reviewed in Section 3.3. The hypothesis is that, within brain, MRs and GRs control gene expression in a co-ordinated manner.

### 2.1   Binding properties of neuronal corticosteroid receptors

MRs and GRs in brain differ in their affinity for natural and synthetic corticosteroids *in vitro*. This conclusion has been derived from radioligand-binding experiments performed with the soluble receptors in cytosol prepared from rat brain regions. The binding assay requires prior adrenalectomy of the animal, since removal of the endogenous corticosteroids makes the receptors in the neuronal cytosol available for exogenously applied radiolabelled corticosteroid ligands. The distinction between MRs and GRs was facilitated when selective glucocorticoid analogues were synthesised. GRs show highest affinity for potent synthetic glucocorticoids such as dexamethasone, RU 26988 and RU 28362, a lower affinity for the naturally occurring corticosterone ($K_d$ approximately 5 nM) and a much lower affinity for aldosterone[22]. By contrast, MR affinity for corticosterone ($K_d$ approximately 0.5 nM) and aldosterone is comparable. MRs show negligible affinity for the RU compounds mentioned above but still show appreciable affinity for dexamethasone.

In the early studies by McEwen[18], tracer doses (0.5 μg) of [³H]-corticosterone and [³H]-aldosterone were administered to adrenalectomised rats. A striking retention of radioactivity was observed in cell nuclei of the hippocampal neurones. The dose of radiolabelled steroid fortuitously happened to be around the $ED_{50}$ for occupancy of hippocam-

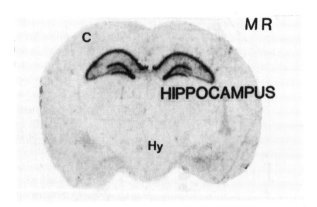

Fig. 8.3. Adrenalectomised rats received an intravenous tracer dose of [³H]-corticosterone *in vivo*, as in the original study by McEwen *et al.*[18]. An autoradiograph of a brain section at the level of the dorsal hippocampus is shown. At the concentration used, the corticosterone has only labelled mineralocorticoid receptors. C, cortex; Hy, hypothalamus. (Courtesy of W. Sutanto.)

pal MRs but was too low for occupancy of the GR ($ED_{50}$ for GRs is 60 μg). It is now accepted that the high retention of the 'glucocorticoid' corticosterone in the hippocampus actually represents binding to MRs and not to GRs; the GRs are only significantly occupied when higher steroid concentrations are used (Fig. 8.3). These observations on the relative binding affinity of MRs and GRs for corticosterone have an important implication. The data suggest that, during the circadian trough when plasma corticosterone levels are below 25 nM and aldosterone levels 1 nM or less, more than 70% of the MRs in the hippocampus would be occupied but only about 10% of the GRs. Variations from basal plasma corticosterone levels up to the peak levels induced by stress or occurring during circadian variation would, thus, affect the degree of MR occupancy (between 70–90%) far less than the degree of GR occupancy (10–90%). The large degree of MR occupancy under physiological conditions has made people wonder about its functional significance. However, as will be pointed out later (Sections 3.2 and 3.3), MR occupation may be an important factor for the maintenance of neuronal excitability in its own right and,

additionally, be a prerequisite for the development of GR-mediated events.

## 2.2 Aldosterone-selective neuronal MRs

In hippocampal neurones, MRs bind aldosterone and corticosterone with comparable affinity. Since the amount of free, circulating corticosterone, even under basal conditions, exceeds the aldosterone concentration by two orders of magnitude, one may doubt whether aldosterone could be an important factor for the control of neuronal function in the hippocampus. While this question needs more investigation, the observation that elsewhere in the brain there are aldosterone-selective actions indicates that at least part of the neuronal MR-containing cell population possesses a mechanism that allows for aldosterone specificity.

Recent work has shown that aldosterone selectivity can be conferred to MRs by the enzyme 11β-hydroxysteroid dehydrogenase (11β-OHSD; see Fig. 8.4). The enzyme converts corticosterone to its 11-oxo metabolite, 11-dehydrocorticosterone, which binds with much lower affinity to MRs or GRs and displays reduced biological activity; the aldo-

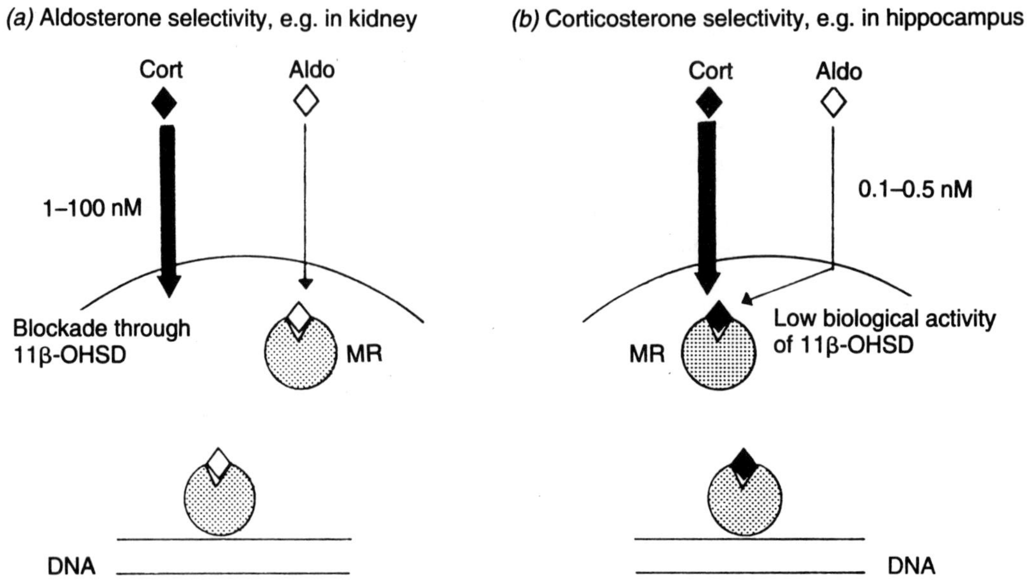

Fig. 8.4. Signal specificity of corticosteroids. The affinity of mineralocorticoid receptors (MR) for corticosterone (Cort) and aldosterone (Aldo) is within the same range (approximately 0.5 nM). Given the excess of circulating corticosterone, mineralocorticoid receptors will be predominantly occupied by corticosterone rather than aldosterone (as in (b), the hippocampus). However, in the presence of the corticosterone converting enzyme 11β-OHSD that produces a corticosterone metabolite with low affinity for mineralocorticoid receptors, these can then be activated by aldosterone. Such an aldosterone-selectivity has been observed, for example, in kidney tissue (a) and in the anterior hypothalamus (see text).

sterone activity is, thus, revealed. In animals pretreated with the licorice component glycyrrhizic acid, which is a blocker of 11β-OHSD, corticosterone is not metabolised and binds to MRs with high affinity thus obscuring the aldosterone effects. The enzyme 11β-OHSD has been found in abundance in the classical aldosterone target tissues, for example the kidneys and parotid glands, which explains the preference of the renal MRs for aldosterone notwithstanding a 100–1000-fold excess of circulating corticosterone.

In the hippocampus, cortex, cerebellum, hypothalamus and the anterior pituitary, the 11β-OHSD gene is transcribed and an immunoreactive form of the enzyme protein is present. Enzyme activity responsible for the conversion of corticosterone can be demonstrated in vitro, but little evidence is presently available for in vivo conversion in brain. However, in the anterior hypothalamus, [3H]-aldosterone is retained in larger quantities than [3H]-corticosterone, suggesting aldosterone selectivity in this area. The anterior hypothalamus is certainly a target for aldosterone in the control of salt appetite and in cardiovascular regulation.

## 2.3 Neuronal MR and GR receptor topography

The topography of MRs and GRs has been studied with in vivo and in vitro autoradiography of radiolabelled brain sections from adrenalectomised rats (Fig. 8.3). More recently, immunocytochemistry and in situ hybridisation procedures have been used, which can be applied to tissue sections from adrenally intact animals. From such studies, the distribution of GRs has been found to be widespread in neurones and glial cells throughout the brain. High GR concentrations are found in the limbic system (hippocampus, septum) and in the parvocellular neurones of the hypothalamic paraventricular nucleus, where glucocorticoids suppress the synthesis of CRH and vasopressin. GRs are also present in relatively high concentrations in the ascending monoaminergic neurones of the brain stem. Peptides from the tachykinin (neuropeptide Y) and opioid (pro-opiomelanocortin, enkephalin and dynorphin) families are found in these same neurones and are also under glucocorticoid control. Moderate GR levels are found in many thalamic nuclei, in a patch-like distribution in the striatum and in the central amygdaloid nucleus, as well as in the cortex. The distibution pattern of GR mRNA, as detected by *in situ* hybridisation, is the same as that of the GR protein and of the labelled GR sites.

In the brain MR mRNA has a more restricted topography than GR mRNA. Consistent with expectations based on MR mRNA distribution, radioligand-binding studies show high MR densities in the neurones of the hippocampal formation, lateral septum, medial and central amygdala, olfactory nucleus, layer II of the cerebral cortex and in brain stem sensory and motor neurones. The strongest nuclear labelling in hippocampal neurones occurs in area CA2 and in the dorsomedial subiculum, followed by area CA1, then CA3 and CA4. The dentate gyrus contains scattered, strongly labelled cells among cells with intermediate nuclear labelling. While in most limbic regions, [$^3$H]-aldosterone and [$^3$H]-corticosterone are retained equally well, preferential labelling by [$^3$H]-aldosterone has been observed in the induseum griseum, the anterior hypothalamus, in circumventricular areas, such as the chorioid plexus, and brain stem regions.

In most of the hippocampal neurones, GRs and MRs are co-localised and both bind corticosterone, though with differing affinities. The radioligand-binding data imply that low levels of circulating free corticosterone (below 2.5 nM) extensively occupy MRs in the hippocampus. At the circadian peak and during stress, corticosterone progressively occupies GRs. In view of the structural similarity between MRs and GRs, these receptors, if co-localised, may interact with the same gene networks.

In addition to these 'classical' intracellular steroid receptors that act through gene transcription, membrane receptors for steroids have been found in brain tissue of amphibians[20]. The existence of such receptors in rat brain is likely, but has not been demonstrated yet. These membrane receptors, which probably are not directly linked to the genome, could mediate the fast actions of steroids which are described below.

## 3 Cellular actions of steroid hormones in the brain

There are now many indications that corticosteroid hormones interfere with transmitter receptor-mediated events, both at the level of agonist binding, G-proteins, second messengers and evoked changes in ion permeability of the membrane. In some cases (in systems where excitatory amino acids are the transmitters) the steroid actions are comparatively fast but not very prominent; even faster actions are seen with neurosteroids, for example on GABA$_A$-mediated responses. In other cases, there is a slow and long-lasting corticosteroid-mediated modulation of transmitter-evoked responses. The relative MR/GR occupation seems to be of great importance for the nature of the steroid-mediated effects. When there is a predominant occupation of MRs, i.e. during the trough of the circadian cycle, the excitability is enhanced or maintained at a certain level. When GRs are also activated, i.e. at the peak of the circadian cycle and after stress, excitability is, in general, suppressed. Hence, neuronal activity is under continuous modulation by corticosteroid hormones, a modulation that may vary during the day depending on endogenous steroid levels and the ensuing relative MR/GR occupation[13].

## 3.1 Fast, transient actions

Consistent with the general mechanism of action described above, adrenal corticosteroids have usually been found to act only after a considerable time delay, although in some cases fast actions of adrenal steroids have been described. Likewise, the group of brain-generated neurosteroids has been found to exert predominantly fast actions on neuronal activity (for reviews see refs. 1, 2, 15 and 16). The fast and transient cellular actions of neurosteroids and adrenal corticosteroid hormones are summarised below.

### 3.1.1 Fast actions on cell excitability

Early studies, in which steroids were applied *in vivo* by iontophoresis and individual neuronal activity was recorded extracellularly, gave rise to reports of several, in some cases contrasting, steroid actions. Both excitatory and inhibitory effects were observed, and in some studies no effects at all. Nevertheless the steroid-mediated changes in neuronal firing frequency had one certain characteristic: iontophoretic application of the steroids immediately affected the cellular firing rate. The underlying membrane process cannot be elucidated from these extracellular studies. Recent intracellular investigations *in vitro* revealed that relatively high levels of corticosterone can transiently hyperpolarise central neurones, which may explain the inhibitory effects observed *in vivo*. The reduction in membrane resistance that was linked to the hyperpolarisation may point to steroid-dependent increases in $K^+$ conductances, although specific types of $K^+$ channel have not been investigated in this regard. The rapid onset of the responses points to an effect mediated by a membrane receptor for steroids rather than by a classical intracellular steroid receptor acting on gene transcription.

Calcium currents are also subject to rapid steroid-mediated changes[8]. In acutely dissociated hippocampal cells, the neurosteroids allotetrahydro(deoxy)-corticosterone, dehy-droepiandrosterone and pregnenalone all rapidly, and reversibly, decreased high-threshold voltage-sensitive $Ca^{2+}$ currents. Both L- and N-type $Ca^{2+}$ currents are affected by the neurosteroids. However, the nature of the receptors through which these rapid effects are mediated is not known at present.

### 3.1.2 Fast actions on neurotransmitter systems

In addition to the actions of steroids on cell firing and membrane conductances, rapid interactions with various transmitter systems have also been reported. $GABA_A$ receptor-mediated responses have been well studied in this respect[15]. It appeared that GABA or benzodiazepine binding to brain cell membranes was enhanced by steroids with reduced A-rings (Fig. 8.1), i.e. pregnanes. Functionally, the pregnanes also affected the $GABA_A$ receptor complex: low doses of tetrahydroprogesterone, tetrahydrodeoxycorticosterone or androsterone increase the GABA-mediated $Cl^-$ current in central neurones, behaving as allosteric agonists in the same way as barbiturates. At higher doses, the steroids can open the $Cl^-$ channel of the $GABA_A$ receptor even in the absence of GABA itself. Inhibitory postsynaptic potentials, mediated by $GABA_A$ receptors, are increased in duration by these 5α-reduced steroids. Direct effects on glutamate-induced excitatory postsynaptic potentials were not observed, although it can be inferred that the excitatory responses will be diminished, secondary to the increase in inhibitory potentials. Non-competitive antagonistic actions by neurosteroids on the $GABA_A$ receptor complex have also been described, in particular by pregnenolone sulphate and dehydroepiandrosterone sulphate.

The interactions between (neuro)steroids and the $GABA_A$ receptor complex all take place at the postsynaptic membrane. Comparatively little is known about fast, transient actions of (neuro)steroids on presynaptic processes, such as transmitter uptake and release. Nevertheless, the release of at least two transmitters, acetylcholine and

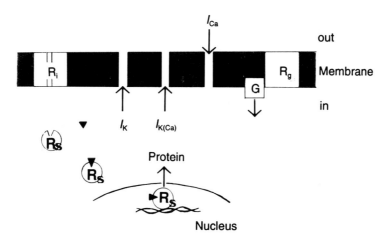

Fig. 8.5. Corticosteroid hormones (▼), bound to intracellular steroid receptors (Rs), act as transcription factors for the genome, inducing alterations in cellular protein synthesis. If, as a result of altered protein synthesis, channel proteins are modified, intrinsic membrane conductances, such as voltage-dependent $K^+$ and $Ca^{2+}$ conductances ($I_K$ and $I_{Ca}$, respectively) or $Ca^{2+}$-dependent $K^+$ conductances ($I_{K(Ca)}$) could be changed. In addition, the steroid-induced effects on protein synthesis could have consequences for the structure and function of the ionotropic ($R_i$) or G-protein-coupled transmitter receptors ($R_g$) in the membrane.

dopamine, is modulated by corticosteroids[9,10,11]. For example, imposed stress or administration of glucocorticoids was found to enhance the release of acetylcholine and dopamine from the hippocampus, as established by the microdialysis technique *in vivo* (see Chapter 12). The increase is apparent within 10 min and reversed within 1 h. *In vitro* too, glucocorticoid administration or imposed stress immediately prior to the preparation of the tissue induced an increase in dopamine and acetylcholine release in limbic areas, while dopamine uptake was diminished. Other studies of steroid actions on transmitter release, particularly with respect to peptide transmitters, have focused on the 'classical' neuroendocrine pathways[5,6]. Thus, stimulus-induced CRH release from hypothalamic synaptosomes is reduced by corticosterone or cortisol pretreatment *in vivo*. Furthermore, in hypothalamic synaptosomes or slices, it was demonstrated that luteinising hormone releasing hormone (LHRH) release is enhanced by progesterone if animals had been primed *in vivo* with oestradiol. While these observations are of relevance for the

endocrine regulatory pathways involved in stress and reproduction, it remains unclear at present whether or not similar steroid effects on peptide release also occur in higher brain areas and, most importantly, what the functional relevance of such interactions could be.

### 3.2 Long-lasting effects on intrinsic membrane properties

The intracellular steroid receptors are known to act as gene transcription factors. Altered gene transcription results in modulation of protein synthesis, which has indeed been shown for central neurones after steroid treatment or stress. The steroid actions mediated by these intracellular receptors are slow ($> 15$ min) in onset and long lasting ($> 1$ h).

Relatively little is known about the nature of the proteins the synthesis of which is affected by steroid hormones. It is conceivable that they could determine membrane properties and thence ionic conductances (see Fig. 8.5). In addition, neurotransmitter-related events, such as synthesis of transmitters, their release and their subsequent receptor-mediated actions, or very general cell properties, like energy processes, could be affected. The evidence for such actions is reviewed briefly below.

In the early 1970s, Pfaff and co-workers[21] found that injection of corticosterone into hypophysectomised rats reduced the extracellular hippocampal single unit activity, with a delay of approximately 30 min. Recent studies *in vitro* have provided insight into which processes may underlie the delayed inhibitory corticosteroid action. These studies were, in most cases, performed in hippocampal slices (prepared from brains taken from adrenalectomised rats) to which selective MR and/or GR ligands were added for 20 min *in vitro*. Whenever possible, neuronal properties were followed in the same neurone before, during, and up to 1 h after the brief steroid application. To study steroid-mediated actions over a more prolonged period of time, another experimental protocol was used in which neurones before steroid application were compared with neurones recorded between 30 min and several hours after termination of the steroid treatment. The general features studied were: (i) the resting membrane potential; (ii) the membrane resistance; (iii) spontaneous electrical activity; and (iv) the accommodation and after-hyperpolarisation (AHP) associated with short depolarisations of the cell. Accommodation describes the phenomenon whereby hippocampal cells, upon depolarisation, do not fire continuously but instead gradually slow down their rate of firing. This characteristic is linked to the activation of a slow $Ca^{2+}$-dependent $K^+$ conductance; at the end of the depolarising input the membrane is briefly hyperpolarised (AHP). The accommodation and AHP may serve to attenuate the transmission of a steady excitatory input in a neuronal circuit.

It appears that activation of MRs does not affect resting membrane potential, input resistance or spontaneous electrical activity of CA1 pyramidal neurones *in vitro,* but brings the accommodation and AHP to a very low setpoint, with a delay between 30 and 60 min[12]. Concurrent occupation of a small fraction of the GRs gradually elevates this level of accommodation and AHP amplitude, approximately to the value observed in the absence of steroid-receptor occupation. Yet, if GRs are fully activated (both in the absence and presence of concurrent MR activation), the accommodation is strong and the AHP amplitude large, suggesting that GR activation in time increases the $Ca^{2+}$-dependent $K^+$ conductance underlying these two phenomena. Functionally, these MR- and GR-mediated events may alter the local excitability: while predominant MR activation maintains or even enhances the excitability in the circuit, additional GR activation results in suppression of neuronal activity.

The GR-dependent increase of the AHP amplitude depends on protein synthesis, supporting a role for the 'classical' intracellular receptor acting on the genome. In this context, there are several pathways by which the steroid-dependent changes in the $Ca^{2+}$-dependent $K^+$ conductance may have been accomplished. Two obvious possibilities are that: (i) the properties of the $K^+$ conductance itself are affected by the steroids or (ii) the intracellular $Ca^{2+}$ levels during short depolarisation of the cell are changed after steroid treatment.

While these two possibilities need to be investigated in detail, some information is already available. For example, it has been shown that corticosteroids can indeed change specific $K^+$ conductances. Recently, it has been observed that the properties of an inwardly rectifying $K^+$ conductance are under control of corticosteroids, while two other $K^+$ conductances (the transient outward current $I_A$ and the delayed rectifier) are not affected by activation of steroid receptors. With respect to $Ca^{2+,}$ it has been shown that relatively high doses of corticosterone, or of selective GR agonists, increase sustained $Ca^{2+}$ currents in CA1 pyramidal cells[14]. The $Ca^{2+}$ current change was sensitive to protein-synthesis inhibitors. In addition, prolonged exposure of hippocampal cultures to high doses of glucocorticoids resulted in a considerable accumulation of $Ca^{2+}$ in the hippocampal neurones.

In summary, it may be concluded that corticosteroid hormones can induce slow- and long-lasting actions on $K^+$ and $Ca^{2+}$ conductances in neurones.

### 3.3  Long-lasting effects on neurotransmitter systems

In addition to the effects on intrinsic properties of neuronal membranes, such as alteration of ionic conductances, transmitter-coupled processes also seem to be subject to modulation by steroids.

There are many indications that enzymes involved in the synthesis or turnover of noradrenaline, dopamine and, particularly, 5-HT are modulated by corticosteroid hormones. For example, tryptophan hydroxylase activity and, therefore, 5-HT formation during stress is enhanced by a permissive GR-mediated action of glucocorticoids. Adrenalectomy reduces the rate of 5-HT biosynthesis, both in the raphe nuclei and the hippocampal target area. This reduction can be restored within 1 h by corticosterone but not by aldosterone.

#### 3.3.1  Long-lasting effects on transmitter release

Indications of long-lasting and persistent steroid-mediated effects on neurotransmitter release are limited. The actions of glucocorticoids on acetylcholine and dopamine release that have been described are generally fast and short-lasting[9,10,11]. However, there are some indications for delayed, genomic effects. Thus, decrease in choline uptake and increase in the acetylcholine release (from a hippocampal synaptosomal preparation) persisted for several days after chronic stress (prior to the *in vitro* study), although they had returned to normal after 1 week. Also, 2 days after adrenalectomy, acetylcholine release from the hippocampus *in vitro* was increased when compared with the control

animals, and the effects of adrenalectomy were reversed by administration of corticosterone.

Although direct steroid effects on transmitter release have not been studied in detail, it is clear that all the steroid-mediated actions on intrinsic membrane properties and interactions with transmitter systems described above and below have sequellae for neurotransmitter release: if the excitability and, therefore, the firing pattern of a neurone is affected by a steroid and the synthesis of transmitter altered, then the ensuing transmitter release at the terminals of the neurone will also be changed. This issue is further discussed in Section 8.4.

#### 3.3.2  Long-lasting effects on signal transduction

There is an increasing amount of information available regarding steroid effects on transduction processes taking place between binding of a ligand to a transmitter receptor and the ion permeability of the membrane. Ligand-binding studies show that changes in circulating corticosteroid levels have little effect on the binding properties of excitatory amino acid receptors, although acute stress (tail shocks) was found to alter significantly ligand binding to AMPA sites. Extracellular action potentials recorded from a population of CA1 hippocampal cells in response to synaptic input carried by excitatory amino acids (the population spike) also revealed relatively small effects of corticosteroid hormones. In general, low concentrations of corticosterone (i.e. a predominant MR occupation) enhanced the amplitude of the population spike while high corticosterone concentrations (MR plus GR occupation) depressed the synaptic response. The GR-mediated effect was amplified when the extracellular $Ca^{2+}$ concentration was raised[23]. In contrast to the effects on the population spike, the extracellularly recorded EPSPs or degree of paired-pulse facilitation, which is a measure of presynaptic processes, were not affected by the steroids. The lack of steroid-mediated actions on the EPSP suggests that the decrease of the population spike amplitude was not caused by a decline in the excitatory amino acid release. This was corroborated by a recent intracellular study showing that activation of GRs decreases the success rate of synaptically induced action potentials, while the effect on the EPSP is relatively small. A similar failure to transmit synaptically evoked action potentials was observed in the absence of corticosteroid hormones (brain slices from adrenalectomised rats) but not when MRs only were activated. The steroid actions on excitatory amino acid-mediated transmission started within 10 min, persisted for 1 h but were no longer apparent after several hours. The time scale of these actions was clearly slower than that observed, for example, with the neurosteroid modulation of $GABA_A$ receptor-mediated responses, but was rather rapid for a gene-mediated process. In fact, in none of the studies was involvement of gene transcription or protein synthesis established. All in all, the steroid effects on excitatory amino acid-mediated transmission seem to be modest, as reflected by the minor changes in the EPSP amplitude. However, these effects may become amplified when the membrane potential is around the threshold for induction of action potentials.

Slow actions of steroids on GABA-mediated transmission are not well documented. One report shows that high corticosterone levels can depress the $GABA_A$ receptor-mediated fast IPSP. However, corticosterone levels within the physiological range did not affect the fast IPSP amplitude, whereas the amplitude of the $GABA_B$ receptor-mediated slow IPSP was reduced by moderate levels of corticosterone. The fact that the fast IPSP and slow IPSP were differentially affected by corticosteroid treatment suggests that post-synaptic GABA responsiveness, particularly the $GABA_B$ receptor-mediated responses, rather than presynaptic GABA release is altered by corticosteroids. However, responses to the exogenously applied $GABA_B$ agonist baclofen in slices from adrenalectomised rats were the same as in sham-operated controls regardless of whether MR were activated.

### 3.3.3 Long-lasting interactions with noradrenaline

Steroid-mediated interactions with monoamines are much more striking. Receptor sites for noradrenaline and also the noradrenaline-coupled formation of cAMP are modulated by corticosteroid hormones. In general, adrenalectomy enhances these parameters, while treatment with glucocorticoid hormones suppresses the noradrenaline-induced activity.

Glucocorticoids appear to affect the G-proteins coupled to adrenergic receptors. Thus, chronic application of corticosterone to adrenalectomised rats enhanced the amount of $G_{s\alpha}$ mRNA and ADP ribosylation in the cerebral cortex while there was a decrease in the amount of $G_{i\alpha}$ mRNA. Perhaps it is as a result of the steroid actions on adrenoceptor-binding properties, G-protein activity and cAMP formation that noradrenaline-induced changes in membrane conductance are affected by glucocorticoid hormones. Noradrenaline depresses the accommodation and AHP amplitude of pyramidal CA1 neurones via a $\beta_1$-adrenoceptor-mediated and cAMP-dependent process. It appeared that noradrenaline-induced responses were large in slices from adrenalectomised rats compared with slices either from sham-operated controls or from adrenalectomised rats treated with corticosterone or a selective glucocorticoid. These effects on noradrenaline actions were quite robust, slow in onset and long lasting.

Effects of corticosteroids on the central adrenergic system are not very well documented. In the adrenal medulla, however, glucocorticoids are required for maintenance of the activity of phenylethanolamine N-methyltransferase (PNMT), the rate-limiting enzyme for adrenaline formation from noradrenaline. This action involves a GR-mediated influence on S-adenosylmethionine, which serves as a methyl donor.

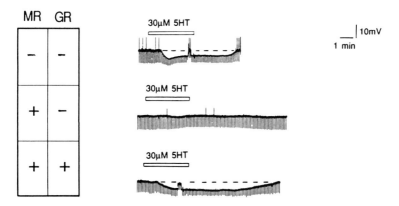

Fig. 8.6. Hyperpolarisation mediated by 5-HT in tissues from adrenalectomised rats. (*a*) A CA1 pyramidal neurone in a slice from an adrenalectomised rat responded to 30 μM 5-HT with a reversible hyperpolarisation of the membrane. The hyperpolarisation was accompanied by a decrease of the cell resistance, as inferred from the diminished down-going voltage deflections (vertical spikes) in response to constant current pulses. (*b*) Several hours after a brief application of 3 nM aldosterone (which would occupy the mineralocorticoid receptors, MR, mainly), the response to 5-HT was markedly reduced. (*c*) When aldosterone was added in the presence of the glucocorticoid receptor (GR) agonist RU 28362, normal 5-HT responses were observed. Therefore, 5-HT responsiveness is specifically decreased by MR occupation only. The putative MR and GR occupation for each of the test situations is indicated at the left.

### 3.3.4  Long-lasting interactions with 5-HT

The density of 5-HT$_1$ receptors in the CA1 hippocampal area is significantly increased after adrenalectomy. Steroid replacement with the mixed MR and GR agonist corticosterone reverses this increase. By contrast, the MR agonist aldosterone is ineffective, while pure glucocorticoids even increase the number of 5-HT$_1$-binding sites. The response mediated by 5-HT$_{1a}$ sites, i.e. a hyperpolarisation of the cell membrane, was found to be similar for adrenalectomised and sham-operated rats. However, in tissue from adrenalectomised rats where only MRs were activated, 5-HT$_{1a}$-mediated hyperpolarisations were (with a delay of approximately 2 h) significantly and persistently decreased (Fig. 8.6). This suppression of 5-HT responses mediated by MRs depends on protein synthesis. If in addition to MRs, GRs are also activated, 5-HT responses were no longer depressed, indicating that there may exist a functional antagonism of MR- and GR-mediated effects on 5-HT responses. At present it is not clear at which step or process between 5-HT binding and membrane hyperpolarisation steroid hormones may interfere.

## 4  Cellular steroid actions: implications for modulation of neurotransmitter release

As may be clear from the account above, direct steroid hormone-mediated actions on neurotransmitter release *per se* are not well documented; in fact, detailed studies on this subject are rather scarce. Nevertheless, the cellular steroid actions described certainly affect transmitter-related processes indirectly. This is evident for the steroid-mediated actions on intrinsic membrane properties. First, when steroids increase or decrease cellular excitability, the net electrical signal that reaches the terminals of the cell will be affected and subsequent transmitter release will change. Second, although steroid-dependent changes in Ca$^{2+}$ conductance have only been established in the cell soma (because of

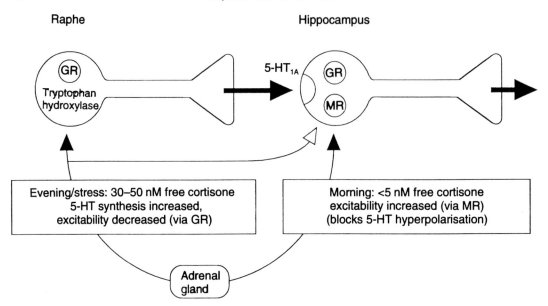

Fig. 8.7. Schematic representation of the control exerted by corticosterone on the 5-HT system in the brain. As illustrated in Fig. 8.6, low levels of corticosterone, resulting in predominant occupation of MRs, depress 5-HT$_{1A}$ receptor-mediated hyperpolarisation in hippocampal CA1 neurones, which may result in enhanced excitability. A rise in the plasma corticosterone level, activating GRs in addition to MRs, reverses the MR-mediated depression of 5-HT$_{1A}$-induced hyperpolarisation in the hippocampus (open arrow) thereby decreasing local excitability. These antagonistic actions on excitability via MR and GR are also observed for other parameters in hippocampal cells, such as after-hyperpolarisation and accommodation. Occupation of GRs not only affects the 5-HT system in the hippocampus but also interferes at the level of the raphe nucleus: 5-HT formation during stress is facilitated by a GR-mediated action (filled arrow). As a result of these interactions between corticosteroid hormones and the 5-HT system, transmitter release from hippocampal afferents and efferents may be altered. Thus, low plasma corticosterone levels (MR occupation) may enhance transmitter release from CA1 hippocampal neurones, while GR-mediated events occurring with higher steroid levels could have a dual effect on release: (i) an enhanced 5-HT release from the raphe fibres (caused by facilitated synthesis) and (ii) decreased transmitter release from hippocampal efferents (caused by depression of local excitability).

technical limitations), they may very well also occur in the synaptic terminal. Clearly, steroid-mediated effects on Ca$^{2+}$ influx in the terminal region would alter transmitter release profoundly.

Interactions between steroid hormones and other aspects of the neurotransmitter economy will also have, indirectly, consequences for transmitter release: first, steroid-mediated changes in neurotransmitter biosynthesis, as described for 5-HT for example, may be reflected later in altered transmitter release, although this link has never actually been established for this particular situation. Second, steroid-induced changes in

neurotransmitter receptor density may not hold only for the postsynaptic site of the membrane, but may also occur for presynaptic transmitter receptors, which would be reflected by changes in release of that particular transmitter and maybe also of other (co-)transmitters released from the same terminal.

The relevance of steroid-mediated (inter)actions in the brain for neurotransmitter release can be illustrated by a well-documented example of steroid activity: the effects exerted by corticosteroid hormones on the 5-HT transmitter system (Fig. 8.7). In the raphe nuclei, 5-HT formation during stress is facilitated by a permissive GR-mediated action of glucocorticoid hormones. The catalytic efficiency rather than the amount of tryptophan hydroxylase, the rate-limiting enzyme in 5-HT biosynthesis, is enhanced by the steroids. The increased availability of 5-HT may result in an increased 5-HT release in the hippocampus, one of the target areas for the 5-HT projection from the raphe nuclei. Neuronal excitability is inhibited by 5-HT, as the result of a $5\text{-HT}_{1A}$-mediated action. Occupation of MRs only reduces this effect of 5-HT, potentially enhancing the electrical activity of the CA1 neurones. However, during situations in which there are higher circulating corticosterone levels, resulting in not only MR but also GR occupation, the decreased 5-HT responsiveness is normalised, thus reducing the cellular excitability again. These MR- and GR-mediated actions on 5-HT responsiveness might be accompanied by other interactive corticosteroid actions, all leading to enhanced excitability during exclusive MR activation and subsequent depression of induced activity when GRs are additionally occupied. If the MR-dependent increase in cellular excitability is accompanied by an increased generation of action potentials in the soma of the CA1 cell, we can expect that the transmitter release in the terminals of the CA1 cells will be increased. The reverse would hold for GR activation. These events would change the transmitter release both in the CA1 hippocampal area and in its projection areas.

## 5  Summary

The characteristics of corticosteroid actions in the brain and their potential significance for the control of neurotransmitter release have been described. Corticosteroid hormones affect the cellular properties of neurones in a way that is, in many respects, quite different from the mechanism of action of neurotransmitters and peptides. First, the distribution pathway for corticosteroids is not confined to an axonal projection, via which

neurotransmitters are transported from their site of synthesis to the site of action. Instead, the steroids are transported as hormones. After synthesis in an endocrine gland, they are released into the circulation and widely distributed, exerting their activity at all sites where they can bind to a steroid receptor. Second, the adrenocortical hormones act as transcription factors for the genome. Consequently, their actions within the cell may be diverse and, most importantly, slow in onset and long lasting. The slow and persisting steroid-induced events provide a unique mechanism by which adaptive processes can occur in the brain, complementary to the fast and transient processes initiated by neurotransmitters and also by the recently described neurosteroids. Finally, adrenocortical steroids induce conditional effects through a co-ordinated, often antagonistic, MR- and GR-mediated control of neuronal excitability. The fact that MRs and GRs bind corticosterone with differing affinities and that consequently the relative MR/GR occupation varies throughout the day, or after stress, means that the net effect of corticosterone on neuronal excitability strongly depends on the endogenous level of free corticosterone.

Investigations of steroid actions on neurotransmitter release have been quite limited. Although there are indications that the release of biogenic amines in particular is altered by stress or manipulations of the hypothalamo–pituitary–adrenal axis, there is still a need for detailed *in vivo* studies, with selective steroid-receptor activation. However, the cellular actions of steroids that have been described so far clearly include alterations of transmitter release, albeit indirectly. First, presynaptic actions of steroids on neurotransmitter biosynthesis and turnover, perhaps also on the density of transmitter autoreceptors or $Ca^{2+}$ influx, will certainly modulate the release of transmitters. But, second, astrocytes and oligodendrocytes have been shown to contain GRs. Although the glial GRs are involved primarily in energy metabolism by enhancing the synthesis of enzymes that are active in the breakdown of glucose to pyruvate, glial cells are also important sites for uptake and storage of neurotransmitters. It is possible that the GRs in glial cells may, therefore, modulate the availability of transmitters for release. Finally, postsynaptic MR- and GR-dependent control of cellular excitability may result in an alteration of neuronal firing patterns, eventually leading to changes of transmitter release at the synaptic terminals. All of these steroid-induced cellular actions potentially can result in a continuing, persistent modulation of neurotransmitter release, complementary to the faster and usually more transient modulatory actions exerted by transmitters, peptides and neurosteroids.

## References

1. Chadwick D and Widdows K (eds) (1990) Steroids and neuronal activity. *Ciba Foundation Symposium 153*. John Wiley, England
2. Costa E and Paul SM (eds) (1991) Neurosteroids and brain function. *Fidia Research Foundation Symposium Series 8*. Thieme Medical, New York
3. Dallman MF, Akana SF, Scribner KA *et al.* (1992) Mortyn Jones Memorial Lecture. Stress, feedback and facilitation in the hypothalamo–pituitary–adrenal axis. *Journal of Neuroendocrinology* **4**: 517–526
4. de Kloet ER (1991) Brain corticosteroid receptor balance and homeostatic control. *Frontiers in Neuroendocrinology* **12**: 95–164
5. Drouva SV, Laplante E and Kordon C (1983) Effects of ovarian steroids on *in vitro* release of LHRH from mediobasal hypothalamus. *Neuroendocrinology* **37**: 336–341
6. Edwardson JA and Bennett GW (1974) Modulation of corticotrophin-releasing factor release from hypothalamic synaptosomes. *Nature* **251**: 425–427
7. Evans RM (1989) A molecular framework for the actions of glucocorticoid hormones in the nervous system. *Neuron* **2**: 1105–1112
8. ffrench-Mullen JHM and Spence K (1991) Neurosteroids block $Ca^{2+}$ channel current in freshly isolated hippocampal CA1 neurons. *European Journal of Pharmacology* **202**: 269–272
9. Gilad GM, Mahon BD, Finkelstein Y, Koffler B and Gilad VH (1985) Stress-induced activation of the hippocampal cholinergic system and the pituitary–adrenocortical axis. *Brain Research* **347**: 404–408
10. Gilad GM, Rabey JM and Gilad VH (1987) Presynaptic effects of glucocorticoids on dopaminergic and cholinergic synaptosomes. Implications for rapid endocrine–neural interactions in stress. *Life Science* **40**: 2401–2408
11. Imperato A, Puglisi-Allegra S, Casolini P, Zocchi A and Angelucci L (1989) Stress-induced enhancement of dopamine and acetylcholine release in limbic structures: role of corticosterone. *European Journal of Pharmacology* **165**: 337–338
12. Joëls M and de Kloet ER (1989) Effects of glucocorticoids and norepinephrine on the excitability in the hippocampus. *Science* **245**: 1502–1505
13. Joëls M and de Kloet ER (1992) Control of neuronal excitability by corticosteroid hormones. *Trends in Neuroscience* **15**: 25–30
14. Kerr DS, Campbell LW, Thibault O and Landfield PW (1992) Hippocampal glucocorticoid receptor activation enhances voltage-dependent $Ca^{2+}$ conductances: relevance to brain aging. *Proceedings of the National Academy of Sciences USA* **89**: 8527–8531
15. Majewska MD, Harrison NL, Schwartz RD, Barker JL and Paul SM (1986) Steroid hormone metabolites are barbiturate-like modulators of the GABA receptors. *Science* **232**: 1004–1007
16. McEwen BS (1991) Non-genomic and genomic effects of steroids on neural activity. *Trends in Pharmacological Sciences* **12**: 141–147
17. McEwen BS, de Kloet ER and Rostene W (1986) Adrenal steroid receptors and actions in the nervous system. *Physiological Reviews* **66**: 1121–1188
18. McEwen BS, Weiss JM and Schwartz LS (1968) Selective retention of corticosterone by limbic structures in rat brain. *Nature* **220**: 911–912
19. Munck A, Guyre PM and Holbrook NJ (1984) Physiological functions of glucocorticoids in stress and their relation to pharmacological actions. *Endocrinology Reviews* **5**: 25–44
20. Orchinik M, Murray TF and Moore FL (1991) A corticosteroid receptor in neuronal membranes. *Science* **252**: 1848–1851

21. Pfaff DW, Silva MTA and Weiss JM (1971) Telemetered recording of hormone effects on hippocampal neurons. *Science* **171:** 394–395

22. Reul JMHM and de Kloet ER (1985) Two receptor systems for corticosterone in rat brain: microdistribution and differential occupation. *Endocrinology* **117:** 2505–2512

23. Talmi M, Carlier E, Rey M and Soumireu-Mourat B (1992) Modulation of the *in vitro* electrophysiological effect of corticosterone by extracellular calcium in the hippocampus. *Neuroendocrinology* **55:** 257–263

24. Tausk M (1951) *Das Hormon 3.* Hat die Nebenniere tatsachlich eine Verteidigungsfunction? Organon, The Netherlands

# 3 Modulation of neurotransmitter release: cellular mechanisms

# 9 Second messenger pathways in the modulation of neurotransmitter release

Henryk Majewski and Michelle Barrington

Thus far the phenomenon of modulation of neurotransmitter release has been described as has some of the range of neurotransmitters, hormones and locally derived factors that can exert a modulatory influence. How is their effect achieved? By what mechanisms are the extracellular stimuli which impinge on cell-surface receptors transduced to an intracellular signal that increases or decreases the amount of neurotransmitter released by an effective action potential that invades the release site? The general view presumes that the amount of neurotransmitter ultimately released depends on the presence of free $Ca^{2+}$ in the immediate vicinity of the exocytotic machinery and suggests that modulation of release occurs by regulating either the availability of free $Ca^{2+}$ or the sensitivity of the release mechanisms to $Ca^{2+}$. In this chapter, Henryk Majewski and Michelle Barrington consider some models for modulation of release that involve intracellular chemical messenger molecules. The pathways they describe are based on a sequence that may be summarised as follows. The extracellular modulator combines with a neuronal cell-surface receptor and the association triggers, via enzymatically catalysed reactions, an increased or decreased production of intracellular second messenger molecules that, in turn, and by a variety of possible mechanisms, either regulate the availability of free $Ca^{2+}$ at the site of neurotransmitter release or alter the sensitivity of the release machinery for $Ca^{2+}$.

## 1    Introduction

The activation of membrane receptors is a common mechanism through which cellular functions, including neurotransmitter release, can be modulated. There are three principal mechanisms to connect receptors to changes in intracellular events. The first involves the activation of GTP-binding proteins (G-proteins) to alter either the conductance of ion channels or the activity of enzymes which form intracellular molecules (second messengers). This is the 'G-protein linked' superfamily of receptors (see Table 9.1). The second is where the receptor complex itself forms an ion channel that can open on activation. This is the 'ligand-gated ion-channel' superfamily of receptors (see Table 9.1). The third mechanism is where the receptor complex has intrinsic enzyme activity and can directly influence cellular proteins. These are the tyrosine kinase-associated receptors, which include receptors for insulin and other growth factors. The tyrosine kinase-associated receptors and the ligand-gated ion-channel receptors will not be considered here (but see Chapter 10 for the latter). For many receptors there are multiple signalling pathways possible (see Table 9.1). However, even the signalling pathways mentioned may

Table 9.1. *Possible signal transduction pathways for G-protein-linked receptors*

| Receptor | | Second messenger link | Ion channel link |
|---|---|---|---|
| Adenosine | $A_1$ | cAMP ↓ | $K^+$ ↑  $Ca^{2+}$ ↓ |
| Adrenoceptors | $\alpha_1$ | $IP_3$/DAG ↑ | $Ca^{2+}$ ↑ |
| | $\alpha_2$ | cAMP ↓ | $K^+$ ↑  $Ca^{2+}$ ↓ |
| | $\beta$ | cAMP ↑ | $Ca^{2+}$ ↑ |
| Angiotensin | | $IP_3$/DAG ↑ | $Ca^{2+}$ ↑ |
| | | cAMP ↓ | |
| Dopamine | $D_1$ | cAMP ↑ | |
| | $D_2$ | cAMP ↓ | $K^+$ ↑  $Ca^{2+}$ ↓ |
| Muscarinic | $M_1$ | $IP_3$/DAG ↑ | |
| | $M_2$ | cAMP ↓ | $K^+$ ↑ |
| | $M_3$ | $IP_3$/DAG ↑ | |
| Neuropeptide Y | | cAMP ↓ | $Ca^{2+}$ ↑ |

Receptor activation of G-proteins can either (i) increase or decrease adenylyl cyclase activity, thereby altering cAMP production; or (ii) alter the activity of phospholipase C, thereby altering $IP_3$ production and, through the mediation of diacylglycerol (DAG), alter protein kinase C activity. The receptors may also be linked through G-proteins to ion channels and can affect both $Ca^{2+}$ entry and $K^+$ efflux from cells. ↑ indicates activation of pathway and ↓ indicates inhibition of pathway.

not encompass all possibilities. Therefore, extrapolation of the signal transduction linkages of a particular receptor from one system to another may sometimes be inappropriate.

This chapter focuses on the receptors that require G-proteins to connect receptor activation with changes to the enzymes that form the second messenger molecules. Examples of these G-protein-linked receptors are shown in Table 9.1 and include receptors for hormones, neurotransmitters and autacoids (see also ref. 37). In general, second messenger molecules that are formed subsequent to receptor activation can affect either ion channels directly or kinase enzymes that are involved in the phosphorylation of proteins. The addition of a highly charged phosphate group can induce a substantial change in protein structure, resulting in a range of events, such as altered enzymatic activity, altered intracellular function or, if the protein constitutes an ion channel, altered permeability to ions which pass through the cell membrane. The aim of this chapter is to discuss the role of second messengers, specifically cAMP, cGMP, inositol phosphates, diacylglycerol and eicosanoids, as mediators in the receptor modulation of neurotransmitter release. (For general reviews on second messengers in neuronal function, see refs. 23 and 34.)

It should be noted that some receptors linked to G-proteins are not associated with enzyme-linked second messenger production, but rather the G-protein directly interacts with ion channels. This is further considered in Chapter 10.

### 1.1 Limitations of methods used to study second messenger-mediated modulation of neurotransmitter release

Although the signal transduction of receptor events has been widely investigated in a variety of cell types, for practical reasons those events at the nerve terminal have been less well studied. The nerve terminal is but a small unit of the peripheral nerve, which, in turn, constitutes a small portion of the effector tissue. Effector tissue consists mainly of other cell types, which complicates biochemical measurement of second messenger generation specifically in the nerve terminals. The same is true for the CNS, where the presence of other cells and multiple transmitter systems limits specific identification of bio-chemical markers. Even when second messengers can be measured, it is difficult to prove that detected changes in second messenger levels are themselves the direct cause of a change in transmitter release.

Although patch-clamp techniques have the capability of investigating signal transduction of single cells, there are still problems with extrapolating the results to receptor events at the nerve terminals since the function of receptors at the cell body may be different to those same receptor types at the nerve terminal. Because of this, studies on receptor modulation of events in whole cells and changes in second messenger levels have been deliberately omitted from the following discussion.

The study of signal transduction at nerve terminals has relied heavily on pharmacological probes to manipulate the second messenger pathways and examine the resultant effect on transmitter release. Pharmacological probes have their limitations. First, some drugs that are used as probes may not be entirely selective for the intended target. Second, activation of signal transduction pathways with exogenous agents may flood the cell with second messengers so that they reach intracellular regions where they are not normally present. In this respect, there is increasing evidence that endogenous second messengers may have highly compartmentalised effects within cells[23]. Third, the experimentally imposed time course of activation may be inappropriate since many second messengers have extremely short half-lives and exogenous activators are often chosen for their prolonged effects. This may not only affect the nature of the response but also the compensatory adjustments that neurones may make, since it is clear that signal-transduction mechanisms form a web of mutually dependent reactions, interacting at many levels. Finally, in the specific case of presynaptic autoreceptors, where signal transduction manipulations change the amount of transmitter released, there may be an inappropriate interference with autoreceptor feedback

processes, not because of specific common biochemical linkings but because of the change in levels of transmitter release *per se*. For example, in the presence of α-adrenoceptor blockade, the release-enhancing effects of phorbol dibutyrate is increased in rabbit hippocampus, probably because of removal of α-autoreceptor feedback inhibition[3]. All of these problems highlight the need for careful and critical evaluation of the pharmacological approach.

## 2 Receptors and G-proteins

### 2.1 Receptor structure

Receptors that are linked to G-proteins are membrane proteins consisting of a single polypeptide chain containing seven hydrophobic membrane-spanning domains connected by hydrophilic extracellular and cytoplasmic loops. The extracellular portions contain the agonist-recognition sites and binding of an agonist to the receptor leads to a conformation change in the protein structure of the receptor. There is an extended cytoplasmic loop between membrane spans five and six which is thought to be the site of interaction between the receptor and G-proteins (see Fig. 9.1).

### 2.2 G-protein activation

G-proteins are heterotrimeric proteins (containing α-, β- and γ-subunits) that are present in cell membranes and transduce the receptor activation event to changes in enzyme or ion-channel activity (see Fig. 9.1). The α-subunit is the largest of the three subunits and has both a site for binding a guanine nucleotide and also an intrinsic GTPase activity capable of converting GTP to GDP. There are more than 20 distinct α-subunits, and these confer considerable heterogeneity to G-proteins. There are several distinct G-proteins[7] including those designated $G_i$, $G_o$, $G_s$, $G_t$, $G_{pla}$, $G_p$, $G_k$, $G_z$ and

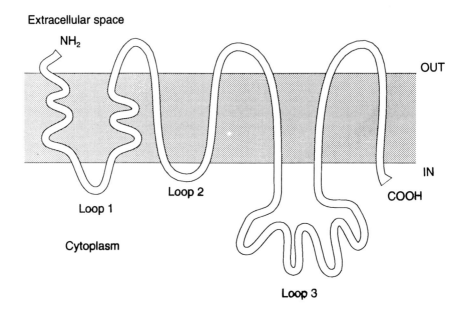

**Fig. 9.1.** Diagrammatic representation of the general structure of a G-protein-linked receptor. There are seven membrane-spanning domains, which produce three cytoplasmic loops. The length of the C-terminus and the size of the loops, particularly the third loop, varies considerably between receptor types. Loop 3 is thought to be the site of interaction with G-proteins. The extracellular portions form the ligand-binding domains and the length of the N-terminus can vary considerably. Some receptors have extracellular glycosylation sites and potential phosphorylation sites in the intracellular domain.

$G_q$. The specificity of receptor coupling to G-proteins and their subsequent coupling to various effector systems is also conferred by the $\alpha$-subunits. The $\beta$- and $\gamma$-subunits are more conserved than the $\alpha$-subunits and are found tightly associated as a complex.

The binding of an agonist to the receptor leads to a structural change in the receptor so that it interacts with the G-protein in a way that facilitates the exchange of GDP, which is bound to the $\alpha$-subunit of the G-protein, with cytosolic GTP. Once GTP is bound to the $\alpha$-subunit, the G-protein dissociates from the receptor and then itself dissociates into $\alpha$- and $\beta\gamma$-subunits. The $\alpha$-subunit then interacts with an enzyme or ion channel to cause changes that ultimately alter the effector's activity (Fig. 9.2). Since several G-protein complexes can associate with a single receptor, there may be amplification of the receptor signal. Although the $\alpha$-subunit is the major transducer of receptor activation, it has been proposed that the $\beta\gamma$-subunits also have some actions on enzymes or ion channels, either directly or indirectly by binding free $\alpha$-subunits. The action of the $\alpha$-subunit is terminated by the conversion of the bound GTP to GDP by the intrinsic GTPase activity of the subunit. This results in the reassociation of the three subunits. Studies from a wide variety of cells suggest that specific receptors are associated with distinct G-proteins, although the associations are far from completely characterised. In addition, it has been found that certain G-proteins are associated with multiple receptor types.

### 2.3 Tools in G-protein research

Research into G-protein involvement in presynaptic receptor modulation of neurotransmitter release has, to date, been indirect

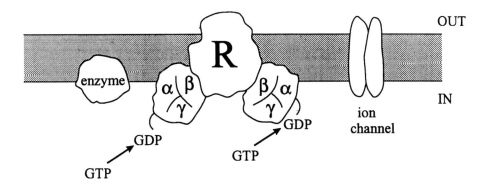

2. Dissociated α-subunit influences ion channels or enzymes

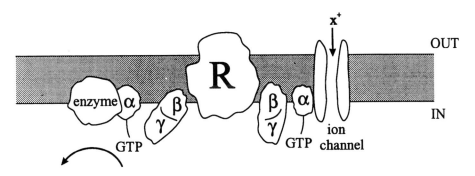

3. Intrinsic GTPase of α-subunit converts GTP to GDP and the reassociation of the subunits occurs

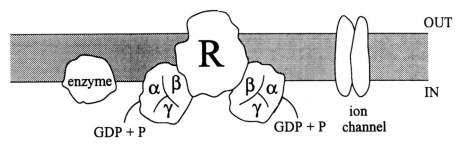

**Fig. 9.2.** Activation of the receptor (R) leads to G-protein activation and either activation or inhibition of an effector (either an enzyme or an ion channel). G-proteins are activated by GTP exchange with GDP on the α-subunit, which leads to the dissociation of the α-subunit from the βγ complex (1). The α-subunit can then interact with either an enzyme or ion channel to alter its activity (2). An intrinsic GTPase activity in the α-subunit dephosphorylates GTP to GDP and the subunits reunite to form a stable inactive complex.

and has used pharmacological probes, such as pertussis toxin, cholera toxin and *N*-ethyl-maleimide.

Pertussis toxin is derived from *Bordatella pertussis* and can catalyse the transfer of ADP-ribose from $NAD^+$ (ADP ribosylation) onto cysteine side chains of the α-subunits of $G_i$ and $G_o$ (and perhaps other G-proteins such as $G_k$ and $G_{pla}$, but not $G_s$). This inhibits the dissociation of the subunits, thereby preventing signal transduction. In whole cells, pertussis toxin must be taken up by a specific transport process before it can ADP-ribosylate G-proteins. Therefore, either *in vivo* (up to 4 days) or long-term (2–20 h) *in vitro* pre-treatment is necessary for the full effect of the toxin to develop. The actions of pertussis toxin are thought to be relatively selective for G-proteins.

Cholera toxin can ADP-ribosylate arginine side chains of the α-subunit of $G_s$ thereby preventing intrinsic GTPase activity. The result is permanent activation of $G_s$.

*N*-ethylmaleimide alkylates sulphydryl groups on proteins. Although this is a relatively non-selective action, it has been suggested that, at appropriate concentrations and duration of contact, G-proteins can be selectively alkylated and thus inactivated[24]. It has been suggested that *N*-ethylmaleimide has a similar spectrum of action to pertussis toxin[24], but some workers suggest that it actually targets a wider range of G-proteins[15].

# 3   Cyclic nucleotides and modulation of neurotransmitter release

## 3.1   Adenylyl cyclase and cAMP

The adenylyl cyclase–cAMP signal transduction pathway has been one of the most widely studied. Several receptors stimulate adenylyl cyclase activity through the mediation of the G-protein $G_s$ (see Table 9.1). Inhibitory receptor modulation of adenylyl cyclase activity occurs through a separate G-protein ($G_i$). In some systems, this inhibition is only seen if the adenylyl cyclase is first activated

by the $G_s$ pathway. Adenylyl cyclase converts ATP to cAMP, which in turn activates protein kinase A. The cAMP formed is degraded by phosphodiesterase enzymes to 5′-AMP. Protein kinase A has a widespread distribution within cells in both membrane and cytosolic compartments and phosphorylates serine and threonine residues on a wide variety of proteins, including receptors, ion channels, enzymes and cytoskeletal proteins, which results in changes in their activity or function[34].

## 3.2   Neuronal function and cAMP

It has been shown that activation of the adenylyl cyclase–cAMP system enhances action potential-evoked neurotransmitter release from a variety of neurones, as well as having other effects on neuronal function including growth, development and transmitter biosynthesis[34] (Fig. 9.3). Therefore, cell permeable analogues of cAMP, such as 8-bromo-cAMP and dibutyryl cAMP, the adenylyl cyclase activator forskolin and phosphodiesterase inhibitors, which prevent the breakdown of cAMP, all enhance neurotransmitter release from a variety of neurone types including noradrenergic[26,41], cholinergic[41] and serotonergic[41] neurones. The specific linking of release-modulating receptors to adenylyl cyclase is described below.

## 3.3   Guanylyl cyclase and cGMP

Cyclic GMP is produced by two different enzymes, particulate and soluble guanylyl cyclase. Both forms convert GTP to cGMP, which can activate a cGMP-dependent protein kinase that then phosphorylates proteins. Soluble guanylate cyclase can be activated by nitric oxide or nitric oxide-containing compounds, such as sodium nitroprusside. Soluble guanylate cyclase, however, is not linked to membrane receptors. Nevertheless, receptors may increase guanylate cyclase activity through the generation of fatty acids, particularly lipoxygenase metabolites of

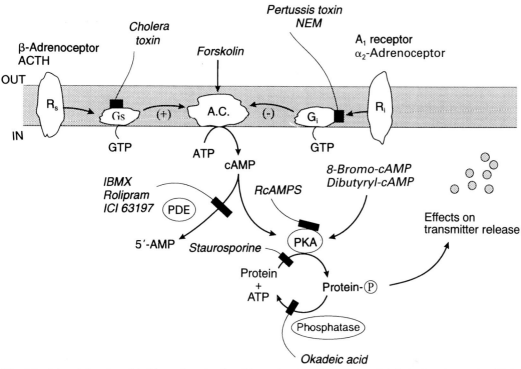

**Fig. 9.3.** Adenylyl cyclase (A.C.) can be stimulated by activation of receptors ($R_s$) linked to G-proteins ($G_s$) and inhibited by receptors ($R_i$) linked to other G-proteins ($G_i$). The effects of $G_s$ can be potentiated by cholera toxin, which ADP-ribosylates the $\alpha_s$-subunit to prevent the intrinsic GTPase activity. Effects of $G_i$ can be prevented by either pertussis toxin, which ADP-ribosylates the $\alpha_i$-subunit thereby inhibiting dissociation, or N-ethylmaleimide (NEM), which alkylates the $\alpha_i$-subunits. Adenylyl cyclase activity can be directly increased by forskolin. The production of cAMP by adenylate cyclase can activate protein kinase A (PKA) to phosphorylate target proteins that may then have effects on transmitter release. The actions of cAMP can be enhanced by drugs (e.g. IBMX, rolipram, ICI63197) that inhibit phosphodiesterase (PDE) and prevent the breakdown of cAMP. The effects of cAMP can be mimicked by permeable analogues (8-bromo-cAMP, dibutyryl-cAMP) and blocked by (R)-p-cyclic adenosine monophosphothioate (RcAMPS) and a non-selective protein kinase inhibitor staurosporine. The effects of the phosphorylated protein can be prolonged by the phosphatase inhibitor okadeic acid.

arachidonic acid (see Section 4), or activation of other enzymes such as protein kinase C. Particulate guanylate cyclase activity, however, appears to be an intrinsic part of the atrial natriuretic peptide (ANP) receptor protein structure and is activated by ANP.

### 3.4    Neuronal function and cGMP

The action of cGMP within neurones is controversial and no clear picture has yet emerged. It has been suggested that drugs that stimulate guanylyl cyclase, such as sodium nitroprusside, inhibit action potential-evoked noradrenaline release from sympathetic nerves of dog mesenteric artery[22], but this is not seen with those of rat tail artery[42]. However, substantive argument against an inhibitory role for cGMP stems from observations that cGMP analogues increase, or have no effect on, noradrenaline release from many sympathetically innervated tissues.

The enhancing effects on transmitter release may be because the guanylyl cyclase system has a high degree of reactivity with the adenylyl cyclase system. In the cat spleen, 8-bromocyclic-GMP, a cell permeable cGMP analogue, enhanced the action potential-evoked release of noradrenaline. However, the action of cGMP was suggested to be caused by inhibition of phosphodiesterase, which would lead to a reduction in endogenous cAMP breakdown[12].

# 4 Phospholipases and modulation of neurotransmitter release

In many cases, receptors are linked via G-proteins to phospholipases (see Table 9.1). These are a variety of membrane-located enzymes that cleave plasma membrane phospholipids, yielding a range of second messenger molecules. Three phospholipases in particular generate second messengers that may be important in the regulation of neurotransmission: phospholipase C, phospholipase D and phospholipase $A_2$.

## 4.1 Phospholipase C

Activation of phospholipase C, either through receptors or simply by membrane depolarisation, results in breakdown of the membrane phospholipid phosphatidylinositol bisphosphate into two second messengers: $Ins(1,4,5)P_3$ and diacylglycerol. The $Ins(1,4,5)P_3$ releases $Ca^{2+}$ from storage sites in the endoplasmic reticulum and is subsequently broken down into other inositol phosphates to be reincorporated into membrane phospholipids. The appearance of diacylglycerol in the membrane results in movement of cytoplasmic protein kinase C to the membrane (translocation), which is then activated by the diacylglycerol (Fig. 9.4). Protein kinase C can phosphorylate a variety of proteins involved in cellular function and has been implicated in cellular growth and differentiation, smooth muscle contraction as well as in neurotransmitter release[35]. The protein kinase C family

of enzymes consists of at least nine isoenzymes and, in general, they all require diacylglycerol, $Ca^{2+}$ and phosphatidylserine for activity, although some forms can be activated by arachidonic acid and some appear not to require $Ca^{2+}$ (see ref. 35). Diacylglycerol is broken down principally by diacylglycerol kinase to phosphatidic acid and to a lesser extent by diacylglycerol lipase to arachidonic acid.

### 4.1.1 Neurotransmitter release and $Ins(1,4,5)P_3$

The derivative $Ins(1,4,5)P_3$ can be considered as a second messenger since it influences intracellular function directly. In addition, $Ins(1,4,5)P_3$ mobilises $Ca^{2+}$ from intracellular stores. Mobilised $Ca^{2+}$ activates a variety of $Ca^{2+}$-dependent enzymes, including kinases and phosphatases, either directly or through its association with $Ca^{2+}$-binding proteins such as calmodulin. In many systems, $Ins(1,4,5)P_3$ is of great importance, for example in receptor-mediated smooth muscle contraction. In nerves, however, there is little evidence that the intracellular $Ca^{2+}$-releasing actions of $Ins(1,4,5)P_3$ alter transmitter release and even less evidence for $Ins(1,4,5)P_3$ being involved in receptor-mediated modulation of transmitter release (see also Chapter 1). Agents such as acetylcholine and 5-HT, which activate muscarinic and serotonergic receptors, respectively, increase $Ins(1,4,5)P_3$ production in sympathetic nerves in culture but do not increase intraneuronal $Ca^{2+}$ by themselves, nor do they induce transmitter release[44].

### 4.1.2 Protein kinase C activation and neurotransmitter release

The principal endogenous activator of protein kinase C is diacylglycerol. Conventionally, it has been thought that the principal source of diacylglycerol is from the cleavage of inositol phospholipids by phospholipase C (see above). However, it has been suggested, for sympathetic neurones at least, that breakdown of phosphatidylcholine

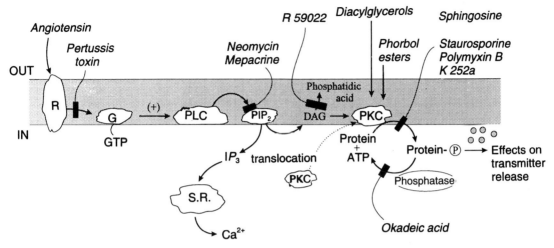

Fig. 9.4. Receptors (R) such as those for angiotensin II can activate phospholipase C (PLC). In some cases the G-protein involved is inactivated by pertussis toxin. Phospholipase C cleaves membrane phosphatidyl inositol bisphosphate ($PIP_2$) to inositol trisphosphate ($IP_3$), which can release $Ca^{2+}$ from internal stores (S.R.) and diacylglycerol (DAG), which causes protein kinase C (PKC) to translocate to the membrane. Neomycin and mepacrine can inhibit phospholipase C. Diacylglycerol breakdown by diacylglycerol kinase to phosphatidic acid can be prevented by R 59022. Protein kinase C translocation and activation can also be brought about by synthetic diacylglycerols and tumour promoting phorbol esters. Protein kinase C can phosphorylate target proteins involved in neurotransmitter release. This phosphorylation is inhibited by protein kinase C inhibitors, such as sphingosine, staurosporine, polymyxin B or K 252a. Okadeic acid can inhibit the protein phosphatases that dephosphorylate the target proteins.

by phospholipase D may also be an important source of diacylglycerol[44]. Arachidonic acid (see below) has also been shown to activate some forms of protein kinase C. Activators of protein kinase C, such as tumour-promoting phorbol esters (e.g. phorbol myristate acetate and phorbol dibutyrate) that mimic the effects of endogenous diacylglycerol, enhance neurotransmitter release from a variety of neurones, including noradrenergic, cholinergic, dopaminergic, GABAergic and serotonergic types (see, for example, the effects on noradrenaline release[32]). In some systems, inhibitors of protein kinase C (such as staurosporine, K252a, H7, calphostin C and polymyxin B) inhibit neurotransmitter release, suggesting that endogenous activation of protein kinase C is involved in neurotransmitter release (see ref. 4). However, none of these agents has good selectivity for protein kinase C and the specificity of their effects has not always been determined.

It has been suggested for peripheral nor-

adrenergic nerves that protein kinase C has a direct role in transmitter release only when high output of transmitter is induced[17,32]. In support of this, the protein kinase C inhibitor polymyxin B, at a concentration that by itself does not affect noradrenaline release evoked by low-frequency (5 Hz) electrical stimulation, attenuates noradrenaline release when protein kinase C is elevated by higher-frequency stimulation or release-enhancing drugs. Likewise, protein kinase C down-regulation does not affect low-level transmitter release but attenuates the effects of release-enhancing agents and manipulations[17,32]. It may be that to sustain high neurotransmitter release rates, increased vesicle transport and docking is required and this may be the step that involves protein kinase C.

## 4.2   Phospholipase D

It is suggested that phospholipase D is important in diacylglycerol formation in sympathetic

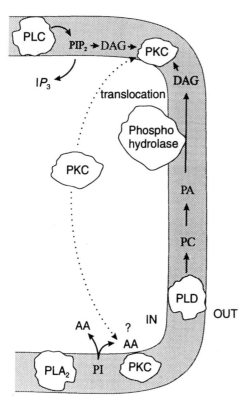

Fig. 9.5. There are many possible routes of protein kinase C (PKC) activation. Some isoforms of protein kinase C are activated by arachidonic acid (AA), which is formed by phospholipase $A_2$ (PLA$_2$)-catalysed breakdown of membrane phospholipids. The principal activator however is diacylglycerol (DAG) formed from phospholipase C (PLC) cleavage of phosphoinositol bisphosphate (PIP$_2$). Another synthetic route of diacylglycerol is via the breakdown of phosphatidyl choline (PC) to phosphatidic acid (PA) which is then converted to diacylglycerol by phosphohydrolase.

nerves during depolarisation[44]. Membrane phospholipids, such as phosphatidylcholine, are metabolised by phospholipase D to phosphatidic acid. Phosphatidic acid may be a second messenger in its own right, but this issue remains to be resolved. In any event, phosphatidic acid can be converted by phosphohydrolase to diacylglycerol, which activates

protein kinase C (see review by Shulka and Halenda[39]) (Fig. 9.5). However, the role of the phospholipase D pathway in neurotransmitter release and any link that it might have to release-modulating receptors is not yet clear.

### 4.3 Phospholipase $A_2$

Phospholipase $A_2$ can cleave membrane phospholipids (phosphatidylinositol, phosphatidylcholine) to yield arachidonic acid. There is a myriad of subsequent oxidation products of arachidonic acid, such as prostaglandins, thromboxanes, leukotrienes and lipoxins, all of which have important biological actions. Phospholipase $A_2$ can be activated as a consequence of anaphylaxis, antigen–antibody reactions, responses to cell injury and by a variety of chemicals. However, it has also been proposed that membrane receptors can activate phospholipase $A_2$ through G-protein mechanisms (see ref. 6). The receptors include $\alpha_1$-adrenoceptors, GABA$_B$ receptors and muscarinic receptors.

Arachidonic acid and its metabolites have been considered to act principally intercellularly, as paracrine factors. In a multitude of neuronal systems, many of the metabolites can apparently modulate transmitter release (see Chapter 6). Arachidonic acid and its metabolites also act as intracellular messengers for postreceptor effects. The differentiation of their roles as intracellular messengers and paracrine factors has not yet been adequately addressed by researchers, but this is a developing area (see ref. 6). At this time, the intracellular second messenger actions of arachidonic acid and its metabolites on neurotransmitter release has not been widely studied.

## 5    Interactions between signal transduction pathways

There is considerable cross-talk between signal transduction pathways in many cellular systems, and the possibility exists that activation of one pathway may interact with another in neurones. For example, increasing intracellular cAMP levels inhibits phorbol ester (protein kinase C)-potentiated $K^+$-evoked noradrenaline release in guinea-pig brain cortical synaptosomes[40]. By contrast, no specific interaction has been found between the adenylyl cyclase system and the protein kinase C system in sympathetic nerves of mouse atria, where the effects of phorbol myristate acetate and 8-bromo-cAMP are additive[25].

# 6 Presynaptic receptors and second messengers

The discussion that follows has been restricted to six presynaptic receptors: $\alpha_2$-adrenoceptors, $\beta$-adrenoceptors, ACTH, angiotensin II, muscarinic, neuropeptide Y and dopamine receptors. These occur in the autonomic nervous system and also in the CNS. The systems discussed represent fairly the current debate on second-messenger mechanisms in presynaptic receptor systems, although the selection reflects the authors' particular interest.

## 6.1 Presynaptic $\alpha_2$-adrenoceptors

Presynaptic $\alpha_2$-adrenoceptors are found on a variety of neurones and when activated inhibit neurotransmitter release.

### 6.1.1 Presynaptic $\alpha_2$-adrenoceptors and G-proteins

It is clear from their structure and pharmacology that $\alpha_2$-adrenoceptors belong to the G-protein linked family and, in most cell types, are coupled to pertussis toxin-sensitive G-proteins. For example, in the CNS, pertussis toxin treatment prevents the $\alpha_2$-adrenoceptor inhibition of stimulation-induced noradrenaline release by $\alpha_2$-adrenoceptor agonists[24]. The absolute level of stimulation-induced noradrenaline release is elevated by

the toxin, presumably because the (autoreceptor-mediated) feedback inhibition of neuronally released noradrenaline is no longer functional[24]. Consistent with this, $\alpha_2$-adrenoceptor antagonists no longer elevate stimulation-induced noradrenaline release after pertussis toxin.

In the sympathetic nervous system, the actions of pertussis toxin are less clear cut. In many sympathetically innervated tissues, pertussis toxin treatment does not affect the action of $\alpha_2$-adrenoceptor agonists and antagonists on stimulation-induced noradrenaline release, nor does it affect the absolute levels of release (see ref. 33). By comparison, in chick sympathetic neurones grown in culture, pertussis toxin does prevent $\alpha_2$-adrenoceptor agonist modulation of noradrenaline release[8]. The mixed results from the different tissues are difficult to explain. It may be that the pertussis toxin was ineffective because the treatment schedules were inappropriate, or that it could not gain access to the G-proteins. However, in many cases, the treatment regimens were tested by using other pertussis toxin-sensitive events and found to be effective. One striking example of this is that $\alpha_1$-but not $\alpha_2$-adrenoceptor inhibition of noradrenaline release from rat kidney cortex slices was inhibited by pertussis toxin[30]. It may be that presynaptic $\alpha$-adrenoceptors are coupled to different G-proteins in different locations. Certainly it appears that there are different presynaptic $\alpha_2$-adrenoceptor subtypes ($\alpha_{2a}$, $\alpha_{2b}$, $\alpha_{2c}$, $\alpha_{2d}$), as determined pharmacologically, in different locations and tissues, which raises the possibility for different coupling mechanisms.

$N$-ethylmaleimide (see above) has been used to examine linking of $\alpha$-adrenoceptors to G-proteins and, where tested, appears to inhibit $\alpha$-adrenoceptor inhibition of noradrenaline release, implying G-protein involvement. It has been suggested that $N$-ethylmaleimide inactivates the same G-proteins as pertussis toxin[24], but this has been disputed. In the case of $\alpha_2$-adrenoceptors, $N$-ethylmaleimide has been shown to inhibit $\alpha_2$-adrenoceptor effects on noradrenaline release in tissues where pertussis toxin was not effective (see for example, ref. 29), which suggests that it has a wider spectrum of action.

### 6.1.2 Presynaptic $\alpha_2$-adrenoceptors and adenylyl cyclase

It is well established that some receptors inhibit adenylyl cyclase through the G-protein $G_i$. The $\alpha_2$-adrenoceptor subtype has been found to inhibit adenylyl cyclase and decrease cAMP levels in many cell types including neurones. Cyclic AMP has a facilitatory effect on many transmitter systems, including the noradrenergic system (see ref. 26). Therefore, it has been hypothesised that $\alpha_2$-adrenoceptors may inhibit noradrenaline release by inhibiting adenylyl cyclase[38]. Manipulations that increase cAMP levels, such as the adenylyl cyclase activator forskolin, phosphodiesterase inhibitors and cell-permeable cAMP analogues, reduced $\alpha$-adrenoceptor inhibition of noradrenaline release from rat cerebral cortex slices, again suggesting that cAMP was the transducing moiety[38]. However, in several studies with sympathetically innervated tissues, and in other noradrenergic neurones in the CNS[20,26], forskolin and phosphodiesterase inhibitors either did not change, or actually augmented, the effects of $\alpha_2$-adrenoceptor ligands on the release of noradrenaline, which contradicts the hypothesis. Drugs that elevate cAMP levels invariably have much smaller facilitatory effects on noradrenaline release than $\alpha$-adrenoceptor antagonists (see refs. 26 and 41 for discussion). This finding is inconsistent with the adenylyl cyclase hypothesis, since this requires that disruption of $\alpha$-adrenoceptor automodulation by $\alpha$-adrenoceptor-blocking drugs, such as phentolamine, should enhance noradrenaline release because of increased cAMP levels. Additionally, when cAMP mechanisms in mouse atria sympathetic nerves were supra-maximally activated by 8-bromo-cAMP to elevate stimulation-induced noradrenaline release, the facilitatory effect of activation of presynaptic $\beta$-

adrenoceptors or presynaptic ACTH receptors (both of which are coupled to adenylyl cyclase, see below) was abolished, but the facilitatory effect of the $\alpha$-adrenoceptor antagonist phentolamine on noradrenaline release was not affected[26]. This result strongly suggests that cAMP is not involved in $\alpha$-adrenoceptor modulation of noradrenaline release, but more definitive experiments are required, particularly in the CNS.

### 6.1.3 Presynaptic $\alpha_2$-adrenoceptors and protein kinase C

Given the enhancing effect of protein kinase C activation on neurotransmitter release, attention has been given to interactions between presynaptic $\alpha_2$-adrenoceptors and protein kinase C in the noradrenergic system. There has been complications in interpreting the results of studies, since the demonstration of whether $\alpha_2$-adrenoceptor feedback modulation has occurred is based on the measured level of transmitter release, but this is itself altered by protein kinase C modulators. Thus in the CNS, protein kinase C-activating phorbol esters reduce the level of inhibition of stimulation-induced noradrenaline release caused by clonidine. This is thought to result from the increased level of noradrenaline release prevailing in the presence of the phorbol esters, a condition under which clonidine would be a less effective inhibitor since it is only a partial agonist at $\alpha_2$-adrenoceptors (see ref. 3).

Protein kinase C itself may have an endogenous role in a general mechanism by which drugs elevate transmitter release in the noradrenergic system (see Section 4.1.2 above and also refs. 17 and 32). Thus, in mouse atria, the inhibitory effect of clonidine on stimulation-induced noradrenaline release is unaffected by protein kinase C inhibition or down-regulation, whereas the facilitatory effect of $\alpha$-adrenoceptor antagonists is attenuated[17,32]. The interaction between $\alpha$-adrenoceptor modulation and protein kinase C is complex and, whilst explanations are offered, these have not been fully tested and may vary between systems. There are still many discrepancies in the literature concerning interactions between α-adrenoceptors and protein kinase C, even when similar experimental protocols have been used. For example, the release-enhancing effects of phorbol esters that activate protein kinase C and of α-adrenoceptor-blocking drugs are more than additive in rabbit hippocampus[5], simply additive in mouse atria[32] and less than additive in rat hippocampus[20]. This could indicate interactions between α-adrenoceptors and protein kinase C at many levels. It may also illustrate the multiple roles of protein kinase C in the neurotransmitter release process: from ion channel and G-protein phosphorylation through to an involvement in regulating vesicle dynamics. Protein kinase C may turn out to have no specific involvement in α₂-adrenoceptor signal transduction. Certainly, there is little evidence to indicate that α₂-adrenoceptors are directly coupled to phospholipase C in any cell type.

## 6.2 Presynaptic β-adrenoceptors

Presynaptic β-adrenoceptors, which facilitate stimulation-induced noradrenaline release, have been extensively studied in the sympathetic nervous system (see review by Majewski[25]). The most probable signal transduction pathway utilised by the neuronal presynaptic β-adrenoceptor is that involving adenylyl cyclase, which is the signal transduction pathway that mediates the effects of β-adrenoceptor activation in many other cell types. Activation of the adenylyl cyclase system enhances noradrenaline release in sympathetic nerves (see ref. 26). There are many complementary studies supporting the participation of the adenylyl cyclase system in the presynaptic β-adrenoceptor pathway. These have been based mainly on measuring interactions between β-adrenoceptor agonists and either adenylyl cyclase activators or cAMP mimetics. For example, when noradrenaline release in mouse atria is elevated by maximally effective concentrations of 8-bromo-cAMP, then β-adrenoceptor facilitation of

noradrenaline release is no longer obtained, although other facilitatory processes such as the enhancement by angiotensin II are still evident[26].

The G-protein associated with β-adrenoceptor facilitation of noradrenaline release has not been studied specifically, but, based on findings in most other cell types studied, it is probably $G_s$. Consistent with this is the observation that the facilitatory effects of the β-adrenoceptor agonist isoprenaline on noradrenaline release is not pertussis toxin sensitive[33] but is attenuated by N-ethylmaleimide[15].

## 6.3 Presynaptic ACTH receptors

ACTH is a polypeptide synthesised by the anterior lobe of the pituitary gland and has a facilitatory effect on noradrenaline release from sympathetic nerve terminals[21,26]. Studies have demonstrated that this effect of ACTH can be eliminated when intraneuronal cAMP levels are maximally activated using phosphodiesterase inhibitors and cAMP analogues. This suggests that the facilitatory effect of ACTH, like that for prejunctional β-adrenoceptors, is mediated through the adenylyl cyclase system. This signal transduction process is in accord with the signal transduction process for ACTH receptors in other cell types.

## 6.4 Presynaptic angiotensin II receptors

Angiotensin II, acting through specific presynaptic receptors, enhances stimulation-induced noradrenaline release from sympathetic nerves. Angiotensin II receptors belong to the G-protein-linked family. In sympathetic nerves, the facilitatory effects of angiotensin II on noradrenaline release appear to be resistant to pertussis toxin[16] but are reduced by N-ethylmaleimide (see ref. 15). In some non-neuronal systems, the effects of angiotensin II are inhibited by pertussis toxin, but this is not always observed. Angiotensin II facilitation of noradrenaline release is not mediated by the adenylyl cyclase system since, even in the presence of phentolamine and 8-bromo-cAMP, the facilitatory effects of angiotensin II in rabbit pulmonary artery are not inhibited[10]. However, there are several lines of evidence to suggest that protein kinase C is involved in the pathway. First, in sympathetic nerves, inhibition of protein kinase C with polymyxin B and K252a abolished the facilitatory effect of angiotensin II on noradrenaline release[25,31]. Second, maximal activation of protein kinase C with phorbol dibutyrate prevented the facilitatory effect of angiotensin II[25.] Finally, protein kinase C down-regulation by prolonged exposure of mouse atria to phorbol dibutyrate also abolished the facilitatory effect of angiotensin II on noradrenaline release from the sympathetic nerves in the tissue[17,25]. The conclusion that this signal transduction pathway involves protein kinase C is given further support by studies in non-neuronal systems where angiotensin II receptors are coupled to the phospholipase C/protein kinase C pathway.

## 6.5  Muscarinic receptors

Activation of muscarinic receptors inhibits transmitter release from a variety of neurone types in the central and peripheral nervous systems, although there are also reports of muscarinic receptors enhancing transmitter release.

There are (at least) three muscarinic receptor subtypes ($M_1$, $M_2$, $M_3$) all of which have been shown to be involved in the modulation of transmitter release. This receptor diversity may to some extent explain the diverse range of signal transduction mechanisms proposed. These include inhibition of adenylyl cyclase, stimulation of guanylyl cyclase, activation of phospholipase C as well as direct inhibition of $Ca^{2+}$ channels and activation of $K^+$ channels. It is, therefore, difficult to form a unitary hypothesis of muscarinic signal transduction and each system and receptor subtype must be considered separately.

In sympathetic noradrenergic nerves, the inhibitory presynaptic muscarinic receptor

resembles the $M_2$ subtype. In mouse and rat atria, release-inhibiting presynaptic muscarinic receptors are not linked to pertussis toxin-sensitive G-proteins[11]. Likewise, in the noradrenergic nerves of rat stomach, the inhibitory effect of the muscarinic agonist oxotremorine on noradrenaline release was not affected by pertussis toxin[45].

In sympathetic nerves, the muscarinic receptor-mediated inhibition of noradrenaline release does not involve either adenylyl cyclase or protein kinase C, since the effect is not attenuated by high concentrations of 8-bromo-cAMP or the potent, but non-selective, protein kinase-inhibitor staurosporine[11]. This latter result suggests that protein kinases in general are not involved.

In cholinergic neurones, enzyme-linked signal transduction pathways have been implicated in muscarinic receptor-mediated inhibition of transmitter release. For example in guinea-pig myenteric neurones, the facilitatory effects of forskolin and 3-isobutyl-methyl-xanthine were not additive with that of the muscarinic receptor antagonist atropine[1]. However, the facilitation of acetylcholine release by atropine was far greater than the maximal facilitatory effect produced by the adenylyl cyclase activator forskolin[1], which argues against an important involvement of cAMP.

It has also been proposed that muscarinic inhibition of neurotransmitter release from cholinergic neurones may be mediated by increased cGMP levels, since muscarinic agonists increase cGMP levels. However, this presumably is by an indirect pathway since there is no evidence that muscarinic receptors are linked to guanylyl cyclase. The evidence in support of the hypothesis has been that cGMP analogues prevent the increase in acetylcholine release by atropine in CNS tissues[36]. However, no such effect has been found in peripheral tissues (see ref. 41 for discussion). This hypothesis has not been actively tested, presumably because of more compelling evidence for the direct involvement of ion channels (rather than second messengers) in mediating muscarinic receptor-stimulated events in the CNS.

Finally, although protein kinase C activation can enhance acetylcholine release, this appears not to affect the range of muscarinic modulation of acetylcholine release in the CNS[2].

In summary, the bulk of the evidence suggests that muscarinic receptor-mediated inhibition of neurotransmitter release does not involve enzyme-linked second messenger systems and the possibility of ion-channel modulation ($Ca^{2+}$, $K^+$), perhaps by direct G-protein linking, has to be seriously considered (see ref. 41).

## 6.6 Neuropeptide Y receptors

Neuropeptide Y is co-stored with noradrenaline in peripheral sympathetic neurones and may also be a CNS neurotransmitter. Postsynaptically, neuropeptide Y has potent vasoconstrictor properties and is suggested to be involved in sympathetic vascular control. Activation of presynaptic neuropeptide Y receptors causes inhibition of neurotransmitter release from several neurone types.

The effects of neuropeptide Y on non-neuronal systems appear to be mediated through pertussis toxin-sensitive G-proteins; the structure of its receptor also suggests that it is G-protein linked. However, the inhibitory effect of neuropeptide Y on noradrenaline release from sympathetic nerves is not affected by pertussis toxin[14]. Nevertheless, low concentrations of N-ethylmaleimide were found to attenuate the effects of neuropeptide Y on noradrenaline release from sympathetic nerves of mouse atria, suggesting that pertussis toxin-insensitive G-proteins are involved[14].

It has been proposed that the inhibitory effect of neuropeptide Y on neurotransmitter release may be mediated through inhibition of adenylyl cyclase[43], but the evidence for this hypothesis is highly circumstantial and is based mainly on the ability of neuropeptide Y to decrease cAMP levels in the brain and other tissues. In peripheral sympathetic nerves, the inhibitory effect of neuropeptide Y was found to be independent of the effects of cAMP analogues[14]. Furthermore, the non-selective protein kinase inhibitor K252a did not block the effect of neuropeptide Y on noradrenaline release[16]. This suggests that cAMP is not involved and also that the inhibitory effect of neuropeptide Y probably is not transduced through protein phosphorylation events.

Neuropeptide Y receptors have been found to be linked to inhibition of $Ca^{2+}$ channels, and opening of $K^+$ channels, and this may be a more likely mechanism for the inhibition of transmitter release[13].

## 6.7 Dopamine receptors

Activation of $D_2$ receptors inhibits the release of dopamine from dopaminergic nerves as well as the release from their respective nerve terminals of other neurotransmitters, such as noradrenaline and acetylcholine. Whilst $D_2$ receptors are coupled to inhibition of adenylyl cyclase in some cell types, this pathway is unlikely to be involved in the auto-inhibition of dopamine release. In this regard, it is questionable whether cAMP mimetics enhance dopamine release (see ref. 41). However there are some positive results, such those obtained in rat striatum (see ref. 28). Even in these positively responding tissues, however, the inhibitory effect of $D_2$ receptors appears not to involve adenylyl cyclase, since the presence of forskolin and 3-isobutyl-1-methylxanthine did not affect $D_2$ receptor-mediated inhibition of [$^3$H]-dopamine release from superfused rat striatal slices[9]. Similarly, the inhibition of acetylcholine release by dopamine was not affected by forskolin or by phosphodiesterase inhibition in the striatum[27], further indicating lack of involvement of adenylyl cyclase.

Activation of protein kinase C enhances action potential-evoked dopamine release from rat and rabbit brain slices. It is possible that dopamine may inhibit this pathway but, to date, appropriate interaction experiments to yield a definitive answer have not been conducted.

Again, as with the other inhibitory receptors, the balance of evidence suggests direct ion channel involvement in inhibitory dopamine $D_2$ modulation of neurotransmitter release, rather than mediation by second messengers (see refs. 28 and 41).

## 6.8  Adenosine receptors

Adenosine inhibits evoked release of many neurotransmitters from both peripheral nerves and in the CNS[19]. The inhibitory effect of adenosine on noradrenaline release and noradrenergic neuro-effector transmission has been particularly well described (see also Chapter 7) and is thought to be mediated by adenosine $A_1$ receptors. Adenosine receptors have the general structure expected of G-protein-linked receptors and there is evidence that G-proteins are involved in the inhibitory effects of adenosine on neurotransmitter release. For example, preincubation with *N*-ethylmaleimide reduced the inhibitory effect of adenosine and $A_1$ receptor agonists on noradrenaline and acetylcholine release from rat hippocampus slices (see ref. 18). A similar effect was seen with pertussis toxin[24], although it has been suggested that pertussis toxin-insensitive G-proteins may also be involved in some adenosine effects on transmitter release[18].

Adenosine $A_1$ receptors are often negatively coupled to adenylyl cyclase to reduce the production of cAMP. However, the presynaptic inhibitory effects of adenosine were not modified in rat hippocampal slices when intracellular levels of cAMP were elevated (see ref. 18). Similarly, inhibition of adenylyl cyclase by other means did not affect the inhibitory effect of adenosine on neurotransmitter release (see ref. 18). These results suggest that a decrease in cAMP levels is not the fundamental route through which presynaptic $A_1$ receptors mediate the inhibition of noradrenaline release.

The protein kinase inhibitor staurosporine did not modify inhibition of acetylcholine release by adenosine agonists in the rat hippocampus[18]. This tends to contraindicate the postulated involvement of protein kinase, C and probably other protein kinases given the wide spectrum of kinase inhibition by staurosporine.

In summary, second messenger enzyme-linked signal transduction appears not to be wholly responsible for mediating the inhibitory effects of adenosine on transmitter release and, again, an ion channel mechanism has been postulated[18], particularly voltage-sensitive $Ca^{2+}$ channels. Inhibition of voltage-sensitive $Ca^{2+}$ channels may be indirect, occurring secondarily as a consequence of membrane hyperpolarisation caused by an increase in $K^+$ conductance (see also Chapter 10). The exact mechanism has yet to be elucidated.

## 7  Interactions between presynaptic receptors

There is evidence that presynaptic receptor systems interact with one another. For example, blockade of autoinhibitory α-adrenoceptors is necessary to reveal opioid inhibition of transmitter release in some tissues. This has been explained in terms of the two systems sharing signal transduction mechanisms, or at least G-proteins, such that the appearance of one receptor's effect is limited by the pre-existing activation of the common pathway by the other receptor[24]. Identification of signal transduction mechanisms may ultimately explain these types of interaction. For example, in sympathetic nerves, the non-additive nature of the enhancing effects of ACTH and isoprenaline but the additive effects of ACTH and angiotensin II on noradrenaline release can be explained as follows. In the former case, the pair of agents compete for the adenylyl cyclase pathway while, in the latter case, the angiotensin II recruits also the parallel protein kinase C pathway[10].

## 8  Summary

In three specific cases, β-adrenoceptors, ACTH receptors and angiotensin II receptors, the signal transduction pathways between receptor and release process have been identified as enzyme-linked mechanisms (adenylyl cyclase for the first two, and protein kinase C for angiotensin II). It is interesting to note that all three systems are hormone-initiated systems in which circulating levels of hormones (adrenaline, ACTH and angiotensin II) may activate these receptors over a prolonged period. Furthermore they are all facilitatory systems.

By comparison, from studies so far conducted, the release-inhibiting receptors ($\alpha$-adrenoceptor, dopamine, neuropeptide Y, serotonin, adenosine and muscarinic) appear not to involve enzyme-linked signal transduction processes. However, the focus has generally been on adenylyl cyclase and protein kinase C systems, and it may be that there are as yet undiscovered pathways that play a crucial role. Notwithstanding, it is clear that if the concept of pulse-to-pulse modulation of transmitter release is to be sustained, a fast activation rate and deactivation rate of modulation is required. This may be better served by direct modulation of ion channels without an intervening slow enzyme step, particularly in the case of modulation through presynaptic receptors that are autoreceptors, since the requirement in these cases is to provide a fast feedback of information to the neurone (see Chapters 4 and 5). Another indication against the involvement of second messengers mediating inhibition of neurotransmitter release is that the second messengers known to be involved in neuronal function, cAMP, diacylglycerol and $Ca^{2+}$, all tend to enhance transmitter release. Accordingly, for inhibitory pathways involving second messengers to function, there would need to be a pre-existing high basal production of second messenger, which is then inhibited. This is not an economical mechanism. In addition, existing evidence does not support the notion that there is a normal component of transmitter release that is maintained by second messengers. It is not unexpected, therefore, that the balance of evidence does not favour the involvement of enzyme-linked signal trans-

duction processes in the modulation of neurotransmitter release by inhibitory receptors. Direct ion channel involvement is perhaps more likely (see Chapter 10).

## References

1. Alberts P and Ögren VR (1988) Interaction of forskolin with the effect of atropine on [$^3$H]-acetylcholine secretion in guinea-pig ileum myenteric plexus. *Journal of Physiology* **395:** 441–453

2. Allgaier C, Daschmann B, Huang HY and Hertting G (1988) Protein kinase C and presynaptic modulation of acetylcholine release in rabbit hippocampus. *British Journal of Pharmacology* **93:** 525–534

3. Allgaier C, Daschmann B, Sieverling J and Hertting G (1989) Protein kinase C activation and $\alpha_2$-autoreceptor-modulated release of noradrenaline. *British Journal of Pharmacology* **92:** 161–172

4. Allgaier C and Hertting G (1986) Polymyxin B, a selective inhibitor of protein kinase C diminishes the release of noradrenaline and the enhancement of release caused by phorbol 12,13-butyrate. *Naunyn-Schmiedeberg's Archives of Pharmacology* **334:** 218–221

5. Allgaier C, Hertting G, Huang HY and Jackish R (1987) Protein kinase C activation and $\alpha_2$-autoreceptor modulated release of noradrenaline. *British Journal of Pharmacology* **92:** 161–172

6. Axelrod J, Burch RM and Jelsma CL (1988) Receptor-mediated activation of phospholipase $A_2$ via GTP binding proteins: arachidonic acid and its metabolites as second messengers. *Trends in Neuroscience* **11:** 117–123

7. Bockaert J (1991) G-proteins and G-protein coupled receptors: structure, function and interactions. *Current Opinions in Neurobiology* **1:** 32–42

8. Boehm S, Huck S, Drobny H and Singer EA (1992) Pertussis toxin abolishes the inhibition of $Ca^{2+}$ currents and of noradrenaline release via $\alpha_2$-adrenoceptors in chick sympathetic neurons. *Naunyn-Schmiedeberg's Archives of Pharmacology* **345:** 606–609

9. Bowyer JF and Weiner N (1989) $K^+$-channel and adenylyl cyclase involvement in regulation of $Ca^{2+}$ evoked release of [$^3$H]-dopamine from

synaptosomes. *Journal of Pharmacology and Experimental Therapeutics* **248:** 514–520

10. Costa M and Majewski H (1988) Facilitation of noradrenaline release from sympathetic nerves through activation of ACTH receptors, β-adrenoceptors and angiotensin II receptors. *British Journal of Pharmacology* **95:** 993–1001

11. Costa M and Majewski H (1990) Inhibitory prejunctional muscarinic receptors at sympathetic nerves do not operate through a cAMP dependent pathway. *Naunyn-Schmiedeberg's Archives of Pharmacology* **342:** 630–639

12. Cubeddu LX, Barnes E and Weiner N (1975) Release of norepinephrine and dopamine-β-hydroxylase by nerve stimulation. IV. An evaluation of a role for cyclic adenosine monophosphate. *Journal of Pharmacology and Experimental Therapeutics* **193:** 105–127

13. Ewald DA, Sternweiss PC and Miller RJ (1988) Guanine nucleotide-binding protein $G_o$-induced coupling of neuropeptide Y receptors to $Ca^{++}$ channels in sensory neurones. *Proceedings of the National Academy of Sciences, USA* **85:** 3633–3637

14. Foucart S and Majewski H (1989) Inhibition of noradrenaline release by neuropeptide Y in mouse atria does not involve inhibition of adenylyl cyclase or a pertussis toxin susceptible G-protein. *Naunyn-Schmiedeberg's Archives of Pharmacology* **340:** 658–665

15. Foucart S, Murphy TV and Majewski H (1990) Prejunctional β-adrenoceptors, angiotensin II and neuropeptide Y receptors on sympathetic nerves in mouse atria are linked to *N*-ethylmaleimide-susceptible G-proteins. *Journal of the Autonomic Nervous System* **30:** 221–232

16. Foucart S, Musgrave IF and Majewski H (1990) Inhibition of noradrenaline release by neuropeptide Y does not involve protein kinase C in mouse atria. *Neuropeptides* **15:** 179–185

17. Foucart S, Musgrave IF, Majewski H (1991) Long term treatment with phorbol esters suggests a permissive role for protein kinase C in the enhancement of noradrenaline release. *Molecular Neuropharmacology* **1:** 95–101

18. Fredholm BB, Duner-Engstrom M, Fastbom J, Ping-Sheng H and van der Ploeg I (1990) Role of G-proteins, cyclic AMP, and ion channels in the inhibition of transmitter release by adenosine. *Annals of the New York Academy of Sciences* **604:** 237–249

19. Fredholm BB and Dunwiddie TV (1988) How does adenosine inhibit transmitter release? *Trends in Pharmacological Sciences* **9:** 130–134

20. Fredholm BB and Lindgren E (1987) Effects of *N*-ethylmaleimide and forskolin on noradrenaline release from rat hippocampal slices. evidence that prejunctional adenosine and α-receptors are linked to *N*-proteins, but not to adenylyl cyclase. *Acta Physiologica Scandinavica* **130:** 95–105

21. Göthert M and Hentrich F (1984) Role of cAMP for regulation of impulse-evoked noradrenaline release from the rabbit pulmonary artery and its possible relationship to presynaptic ACTH receptors. *Naunyn-Schmiedeberg's Archives of Pharmacology* **328:** 127–134

22. Greenberg SS, Diecke FPJ, Curro FA, Peevy K and Tanaka TP (1988) Presynaptic modulation of sympathetic neurotransmitter release by modulators of cyclic 3′,5′-guanosine monophosphate in canine vascular smooth muscle. *Annals of the New York Academy of Sciences* **604:** 305–322

23. Harper JF (1988) Stimulus–secretion coupling: second messenger-regulated exocytosis. *Advances in Second Messenger and Phosphoprotein Research* **22:** 193–318

24. Hertting G, Wurster S and Allgaier C (1990) Regulatory proteins in presynaptic function. *Annals of the New York Academy of Sciences* **604:** 289–304

25. Majewski H (1983) Modulation of noradrenaline release through prejunctional β-adrenoceptors. *Journal of Autonomic Pharmacology* **3:** 47–60

26. Majewski H, Costa M, Foucart S, Murphy TV and Musgrave IF (1990) Second messengers are involved in facilitatory but not inhibitory receptor actions at sympathetic nerve ending. *Annals of the New York Academy of Sciences* **604:** 266–275

27. Memo M, Missale C, Carruba MO and Spano PF (1986) D-2 dopamine receptors associated with inhibition of dopamine release from rat striatum are independent of cAMP. *Neuroscience Letters* **71:** 192–196

28. Mulder AH, Schoffelmeer AN and Stoof JC (1990) On the role of adenylyl cyclase in presynaptic modulation of neurotransmitter release mediated by monoamine and opioid receptors in the brain. *Annals of the New York Academy of Sciences* **604:** 237–249

29. Murphy TV, Foucart S and Majewski H (1992)

Prejunctional $\alpha_2$-adrenoceptors in mouse atria function through G-proteins which are sensitive to $N$-ethylmaleimide, but not pertussis toxin. *British Journal of Pharmacology* **106:** 871–876

30. Murphy TV and Majewski H (1990) Pertussis toxin differentiates between $\alpha_1$ and $\alpha_2$-adrenoceptor mediated inhibition of noradrenaline release from rat kidney cortex. *European Journal of Pharmacology* **179:** 435–439

31. Musgrave IF, Foucart S and Majewski H (1991) Evidence that angiotensin II enhances noradrenaline release from sympathetic nerves in mouse atria by activating protein kinase C. *Journal of Autonomic Pharmacology* **11:** 211–220

32. Musgrave IF and Majewski H (1989) Effect of phorbol esters and polymyxin B on modulation of noradrenaline release in mouse atria. *Naunyn-Schmiedeberg's Archives of Pharmacology* **339:** 48–53

33. Musgrave IF, Marley P and Majewski H (1987) Pertussis toxin does not attenuate $\alpha_2$-adrenoceptor mediated inhibition of noradrenaline release in mouse atria. *Naunyn-Schmiedeberg's Archives of Pharmacology* **336:** 280–286

34. Nestler EJ and Greengard P (1989) Protein phosphorylation and regulation of neuronal function. In: Siegel GJ, Agranoff BW, Albers RW and Molinoff PB (eds), *Basic Neurochemistry: Molecular, Cellular and Medical Aspects*, 4th edn, pp 373–398, Raven Press, New York

35. Nishizuka Y (1989) Studies and prospectives of the protein kinase C family for cellular regulation. *Cancer* **63:** 1892–1903

36. Nordström Ö and Bartfai T (1981) 8-Br-cyclic GMP mimics activation of muscarinic autoreceptors and inhibits acetylcholine release from rat hippocampal slices. *Brain Research* **213:** 467–471

37. Receptor Nomenclature Supplement (1993) *Trends in Pharmacological Sciences* **14** (Suppl)

38. Schoffelmeer ANM, Wierenga EA and Mulder AH (1986) Role of adenylyl cyclase in presynaptic $\alpha_2$-adrenoceptor and $\mu$-opioid receptor mediated inhibition of [$^3$H]-noradrenaline release from rat brain cortex slices. *Journal of Neurochemistry* **46:** 1711–1717

39. Shulka SD and Halenda SP (1991) Phospholipase D in cell signalling and its relationship to phospholipase C. *Life Science* **48:** 851–866

40. Shuntoh H, Taniyama K, Fukuzaki H and Tanaka C (1988) Inhibition by cAMP of phorbol ester-potentiated norepinephrine release from guinea-pig brain cortical synaptosomes. *Journal of Neurochemistry* **51:** 1565–1572

41. Starke K, Göthert M and Kilbinger H (1989) Modulation of neurotransmitter release by presynaptic autoreceptors. *Physiological Reviews* **69:** 864–989

42. Vo PA, Reid JJ and Rand MJ (1992) Attenuation of vasoconstriction by endogenous nitric oxide in rat caudal artery. *British Journal of Pharmacology* **107:** 1121–1128

43. Wahlestedt C, Edvinsson L, Ekblad E, Håkanson R (1987) Effects of neuropeptide Y at sympathetic neuroeffector junctions: existence of Y1 and Y2-receptors. In: Nobin A, Owman C, Arneklo-Nobin B (eds), *Neuronal Messengers in Vascular Function,* pp 231–242, Elsevier, Amsterdam,

44. Wakade TD, Bhave SV, Bhave AS, Malhotra RK and Wakade AR (1991) Depolarizing stimuli and neurotransmitters utilize separate pathways to activate protein kinase C. *Journal of Biological Chemistry* **266:** 6424–6428

45. Yokotani K and Osumi Y (1993) Cholinergic $M_2$ muscarinic receptor-mediated inhibition of endogenous noradrenaline release from the isolated vascularly perfused rat stomach. *Journal of Pharmacology and Experimental Therapeutics* **264:** 54–60

# 10 Regulation of calcium influx as a basis for modulation of neurotransmitter release

David Bleakman and Richard J. Miller

Following on from the previous chapter, Richard Miller and David Bleakman consider the possible mechanisms of regulating intracellular free $Ca^{2+}$ availability that do not involve a biochemical second messenger molecule as an intermediate. The basic scheme here is that combination of the extracellular modulator molecule with the neuronal cell-surface receptor results in a series of events restricted to the neuronal cell membrane itself that results in more or less $Ca^{2+}$ influx through $Ca^{2+}$ channels. This then regulates directly the availability of free $Ca^{2+}$ at the site of neurotransmitter release.

## 1  Introduction

The amount of neurotransmitter released at a nerve terminal following an action potential is not constant and may be modified by several processes. For example, most neurones have receptors located on their presynaptic terminals, activation of which has frequently been observed to reduce the evoked release of transmitter, a process known as 'presynaptic inhibition'. In some cases, the opposite has been observed and the amount of transmitter released per impulse is enhanced. How can these events be explained at the molecular level? It is $Ca^{2+}$ influx via $Ca^{2+}$-permeable conductances (voltage-sensitive $Ca^{2+}$ channels (VSCC) or ligand-gated conductances) following an action potential that is thought to be the crucial trigger for neurotransmitter release[4] (see also Chapter 1).

The extracellular $Ca^{2+}$ concentration is approximately 2 mM, whereas the intracellular free $Ca^{2+}$ concentration is approximately 100 nM, and is kept at this low level by a variety of $Ca^{2+}$ buffering and extrusion mechanisms[23]. In response to depolarisation, VSCC open and $Ca^{2+}$ entry into the nerve terminal occurs down the large electrochemical gradient. Experiments in a variety of preparations have shown that the amount of transmitter released following an action potential increases in a non-linear manner with changes in the extracellular $Ca^{2+}$ concentration[3]. In fact, the amount of transmitter released has been estimated to be related to the fourth power of the extracellular $Ca^{2+}$ concentration. Since many $Ca^{2+}$-dependent processes are regulated by $Ca^{2+}$ influx in a non-linear manner, even relatively small changes in the amount of $Ca^{2+}$ influx can be expected to have profound effects on neuronal function.

In this chapter, the routes of $Ca^{2+}$ influx into neurones via both voltage-sensitive and ligand-gated $Ca^{2+}$ channels in vertebrate neurones are described. How modulation of $Ca^{2+}$ entry via the different routes can lead to changes in the degree of evoked neurotransmitter release is also considered.

## 2 Modulatory mechanisms directly involving $Ca^{2+}$ conductances

### 2.1 Voltage-sensitive $Ca^{2+}$ channels

The primary pathway for $Ca^{2+}$ influx into neurones following depolarisation is via VSCC. As indicated above, it is this influx that triggers neurotransmitter release and also provides $Ca^{2+}$ for the control of other neuronal functions, such as the control of cellular metabolism and excitability. The control of neuronal excitability can be short term, as exemplified by modulation of $Ca^{2+}$-activated ionic conductances, or longer term, as exemplified by changes in synaptic efficacy manifest in phenomena such as long-term potentiation or long-term depression.

Several recent reviews have appeared that address the topics of structure and regulation of these channels[5,9,25]. Although much progress has been made in understanding the role of $Ca^{2+}$ influx pathways in the process of triggering neurotransmitter release, in most instances considerable uncertainty remains concerning the channel types that modulate release.

#### 2.1.1 Classification and localisation of VSCC

One of the first attempts to characterise vertebrate neuronal VSCC was made by Nowycky et al.[29], using chick dorsal root ganglion neurones. Their classification was based on the biophysical properties of the channels and their sensitivity to pharmacological antagonists. This initial characterisation has proved to have considerable general utility and has now been expanded in several respects.

Nowycky et al. described three channel types. One low-voltage-activated (LVA) and two high-voltage-activated (HVA) types. Most neurones at rest have membrane potentials which range between $-90$ and $-60$ mV and it is a change in this potential that results in the opening of VSCC. Low-voltage activated, or T-type VSCC, have a low threshold of activation and are activated at a membrane potential of $-70$ mV. They inactivate rapidly when the depolarisation is maintained hence the name 'T', which denotes transient. The T-type VSCC have a single-channel conductance of 8 pS (in 100 mM $Ba^{2+}$) and are relatively insensitive to ω-conotoxin GVIA, a peptide toxin from the cone snail mollusc *Conus geographus* and dihydropyridines, blockers of N- and L-type VSCC, respectively (see below). The T-type VSCC are distributed widely in the central and peripheral nervous system and are thought to be involved in the generation of burst-firing patterns in neurones[37].

Nowycky et al.[29] also described two HVA $Ca^{2+}$ channels in dorsal root ganglion neurones which they called L- and N-type VSCC. The separation of these channel types on the basis of their biophysical characteristics is less clear, and they are probably better separated on the basis of the effects of selective drugs. The L-type VSCC are the targets of dihydropyridine agonists and antagonists (Table 10.1), as well as various phenylalkylamine and dibenzothiazepine $Ca^{2+}$-channel blockers. The L-type VSCC in neurones appear similar to those found in cardiac and smooth muscle, where they control contractility by regulating $Ca^{2+}$ influx. The L-type VSCC have a large single-channel conductance (25 pS). Voltage-dependent inactivation is slow or absent, hence 'L' which denotes long lasting. However, L-type VSCC do tend to inactivate as a consequence of $Ca^{2+}$-dependent processes within the cell (see Section 10.2.1.6).

The N-type VSCC is another type of HVA $Ca^{2+}$ channel, with a single-channel conductance of approximately 13 pS. Unlike L-type VSCC, N-type VSCC do undergo relatively slow voltage-dependent inactivation in some cases. The N-type VSCC are specifically blocked by ω-conotoxin GVIA. The block produced by this toxin is functionally irreversible (the off-rate is extremely slow, taking hours to reverse), although similar toxins from related cone snails sometimes block 'reversibly'.

In general, a rigid classification of VSCC is

Table 10.1. *Classes of voltage-sensitive $Ca^{2+}$ channel and agents that facilitate or inhibit flux of $Ca^{2+}$*

|  | T | N | L | P |
|---|---|---|---|---|
| Inorganic ion block | $Ni^{2+} > Cd^{2+}$ | $Cd^{2+} > Ni^{2+}$ | $Cd^{2+} > Ni^{2+}$ | $Cd^{2+} > Ni^{2+}$ |
| Pharmacological inhibition | Dihydropyridines $(>10\ \mu M)$[13] |  | Dihydropyridines; nimodipine, nifedipine, nicardipine |  |
|  | Octanol $(>100\ \mu M)$ |  | Phenylalkyamine: verapamil |  |
|  | Amiloride $(>100\ \mu M)$ |  | Benzothiazepine: diltiazem |  |
| Pharmacological facilitation |  |  | Dihydropyridines: BAY K 8644 |  |
| Toxin sensitivity | sFTX | ω-CgTx GVIA ω-CmTx MVIIC | Calciceptin | ω-Aga IVA, FTX ω-CmTx MVIIC |

sFTX, synthetic funnel web spider polyamine; FTX, polyamine fraction of funnel web spider venom; ω-CgTx GVIA, ω-conotoxin, polypeptide toxin from *Conus geographicus;* ω-CmTx MVIIC, ω-conotoxin, polypeptide from *Conus magnus;* ω-aga IVA, polypeptide toxin isolated from venom of *Agelenopsis aperta.*

probably an oversimplification. The 'classes' discussed above probably represent closely related families of proteins, subunit combinations and splice variants, which would be expected to exhibit many subtle differences in channel properties in individual instances. Indeed, it is already known that two separate genes, both found in the nervous system, produce L-type VSCC when expressed in frog oocytes (see Section 10.2.1.3). Already, the classification originally proposed by Nowycky *et al.* has needed some revision. For example, recently, other types of VSCC have been identified in the nervous system. The P-type VSCC was first described in mammalian Purkinje neurones[19]. The insensitivity of this HVA $Ca^{2+}$ channel to any of the 'classical' antagonists of L- or N-type VSCC has led to its acceptance as a new channel type. The P-type VSCC have single-channel conductances of 9–19 pS in Purkinje cells and the currents obtained are sustained during depolarisation. This type of channel may be selectively blocked by components of the venom of the funnel web spider, *Agelenopsis aperta,* such as ω-agatoxin IVA or FTX (Table 10.1). On

the basis that they are insensitive to the range of pharmacological agents used to classify N-, T- and L-type $Ca^{2+}$ channels, other types of HVA VSCC clearly also exist. However, their biophysical properties and pharmacology are as yet poorly defined[21].

The various types of VSCC are heterogeneously distributed among different types of neurone. For example, T-type VSCC have been described in many central and peripheral neurones, such as inferior olive[20], hippocampal[26] and dorsal root ganglion neurones[14]. Myenteric and sympathetic neurones possess both N- and L-type but no T-type VSCC[17], whereas chick and rat sensory neurones contain all three types[33]. In the CNS, CA3 hippocampal neurones appear to possess T-, L-, N- and P-type VSCC[26].

It is important to realise that most electrophysiological studies in neurones have been performed on the cell body, mainly because of size considerations. However, when transmitter release is considered, it is clearly the nerve terminal that is the important region. Relatively little is known about the types of $Ca^{2+}$ channels that are found in nerve terminals. The use of site-directed antipeptide antibodies that recognise $Ca^{2+}$-channel subunits specific for N- and L-type VSCC have suggested that L-type VSCC are distributed primarily in neuronal cell bodies and proximal dendrites of central neurones. By comparison, N-type VSCC appear to be predominantly localised on dendritic shafts and punctate synaptic structures, which may represent presynaptic terminals. In the periphery, both L-type (dihydropyridine-sensitive) and non-L-type (dihydropyridine-insensitive) VSCC have been found in somata, along neurites and in growth cones of sympathetic neurones. The $Ca^{2+}$ channels that have been recorded in the presynaptic terminals of chick ciliary ganglion neurones are insensitive to dihydropyiridines but are blocked by $\omega$-conotoxin GVIA, which suggests that they are N-type VSCC. Indeed, transmitter release from sympathetic neurones is selectively blocked by $\omega$-conotoxin GVIA. This observation has encouraged the view that N-type VSCC in particular might normally be those associated with neurotransmitter release[33]. This is addressed below.

### 2.1.2  Pharmacological antagonism and the effects of toxins on VSCC

Table 10.1 summarises some of the discussion so far on the effects of agents that are purported to act selectively at the different classes of VSCC. Dihydropyridines appear to be selective for L-type VSCC (see Fleckenstein[13], for review), although certain reports have suggested that these may also block T-type VSCC. No information is available yet about the pharmacology of individual L-type clones (C and D, see below) but subtle differences may be expected. The toxin $\omega$-conotoxin GVIA has become a useful tool for investigating N-type VSCC. However, related $\omega$-conotoxins show interesting differences in their blocking profiles, suggesting that some heterogeneity in the class of N-type VSCC may also exist. The funnel web spider *Agelenopsis aperta* produces toxins such as the polyamine FTX and

the polypeptide $\omega$-agatoxin IVA, which have been shown to act on P-type $Ca^{2+}$ channels. For $\omega$-agatoxin IVA, the block of P-type VSCC appears to result from binding to the closed state of the channel. There are other toxins also found in spider venom that may block L- or N-type channels as well (e.g. $\omega$-agatoxin IIIA) and the venom of the black mamba contains a 60 amino acid residue peptide called calciseptin that blocks L-type $Ca^{2+}$ channels. A synthetic FTX has been shown to block T-type VSCC at low concentrations[31]. Other agents such as octanol and amiloride also block T-type VSCC. However, their usefulness may be limited because of their lack of specific selectivity towards VSCC.

### 2.1.3  Molecular biology of VSCC

The heterogeneity of VSCC detected in electrophysiological studies is further supported by molecular biological studies[24]. Most data available at present concern the L-type $Ca^{2+}$ channels isolated from skeletal muscle, a tissue that contains an unusually high concentration of high-affinity dihydropyridine-binding sites. The subunit structure of the skeletal muscle dihydropyridine-binding site has been taken as the archetype for other VSCC. Recent studies of L-type VSCC from other tissues, including brain, as well as of N- and P-type VSCC have indicated the validity of this assumption. Therefore, functional expression of all these channels appears to require subunit combinations that are similar to those found in skeletal muscle.

Solubilisation and reconstitution studies on the skeletal muscle dihydropyridine-binding site originally suggested that it is a multisubunit complex consisting of four major and distinct subunits: $\alpha_1$ (170 kDa), $\alpha_2/\delta$ (175 kDa), $\beta$ (52 kDa) and $\gamma$ (32 kDa). The $\alpha_1$-subunit shows high sequence homology to previously cloned and isolated voltage-gated $Na^+$ and $K^+$ channels. The $\alpha_1$-subunit from skeletal muscle appears to contain the dihydropyridine-binding site. Expression studies using this protein in the skeletal muscles of mutant mice suggest that it can reconstitute

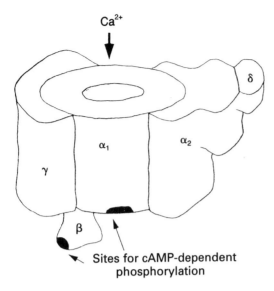

Fig. 10.1. Proposed model of Ca$^{2+}$-channel structure. Sites of cyclic nucleotide-dependent phosphorylation are indicated. The $\alpha_1$-subunit contains four homologous transmembrane domains (analogous to the rat brain Na$^+$ channel $\alpha$-subunit) and is the site for Ca$^{2+}$-antagonist binding. Although the $\alpha_1$-subunit alone can form a functional Ca$^{2+}$ channel, the presence of $\alpha_2$ and $\beta$-subunits dramatically enhance current flow through the channel. Alterations in the $\alpha_1$-subunit result in a different Ca$^{2+}$-channel type, e.g. $\alpha_{1B}$ and $\alpha_{1C/D}$ result in an N- and L-type VSCC, respectively.

both the Ca$^{2+}$ channel and other functions of the dihydropyridine receptor in this tissue. A related $\alpha_1$-subunit has been found in cardiac muscle. Interestingly, when this $\alpha_1$-subunit is expressed in mouse muscle, it produces Ca$^{2+}$ channels with properties similar to those normally found in cardiac rather than skeletal muscle. Therefore, it is currently believed that the $\alpha_1$-subunit is responsible for the major functional and pharmacological properties of each Ca$^{2+}$-channel class. There is evidence for at least five types of $\alpha_1$-subunit in brain (denoted A, B, C, D and E), which all differ from the skeletal muscle $\alpha_1$-subunit (see Fig. 10.1). The clone designated C is the same as that found in cardiac muscle.

The $\alpha_2/\delta$- and $\beta$-subunits appear to inter-

act physically with the $\alpha_1$-subunit. There is evidence that they may play a functional role in modifying the kinetic properties of the VSCC and also their functional expression in the plasma membrane. Interestingly, the $\beta$-subunit contains several consensus phosphorylation sites, which would make it a good target for regulatory action. Antisera directed against this subunit have been shown to co-precipitate specifically bound dihydropyridines and/or $\omega$-conotoxin GVIA, suggesting that $\beta$-subunits may form part of the N-type VSCC in brain as well as part of the L-type VSCC.

A particularly important question to answer is which of the $\alpha_1$-subunits cloned by molecular biologists correspond to the various Ca$^{2+}$-channel classes defined by physiologists and pharmacologists? Expression of the different $\alpha_1$-clones in oocytes or cultured cells has been used to examine their functional properties. Williams et al.[38] have demonstrated that co-expression of the human $\alpha_{1B}$-subunit with the $\alpha_2/\delta$- and $\beta$-subunits in HEK 293 cells results in an N-type VSCC, which is irreversibly blocked by $\omega$-conotoxin GVIA. Similarly, expression of the brain $\alpha_{1A}$-subunit produces a channel which is unaffected by dihydopyridines or $\omega$-conotoxin GVIA but is blocked by 'crude' Agelenopsis aperta venom. Such pharmacological characteristics, together with its expression in Purkinje cells, are suggestive of the P-type VSCC, although some differences may exist.

Finally, the $\alpha_1$-subunit clone E (which is also designated by other synonymous labels: BII or X) has recently been expressed in oocytes and HEK 293 cells, although its pharmacology has yet to be fully described. However, its sequence is more homologous to that of dihydropyridine-resistant channels (containing $\alpha_1$-subunit clones A and B) than to that of the dihydropyridine-sensitive channels (clones C and D). As Ca$^{2+}$ currents have been recorded from neurones that are clearly not blocked by the various blockers described above, it is likely that one or more major classes of VSCC still remain to be characterised. It may be that the newly expressed clone E is responsible for such currents.

### 2.1.4 Neurotransmitter release and Ca$^{2+}$ channels

The identities of the VSCC which regulate neurotransmitter release remains elusive. This is partly because of technical problems. Nerve terminals are generally small structures and are, therefore, inaccessible to conventional electrophysiological studies. In rare instances, such as with the large presynaptic terminals of the squid giant synapse, such studies can be performed since their size does not preclude direct recordings.

Notwithstanding, in vertebrates, N-type VSCC have been identified in the presynaptic nerve terminals of the chick cilary ganglion calyx[32]. Lemos and Nowycky[18] have measured Ca$^{2+}$ currents in the large peptide-containing neuronal terminals of the neurohypophysis. These terminals, which release oxytocin and vasopressin, are in the size range 1–10 μm and recordings suggest that they contain both L- and N-type VSCC. In the CNS, Johnston and colleagues[15] have recorded directly from the terminals of mossy fibres innervating the hippocampus and have demonstrated the presence of Ca$^{2+}$ channels with properties of both L- and N-type VSCC. Therefore, the nerve terminals often seem to contain channels with similar characteristics to channels found in the cell soma. The question to be answered is whether all of the channels found in the nerve terminals influence the release of all types of transmitter released from a given terminal or whether a particular channel type is associated with the release of just one transmitter.

Catecholamine release from sympathetic neurones appears to involve mainly N-type VSCC (see review by Anwyl[1]) and is abolished by ω-conotoxin GVIA. In accord with this, transmission at sympathetic neuro-effector junctions is, in general, relatively insensitive to dihydropyridines. The role of N-type VSCC at sympathetic nerve terminals has been indicated by studies using fluorescent derivatives of ω-conotoxin GVIA to show its histological localisation at 'active zones' of transmitter release. In the myenteric plexus of the guinea-pig ileum, the release of acetylcholine produced by nicotinic agonists also appears to be mediated by N-type VSCC. In some studies, N-type VSCC have also been shown to control transmitter release in the vertebrate CNS. For example, in the dorsal horn of the spinal cord of the rat, the release of substance P and CGRP can be reduced by 70% by ω-conotoxin GVIA. This toxin also blocks the release of GABA, glutamate and noradrenaline from the hippocampus and inhibits the synaptic potentials caused by the release of both GABA and glutamate. In general, therefore, there are several instances in which N-type VSCC have been specifically linked to the release of neurotransmitters. Even though N- and L-type VSCC apparently co-exist in some nerve terminals, there is little effect on neurotransmitter release by agents such as dihydropyridines, which block L-type VSCC (but see Chapter 13 for the situation in adrenal medullary chromaffin cells). The reason for this is not clear but may suggest that Ca$^{2+}$ domains which influence Ca$^{2+}$ influx through the different channel types are highly localised within the nerve terminal.

It is clear that N-type VSCC are not always linked to the release of neurotransmitters. The major portion of the depolarisation-induced Ca$^{2+}$ influx into rat brain synaptosomes and the release of some transmitters from this preparation (e.g. glutamate) are not blocked by ω-conotoxin GVIA but are potently blocked by ω-agatoxin IVA[35] (interestingly the opposite situation occurs in the chick). Thus, P-type VSCC apparently can also play a role in neurotransmitter release. In addition, a polyamine fraction of the venom from *Agelenopsis aperta*, FTX, has been shown to abolish transmitter release at some mammalian neuromuscular junctions[36] that are insensitive to ω-conotoxin GVIA and dihydropyridines.

In conclusion, the type of VSCC that controls transmitter release at most synapses has not been clearly defined. The N-type

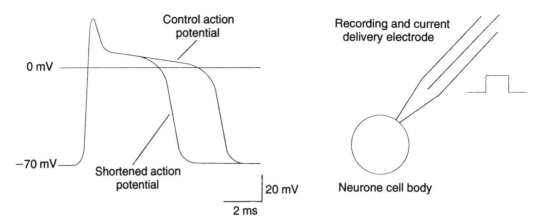

Fig. 10.2. Action potentials may be evoked by passing brief (approximately 1 ms) current pulses through an electrode applied to the neuronal cell body. The trace shows a representative reduction in the duration of the action potential caused by a neuromodulator. Examples of neuromodulators that have this effect include noradrenaline, 5-HT and GABA.

channels certainly seem to play this role in some cases. However, in other instances other channel types may be involved.

### 2.1.5  Receptor-mediated modulation of $Ca^{2+}$ influx through VSCC

Neurotransmitter-induced reductions or increases in $Ca^{2+}$ influx into neurones were originally inferred from electrophysiological studies in which the shape of the action potential was examined. Agents thought to reduce $Ca^{2+}$ influx were found to decrease the duration of the $Ca^{2+}$ spike or the $Ca^{2+}$ component of a mixed $Ca^{2+}/Na^+$ spike (Fig. 10.2).

In dorsal root ganglion neurones, transmitters such as noradrenaline, GABA, dopamine, adrenaline, 5-HT, substance P, opioids and somatostatin were shown to reduce the duration of the $Ca^{2+}$ action potential. Similar effects are produced by noradrenaline, acetylcholine and dopamine in sympathetic neurones and by dopamine and adenosine in the CA1 region of the hippocampus. Such data have supported the view that activation of several types of receptor can lead to inhibition of neuronal VSCC. However, subsequent voltage-clamp record-

ings were necessary to confirm this view, since the shape of the action potential can also be altered by $K^+$-channel activation or inhibition (see below). Therefore, electrophysiological recordings are performed in which currents carried by $Ca^{2+}$ influx through VSCC are measured in relative isolation from other types of channel by using appropriate ionic substitutions and stimulation paradigms.

**Inhibitory modulators of VSCC.** There is now a large body of evidence in the literature describing the effects of activating neurotransmitter receptors and the subsequent modulation of $Ca^{2+}$ influx through VSCC[1]. Inhibitory modulation has usually been shown to involve HVA VSCC and in particular the N-type VSCC. Nevertheless, a smaller body of data suggests receptor-mediated modulation of L-, T- and P-type channels. The transduction mechanism of HVA VSCC generally involves a G-protein in the signal transduction mechanism (see Fig. 10.3 and Section 2.1.7). In the case of N-type VSCC, receptor activation results in a shift in the activation characteristics for the channel. This shift and, therefore, inhibition of channel opening can be overcome by

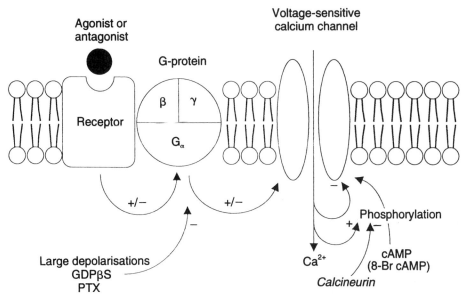

Fig. 10.3. Model showing the possible mechanisms for receptor-mediated modulation of VSCC by neurotransmitters and indicating the sites of interaction of G-proteins, $Ca^{2+}$ and other second messengers.

depolarisation of the cell to very positive membrane potentials or by using a depolarising prepulse[5]. Changes in the channel-gating properties (the opening and closing of the channel) have been demonstrated in single-channel recordings.

In certain cases of inhibitory modulation, second messenger systems have also been implicated, presumably reflecting the change in channel function resulting from a change in the phosphorylation state (see Section 2.1.4). In other cases, a role for second messengers has been excluded. For example, neuropeptide Y has been shown to inhibit $K^+$-depolarisation-induced $Ca^{2+}$ influx through N-type VSCC in myenteric neurones and also to inhibit VSCC currents under whole-cell recording conditions[17]. However, if VSCC currents are recorded in the cell-attached configuration and neuropeptide Y is applied outside the pipette, an inhibition is no longer seen. This suggests that a readily diffusible second messenger is unlikely to be involved in the observed inhibition.

The actions of neuropeptide Y and noradrenaline at a number of peripheral neuro-effector junctions have been particularly well studied. These two transmitters are co-stored in sympathetic neurones and both produce (presynaptic) inhibition of neurotransmitter release. The effects of neuropeptide Y are given as an example, although similar data exist for a number of other modulators. Neuropeptide Y potently inhibits VSCC in neuronal somata of the dorsal root ganglion, myenteric and sympathetic neurones (Fig. 10.4). It also blocks the $Ca^{2+}$ influx that results from the firing of a train of action potentials[7] (see Fig. 10.4b). In dorsal root ganglion neurones, these effects of neuropeptide Y can be blocked by pretreatment with pertussis toxin, indicating the involvement of a G-protein. In addition, infusion of the $G_o$ subunit of the G-protein into dorsal root ganglion neurones pretreated with pertussis toxin recouples the neuropeptide Y receptor to the VSCC[8]. Using combinations of patch clamping and $Ca^{2+}$ imaging[34] (Fig. 10.5, Plate 10.I), the rise in intracellular free $Ca^{2+}$ concentration in individual nerve terminal varicosities produced by firing trains of action potentials has been examined. Atrial

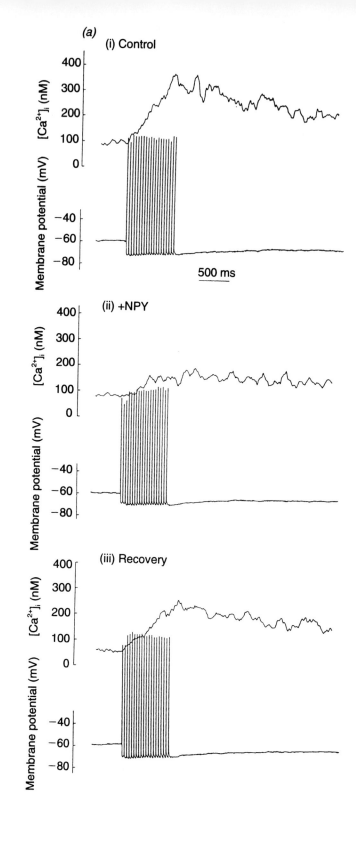

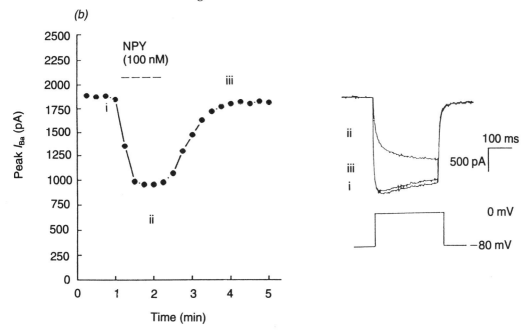

Fig. 10.4. (*a*) Inhibition by neuropeptide Y (NPY, 100 nM) of the action potential-evoked increases in $[Ca^{2+}]_i$ in a single dorsal root ganglion cell. Single cell microfluorimetry using the $Ca^{2+}$-sensitive dye, fura-2, which was present in a patch pipette, was used to measure $[Ca^{2+}]_i$. The cell was stimulated by applying brief depolarising current pulses, under whole-cell recording conditions, which evoked a train of 20 action potentials. This train was repeated every 30 s. The figure shows: (i) a control trace; (ii) a trace recorded 1 min after application of neuropeptide Y (100 nM); and (iii) recovery: a recording made 2.5 min after washout of neuropeptide Y. (*b*) Neuropeptide Y inhibition of VSCC (measured using $Ba^{2+}$ as the charge carrier) in a single dorsal root ganglion neurone. The figure shows the time course of inhibition by neuropeptide Y (100 nM) and the inset shows the individual current traces in the absence and presence of neuropeptide Y. Currents were evoked by depolarising the cell from a holding potential of $-80$ mV to 0 mV under voltage-clamp conditions.

myocytes were co-cultured with sympathetic neurones obtained from the superior cervical ganglia. Functional synapses developed in these cultures and synaptic transmission between neurone and muscle was inhibited by neuropeptide Y. The evoked rise in intracellular free $Ca^{2+}$ concentration in the nerve terminals of these neurones was reduced by both neuropeptide Y and ω-conotoxin GVIA. In the presence of ω-conotoxin GVIA, neuropeptide Y no longer reduced the evoked rise in the intracellular free $Ca^{2+}$ concentration (Plate 10.1). Such results illustrate several important points about $Ca^{2+}$ influx into nerve terminals. First, it is apparent that, in sympathetic nerve terminals, the majority of physiologically evoked $Ca^{2+}$

influx is mediated by the N-type VSCC. Second, presynaptic inhibition produced by neuropeptide Y is associated with inhibition of nerve terminal $Ca^{2+}$ influx. Furthermore, since neuropeptide Y does not inhibit $Ca^{2+}$ influx in the presence of ω-conotoxin GVIA, it appears that the block of the toxin-sensitive channels can entirely explain the ability of neuropeptide Y to produce presynaptic inhibition. If it were to be hypothesised that neuropeptide Y acted to produce presynaptic inhibition by activating $K^+$ channels (see below), then one would have expected to see an inhibition of $Ca^{2+}$ influx by neuropeptide Y, even in the presence of ω-conotoxin GVIA.

Another recent finding is the modulation

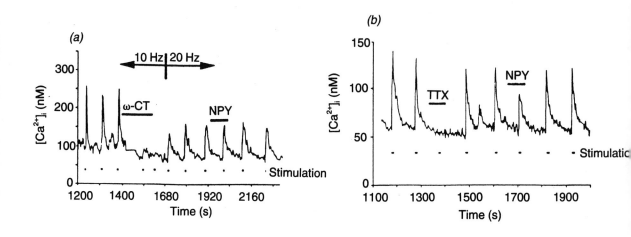

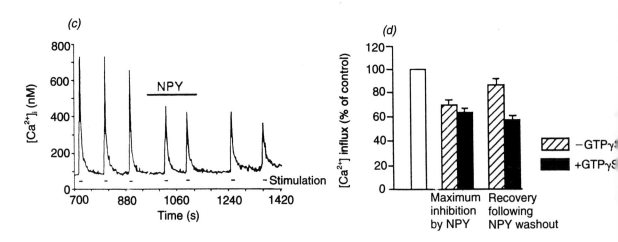

Fig. 10.5. (*a*) Elimination of the effect of neuropeptide Y (300 nM) on $Ca^{2+}$ influx by pretreatment of the culture with ω-conotoxin GVIA (ω-CT). Following toxin treatment, neuropeptide Y had no inhibitory effect on the remaining evoked $Ca^{2+}$ influx. (*b*) A control response, i.e. a promptly reversible decrease in $Ca^{2+}$ influx into nerve terminal varicosities caused by neuropeptide Y. The action potential-evoked rise in $Ca^{2+}$ was also prevented by tetrodotoxin (TTX, 1 μM) which blocks $Na^{+}$ influx. (*c*) The effect of neuropeptide Y (300 nM) on the stimulation-evoked rise in $[Ca^{2+}]_i$ with GTPγS (100 μM) present simultaneously in the patch pipette. Under these conditions, the inhibitory effect of neuropeptide Y was rendered irreversible by the GTPγS. (*d*) The recovery of neuropeptide Y inhibition of $Ca^{2+}$ influx in the presence and absence of GTPγS. The responses have been normalised to the control rise in $[Ca^{2+}]_i$ obtained before addition of neuropeptide Y.

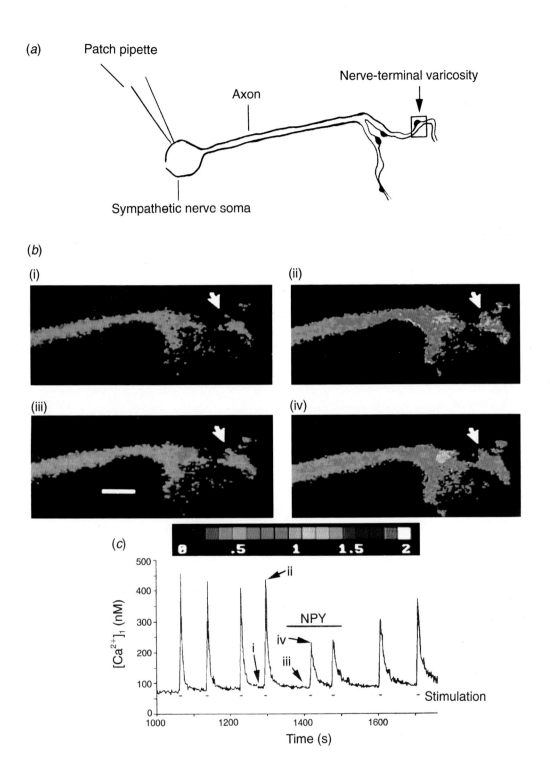

Plate 10.I. (*a*) Schematic diagram of the axon and synaptic varicosities of a sympathetic neurone co-cultured with atrial myocytes. (*b*) The axon was filled with fura-2 via a patch pipette applied to the neurone soma in whole-cell recording configuration and $[Ca^{2+}]_i$ was measured. The arrows in the colour figures (i–iv) indicate the region in which the $[Ca^{2+}]_i$ was measured; the region is identified in (*a*) by the box. Neuropeptide Y (300 nM) reduced the rise in $[Ca^{2+}]_i$ evoked in the terminal region by firing a train of action potentials down the axon via the patch pipette. (*c*) The timecourse of the experiment shown above. The arrows indicate the times at which frames (i–iv) were taken.

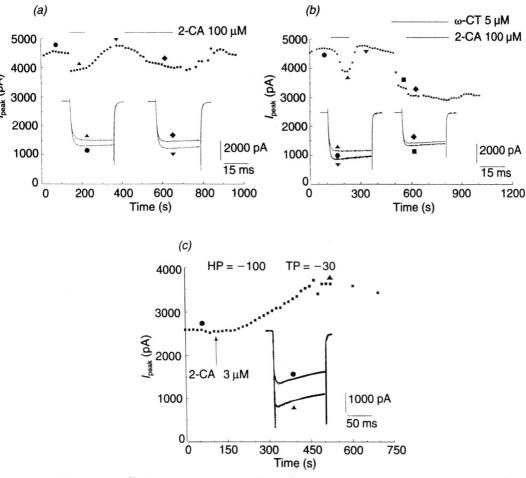

Fig. 10.6. (*a*) Inhibitory effect of 2-chloroadenosine (2-CA, 100 μM, an agonist at the adenosine receptor), on Ca$^{2+}$ currents in acutely isolated rat hippocampal neurones. The CA3 neurone was voltage clamped at −100 mV and depolarised to −10 mV once every 15 s. The timecourse of the peak current ($I_{peak}$) measured in the presence and absence of 100 μM 2-CA is shown. The symbols on the upper trace denote the times during the experiment at which the representative lower traces have been plotted. (*b*) This experiment shows that, after application of the N-type VSCC blocker ω-conotoxin GVIA (ω-CT), there is very little effect of 100 μM 2-CA, indicating that the predominant effect of 2-CA is to inhibit the Ca$^{2+}$ influx through N-type VSCC. (*c*) The influx of Ca$^{2+}$ through VSCC in hippocampal neurones is also potentiated by 2-CA. The upper part of the figure shows the timecourse of the experiment, in which 3 μM 2-CA was added. There was a slow increase in the magnitude of the recorded Ca$^{2+}$ current. The lower part of the figure shows the peak current ($I_{peak}$) measured before and after addition of the adenosine receptor agonist. This up-regulation of the current appears to be mediated by cAMP and is the result of an enhancement of current through P-type VSCC. (From ref. 27, with permission.)

of VSCC by the metabotropic glutamate receptor agonist (1$S$,3$R$)-aminocyclopentane dicarboxylic acid (ACPD). In one study using neocortical neurones, ACPD suppressed the L-type VSCC; whereas in a different study in CA3 hippocampal pyramidal neurones, it was the N-type VSCC that was suppressed, by a process that involved G-proteins. Such receptor-mediated modulation of VSCC may be important in the regulation of glutamate release from the presynaptic terminals, since activation of the metabotropic receptor has been shown to suppress excitatory transmission at CA3–CA1 synapses and also in cortical/striatal synapses (see Schoepp and Conn[30] for review).

Although modulation of N-type VSCC may be a widely occurring mechanism for regulating neurotransmitter release, other mechanisms are clearly also employed at some synapses. For example, as described above, P-type VSCC may be involved in the transmitter-release process at some synapses and these channels may also be modulated by receptors (see Chapter 13). In rare cases, $Ca^{2+}$ currents that appear to be L-type VSCC also seem to be inhibited by a variety of neurotransmitters. It is possible that they too may be able to influence neurotransmitter release in some instances.

**Facilitatory modulators of VSCC.** Some studies have demonstrated that $Ca^{2+}$ currents can be increased rather than decreased by neurotransmitters[1]. For example, experiments using dorsal horn neurones have shown that the $Ca^{2+}$ component of the action potential and the whole-cell $Ca^{2+}$ current are increased by substance P and CGRP. These changes are associated with an increase in neurotransmitter release. Furthermore, 5-HT in rat spinal motor neurones and noradrenaline in the cells of the dentate gyrus have both been shown to increase VSCC currents. In the hippocampus, the $Ca^{2+}$ current in the granule cells is increased by β-adrenoceptor agonists.

Dual effects are seen with certain neurotransmitters. For example, adenosine acting through the adenosine $A_1$ receptors inhibits N-type VSCC in acutely isolated hippocampal pyramidal neurones, whereas activation of the adenosine $A_2$ receptor leads to potentiation of the $Ca^{2+}$ current following a selective increase in currents through P-type VSCC[27] (Fig. 10.6a,b; see also Chapter 7). The increase in $Ca^{2+}$ current appears to be mediated by an increase in intracellular cAMP,

which probably leads to phosphorylation of the channel. However, the role of phosphorylation in the control of neuronal $Ca^{2+}$ channel activity, in general, is not well understood. In cardiac muscle, it is well established that noradrenaline can stimulate $Ca^{2+}$ entry through channels by a cAMP-mediated mechanism. Similar effects are observed in some neurones. For example, in hippocampal neurones, the cell-permeable cAMP analogue 8-bromo-cAMP was shown to increase single-channel N-type VSCC activity and whole-cell $Ca^{2+}$ current. However, this effect is not commonly observed in neurones and may reflect the fact that the VSCC in neurones are normally maximally phosphorylated.

As will be discussed below, the inhibition of neuronal VSCC does not generally appear to be mediated by alterations in channel-protein phosphorylation but rather by a direct action mediated by G-proteins. Nevertheless, there are some reports of inhibition of VSCC by mechanisms that involve protein kinase C, cGMP and other messengers (see Chapter 9).

### 2.1.6   $Ca^{2+}$-dependent inactivation of VSCC

The observation that VSCC can also inactivate following $Ca^{2+}$ entry has established the concept of $Ca^{2+}$-dependent inactivation. Consistent with this proposal is the finding that replacement of $Ca^{2+}$ with $Ba^{2+}$ as a charge carrier, together with buffering any rise in intracellular free $Ca^{2+}$ concentration with $Ca^{2+}$ chelators such as EGTA or BAPTA, dramatically reduces $Ca^{2+}$-dependent inactivation. Agents that block the release of $Ca^{2+}$ from intracellular stores, such as ryanodine, are also effective in reducing the inhibition of VSCC. It was proposed by Eckert and Chad[12] that the inactivation by $Ca^{2+}$ is caused by activation of $Ca^{2+}$-dependent phosphatases and that recovery from inactivation is a consequence of rephosphorylation of the VSCC. It has also been suggested that the dephosphorylation is caused by stimulation by $Ca^{2+}$ of the $Ca^{2+}$-calmodulin-activated phosphatase calcineurin[2].

Certainly it has been observed that calmodulin antagonists enhance $Ca^{2+}$ currents under certain circumstances.

One possible intracellular mechanism for the modulation of VSCC, therefore, may involve $Ca^{2+}$ itself. However, neuromodulators that have been shown to inhibit VSCC can do so independently of agonist increases in intracellular basal free $Ca^{2+}$ concentration[6], although there does appear to be a requirement for $Ca^{2+}$ *per se.*

### 2.1.7 Involvement of G-proteins in the regulation of VSCC

In many cases, the inhibitory modulation of VSCC has been found to be sensitive to pertussis toxin (see reviews by Hille[16] and Dolphin[11]). Since pertussis toxin prevents the receptor/G-protein interaction by ADP-ribosylating a cysteine residue near the N-terminus region of its substrate G-protein, a region associated with binding of the G-protein to the receptor, the data suggest that VSCC activity can be modulated by an interaction with membrane-associated G-proteins. This conclusion is supported by the observation that the introduction of GTP analogues such as GDPβS, which competitively inhibits the binding of GTP to G-proteins, prevents the inhibition of VSCC. In contrast, the introduction of non-hydrolysable GTP analogues such as GTPγS or GppNHp have been shown to slow down the activation kinetics of VSCC opening and also to cause inhibition of VSCC themselves. Sometimes this occurs to such an extent that the receptor-acting neuromodulator becomes ineffective. However in most instances, the presence of GppNHp renders the neuromodulation of VSCC irreversible. Such an example is shown in Plate 10.I in which the inhibitory effect of neuropeptide Y on $Ca^{2+}$ influx into sympathetic nerve terminals is rendered irreversible by GTPγS.

There are several types of G-proteins that exist in the CNS. When neurones are internally perfused with antibodies against the $G_o$-protein, the inhibitory effect is blocked in many cases. In those instances where $G_o$ is not involved in the transduction mechanism, it is possible that $G_i$, or in some cases a non-pertussis toxin-sensitive G-protein such as $G_q$, plays a similar role.

## 2.2 Ligand-gated $Ca^{2+}$ conductances

Besides VSCC, which open in response to changes in the membrane potential of the neurone, there is another family of ion channels that can be activated directly by neurotransmitters in membranes and that could, thus, modulate neurotransmitter release. There are several ligand-gated channels that exist in higher vertebrate neurones. GABA, glycine, glutamate, 5-HT and nicotinic acetylcholine receptors, for example. Glycine and GABA activate anion-permeable channels and are responsible for fast inhibitory synaptic transmission. Glutamate and acetylcholine activate cation-permeable channels and are responsible for fast excitatory transmission.

Most of the neurotransmitters directly linked to ligand-gated conductances utilise two types of receptor. One receptor type causes the direct opening of ion channels, as is the case for $GABA_A$, $5-HT_3$ and nicotinic acetylcholine receptors (nAChR). The other receptor type is linked to a G-protein and thence to various effector molecules, which can include ion channels, enzymes and second messengers. For GABA, 5-HT and acetylcholine, the receptors are $GABA_B$, $5-HT_1$ and $5-HT_2$, and muscarinic acetylcholine receptors, respectively. A similar scenario exists for the glutamate receptors. Kainate/AMPA and NMDA receptors are both subtypes of the glutamate-activated ligand-gated ion channels, whereas a second distinct type of glutamate receptor, the metabotropic glutamate receptor, is G-protein linked and its activation can lead to the production of second messengers and indirect modulation of ion channels.

### 2.2.1 Nicotinic-activated $Ca^{2+}$ channels

The nAChR has been extensively studied particularly at the (postsynaptic) neuromuscular junction. It is known to be permeable not only to monovalent (e.g. $Na^+$), but also to divalent (e.g. $Ca^{2+}$) cations, although for the neuromuscular junction at least it is thought that activation of the nAChR results primarily in $Na^+$ entry. It is thought that $Ca^{2+}$ entry occurs secondarily to depolarisation caused by $Na^+$ entry and consequent opening of VSCC. Certainly in adrenal chromaffin cells, the rise in $[Ca^{2+}]_i$ seen following nAChR activation is thought to occur mainly as a consequence of this mechanism. However, from recent molecular biological studies and expression of various subunits of the nAChR into model cells, it has become apparent that for the nAChR (and for the (postsynaptic) glutamate receptors) there is a large diversity of functional properties dependent upon subunit composition. Indeed for the nAChR, it appears that in several cell types the nAChR channel itself possesses a high permeability to $Ca^{2+}$ and that increases in $[Ca^{2+}]_i$ which occur do not necessarily have to rely upon the presence of functional VSCC[10]. Such $Ca^{2+}$-permeable nAChRs have been demonstrated in the adrenal medullary PC12 tumour cell line, in adrenal chromaffin cells and in medial habenular neurones. It has been postulated that the influx of $Ca^{2+}$ through nAChR is of a similar magnitude to that through VSCC. Since this $Ca^{2+}$ influx would occur at membrane potentials at which activation of the VSCC (or NMDA receptors) had yet to occur, it would contribute in an independent manner to the rise in intracellular free $Ca^{2+}$ concentration in neurones. Since nAChR have a pre- as well as a postsynaptic location, it is tempting to speculate that nicotinic modulation of the $Ca^{2+}$ permeability of the nAChR could confer a role for the nAChR in the presynaptic modulation of transmitter release as well as the postsynaptic modulation of $Ca^{2+}$-dependent conductances (see also Chapter 5).

## 3 Channels other than those for $Ca^{2+}$ that modulate neurotransmitter release

So far the discussion has centred on the proposition that presynaptic VSCC can be directly modulated by neurotransmitters acting at specific receptors. The resulting alterations in $Ca^{2+}$ influx would clearly represent the most parsimonious way of altering the moment-to-moment strength of synaptic transmission. However, the influx of $Ca^{2+}$ could also be altered as a consequence of changes in the activity of other ion channels in nerve terminals. Since the equilibrium potential for both $Cl^-$ and $K^+$ is close to the resting membrane potential of most neurones, opening of these channels would tend to stabilise the cell near to its membrane potential and thereby depress neuronal activity. The consequence of these channels opening would, therefore, be a shorter action potential duration and less $Ca^{2+}$ influx through VSCC.

### 3.1 Inhibitory modulation involving $Cl^-$ channels

The inhibitory amino acids GABA and glycine can activate receptors (GABA and glycine receptors) that lead to the opening of $Cl^-$ permeable channels.

GABA provides an interesting example of a neurotransmitter that can exert multiple effects on neuronal activity. GABA can activate $GABA_A$ channels presynaptically to produce large conductance increases to $Cl^-$, thus reducing the size of the action potential and subsequently reducing transmitter release[28]. In addition, GABA can activate a $K^+$ conductance (see below) which is likely to result from $GABA_B$ receptor activation and be mediated via a G-protein. Finally GABA can act presynaptically, via the $GABA_B$ receptor, to reduce $Ca^{2+}$ influx into cells by inhibition of VSCC through mediation of a pertussis toxin-sensitive G-protein.

## 3.2 Inhibitory modulation involving K⁺ channels

Many neurotransmitters that act as neuro-modulators of VSCC have also been shown to affect neuronal $K^+$ channels[22]. At the presynaptic level, activation of a $K^+$ conductance would tend to stabilise the membrane potential at or near the $K^+$ reversal potential, which, under physiological conditions, is close to the resting membrane potential. As with opened $Cl^-$ channels, the consequence would be a shorter action potential and a smaller $Ca^{2+}$ influx through VSCC. The $K^+$ conductance activated by many neuromodulators has been shown to have properties of the inward, or anomalous rectifier, $K^+$ channel. Such channels have a higher conductance at potentials more negative than the resting membrane potential. Therefore, activation of these channels (depending upon the resting membrane potential) will tend to hyperpolarise the cell and thus counteract the effect of agents which tend to depolarise neurones. In those cases in which this $K^+$ channel has been investigated, it has been shown that modulation of this conductance is both pertussis toxin sensitive and also sensitive to GDPβS[16]. Indeed agents such as enkephalins and 5-HT, which are able to inhibit VSCC, also activate $K^+$ channels simultaneously. In dorsal raphe neurones, for example, $5\text{-HT}_{1A}$ receptors are activated by 5-HT to produce inhibition of VSCC and simultaneous opening of the inwardly rectifying $K^+$ channel.

## 4 Summary

The recent progress towards understanding the structure and function of the diversity of $Ca^{2+}$ channels in neurones has enabled examination of the way in which these influx routes can be regulated at the molecular level and how, in turn, this can produce changes in neuronal function. As discussed above, it is now considered likely that direct modulation of presynaptic VSCC can form a basis of inhibition and facilitation of neurotransmitter release. However, many questions still need to be answered. For example, although N-type VSCC have been shown repeatedly to be important in the process of neurotransmitter release, in several instances it is clear that other VSCC may also be involved. The reasons why, and how, different channels function at different synapses or under different circumstances is obscure.

It is also becoming clear that mechanisms involving the modulation of other ion channels indirectly regulate $Ca^{2+}$ influx and, thus, neurotransmitter release. In addition, it has been shown that neurotransmitter release can be regulated by directly modulating the release apparatus itself, without recourse to altering $Ca^{2+}$ influx at all (see Chapter 11). Again, it is not clear why all these mechanisms exist and, moreover, when each of them is brought to bear under physiological circumstances. Much current research is directed towards trying to find answers to these important questions.

## References

1. Anwyl R (1991) Modulation of vertebrate neuronal calcium channels by transmitters. *Brain Research Reviews* **16**: 265–281
2. Armstrong DI, Rossier MF, Sheherbatko AD and White RE (1991) Enzymatic gating of voltage activated calcium channels. *Annals of the New York Academy of Sciences* **635**: 26–34
3. Augustine GJ and Charlton MP (1986) Calcium dependence of presynaptic calcium current and post-synaptic response in squid giant synapse. *Journal of Physiology* **381**: 619–640
4. Augustine GJ, Charlton MP and Smith SJ (1987) Calcium action in synaptic transmitter release. *Annual Reviews of Neuroscience* **10**: 633–693
5. Bean BP (1989) Classes of calcium channels in vertebrate cells. *Annual Reviews of Physiology* **51**: 367–384
6. Beech DJ, Bernheim L, Mathie A and Hille B (1991) Intracellular $Ca^{2+}$ buffers disrupt muscarinic supression of $Ca^{2+}$ current and M-current in rat sympathetic neurons. *Proceedings of the National Academy of Sciences USA* **88**: 652–656

7. Bleakman D, Colmers WF, Fournier A and Miller RJ (1991) Neuropeptide Y inhibits $Ca^{2+}$ influx into cultured dorsal root ganglion neurons of the rat via a Y2 receptor. *British Journal of Pharmacology* **103:** 1781–1789

8. Bleakman D, Miller RJ and Colmers WF (1993) Actions of neuropeptide Y on the electrophysiological properties of nerve cells. In: Colmers WF and Wahlestedt C (eds), *The Biology of Neuropeptide Y and Related Peptides.* Humana Press, Totowa, NJ

9. Carbone E and Swandulla D (1989) Neuronal calcium channels: kinetics, blockade and modulation. *Progress in Biophysics and Molecular Biology* **54:** 31–58

10. Decker ER and Dani JA (1990) Calcium permeability of the nicotinic acetylcholine receptor; the single channel calcium influx is significant. *Journal of Neuroscience* **10:** 3413–3420

11. Dolphin AC (1990) G-protein modulation of calcium current in neurons. *Annual Reviews of Physiology* **52:** 243–255

12. Eckert R and Chad JE (1984) Inactivation of $Ca^{2+}$ channels. *Progress in Biophysics and Molecular Biology* **44:** 215–267

13. Fleckenstein A (1988) Historical overview. The calcium channel of the heart. *Annals of the New York Academy of Sciences* **522:** 1–15

14. Fox AP, Nowycky MC and Tsien RW (1987) Kinetic and pharmacological properties distinguish three types of calcium currents in chick sensory neurons. *Journal of Physiology* **394:** 149–172

15. Gray R and Johnston D (1988) Recordings of single calcium channels from pre-synaptic mossy fibre terminals in adult guinea pig hippocampus. *Society for Neuroscience Abstracts* **14:** 68

16. Hille B (1992) G-protein coupled mechanisms of nervous signaling. *Neuron* **9:** 187–195

17. Hirning LD, Fox AP and Miller RJ (1990) Inhibition of calcium currents in cultured rat myenteric neurons by neuropeptide Y: evidence for a direct receptor/channel coupling. *Brain Research* **532:** 120–130

18. Lemos J R and Nowycky MC (1989) Two types of calcium channels co-exit in peptide releasing vertebrate nerve terminals. *Neuron* **2:** 1419–1426

19. Llinas R, Sugimori M, Lin JW and Cherksey B (1989) Blocking and isolation of a $Ca^{2+}$ channel from neurons in mammals and cephalapods utilizing a toxin fraction (FTX)

from funnel web spider poison. *Proceedings of the National Academy of Sciences USA* **86:** 1689–1693

20. Llinas R and Yarom Y (1981) Properties and distribution of ionic conductances generating electroresponsiveness of mammalian inferior olivary neurons *in vitro. Journal of Physiology* **315:** 569–584

21. Marubio LM, Philipson LH and Miller RJ (1992). Partial sequence of $\alpha_{1X}$, a putative novel $\alpha_1$ subunit of a voltage sensitive calcium channel. *Society for Neuroscience Abstracts* **18:** 1138

22. Miller RJ (1990) Receptor mediated regulation of calcium channels and neurotransmitter release. *FASEB Journal* **4:** 3291–3299

23. Miller RJ (1991) The control of neuronal $Ca^{2+}$ homeostasis. *Progress in Neurobiology* **37:** 255–285

24. Miller RJ (1992) Voltage sensitive $Ca^{2+}$ channels. *Journal of Biological Chemistry* **267:** 1403–1406

25. Miller RJ and Fox AP (1990) Voltage sensitive calcium channels. In: Bronner F. (ed), *Intracellular Calcium Regulation*, pp 97–138, Alan R. Liss, New York

26. Mogul DJ and Fox AP (1991) Evidence for multiple types of $Ca^{2+}$ channels in acutely isolated hippocampal CA3 pyramidal neurons of the guinea-pig. *Journal of Physiology* **433:** 259–281

27. Mogul DJ, Adams ME and Fox AP (1993) Differential activation of adenosine receptors decreases N-type but potentiates P-type $Ca^{2+}$ current in rat hippocampal CA3 neurons. *Neuron* **10:** 327–334

28. Nicoll RA and Algers BE (1979) Presynaptic inhibition: transmitter and ionic mechanisms. *International Review of Neurobiology* **21:** 217–258

29. Nowycky MC, Fox AP and Tsien RW (1985) Three types of neuronal calcium channels with different calcium agonist sensitivity. *Nature* **316:** 440–443

30. Schoepp DD and Conn PJ (1993) Metabotropic glutamate receptors in brain function and pathology. *Trends in Pharmacological Sciences* **14:** 13–20

31. Scott RH, Sutton KG and Dolphin AC (1993) Interactions of polyamines with neuronal ion channels. *Trends in Neurosciences* **16:** 153–160

32. Stanley EF and Goping G (1991) Characterization of a calcium current in a

vertebrate cholinergic presynaptic nerve terminal. *Journal of Neuroscience* **11:** 985–993

33. Thayer SA, Hirning LD and Miller RJ (1987) Distribution of multiple types of $Ca^{2+}$ channels in rat sympathetic neurons *in vitro*. *Molecular Pharmacology* **32:** 579–586

34. Toth PT, Bindokas VP, Bleakman D, Colmers WF and Miller RJ (1993) Mechanism of presynaptic inhibition by neuropeptide Y at sympathetic nerve terminals. *Nature* **364:** 635–639

35. Turner JT, Adams ME and Dunlap K (1992) Calcium channels coupled to glutamate release identified by ω-Aga IVA. *Science* **258:** 310–313

36. Uchitel OD, Protti DA, Sanchez V, Cherksey BD, Sugimori M and Llinas R (1992) P-type voltage dependent calcium channel mediates presynaptic calcium influx and transmitter release in mammalian synapse. *Proceedings of the National Academy of Sciences USA* **89:** 3330–3333

37. White G, Lovinger DM and Weight FF (1989) Transient low threshold $Ca^{2+}$ current triggers burst firing through an after depolarization potential in adult mammalian neuron. *Proceedings of the National Academy of Sciences USA* **86:** 6802–6806

38. Williams ME, Brust PF, Feldman DH *et al.* (1992) Structure and functional expression of an ω-conotoxin sensitive human N-type calcium channel. *Science* **257:** 389–395

# 11 Calcium-independent modulation of neurotransmitter release

Arun R. Wakade and Dennis A. Przywara

A conclusion that may reasonably be drawn from the previous two chapters is that it is ultimately the concentration of free $Ca^{2+}$ at the site of exocytosis that determines the amount of neurotransmitter released, and that modulation is achieved by increasing or decreasing the availability of $Ca^{2+}$. However, although it is clear that the basic conclusion is valid, it remains possible that there are other mechanisms of modulation superimposed. In this chapter Arun Wakade and Dennis Przywara collate the observations which suggest that neurotransmitter release can be modulated in addition by mechanisms that do not involve changes in intracellular free $Ca^{2+}$.

## 1 Introduction

The work of Douglas, Katz, Kirpekar and others firmly established the requirement for $Ca^{2+}$ in the release of neurotransmitters (see also Chapter 1). Experiments with neuro-effector organs led to the hypothesis that $Ca^{2+}$ enters neurones through voltage-sensitive channels then diffuses to, and binds to, a cytosolic factor which triggers transmitter release. This 'Ca$^{2+}$ hypothesis' of transmitter release has been validated by more than 25 years of research on the mechanisms of $Ca^{2+}$ entry and regulation of $[Ca^{2+}]_i$. Modern techniques of cell culture, molecular biology, fluorescence imaging of ions and macromolecules, and single-channel electrophysiology have greatly expanded our understanding of $Ca^{2+}$-dependent transmitter release. Many $Ca^{2+}$-dependent components of the processes involved with synthesis, transport and release of neurotransmitters have been identified, and the mechanisms of exocytosis are being defined (see Chapter 1). Accordingly, the primary focus of research concerning modula-

tion of neurotransmitter release has been on the mechanisms of modulation of $Ca^{2+}$ entry to the neurone and/or $Ca^{2+}$ access to the site of exocytosis. The aim of the present chapter, however, is to consider the evidence for $Ca^{2+}$-*in*dependent mechanisms for modulation of transmitter release. While considering $Ca^{2+}$-independent modulation, it is important to keep in mind that $Ca^{2+}$ is an obligatory factor in the release process. Release of transmitter from normal, intact neurones does not occur without an initial increase in $Ca^{2+}$ concentration near the release site. However, modulation of release may occur independently of any further change, up or down, in $Ca^{2+}$ concentration (see Fig. 11.1). It is in this context that the term $Ca^{2+}$ independent is used. Furthermore, the definition of 'modulation of release' used here includes not only the exocytotic event itself but also the modulation of the preceding steps that control the availability of transmitter and vesicles at the site of exocytosis.

Figure 11.1 shows how the original $Ca^{2+}$ hypothesis (Fig. 11.1*a*, in which transmitter

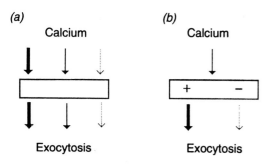

Fig. 11.1. The original 'calcium hypothesis' of neurotransmitter release (*a*) states that exocytosis is controlled by intracellular $Ca^{2+}$ levels. Various components of the exocytotic pathway (box) couple the $Ca^{2+}$ signals to exocytosis. If $Ca^{2+}$ is increased (thick arrow) or decreased (broken arrow) transmitter release is altered accordingly. $Ca^{2+}$-independent modulation of transmitter release (*b*) is an extension of the calcium hypothesis to show that components of the exocytotic pathway can be influenced to increase or decrease transmitter release in the presence of a constant $Ca^{2+}$ signal.

release can be modulated by changes in $[Ca^{2+}]_i$) has been extended to include modulation of transmitter release 'downstream' from $Ca^{2+}$ entry. The extended portion of the model (Fig. 11.1*b*) implies that modulation of release may also occur without further changes in $[Ca^{2+}]_i$.

## 2 Possible sites for $Ca^{2+}$-independent regulation of transmitter release

Much progress has been made in identifying the molecular components involved in the synthesis, storage and exocytotic release of neurotransmitters. How the various components interact to control release is not completely clear, and a specific $Ca^{2+}$-sensitive receptor that triggers exocytosis has yet to be identified (see Chapter 1). Each of the secretory components discussed below, although sensitive to $Ca^{2+}$, also presents a target for $Ca^{2+}$-independent modulation of transmitter release. Protein kinases may play a particu-

larly important role in $Ca^{2+}$-independent modulation of the secretory process (see Chapter 9).

Potential sites for modulation of neurotransmitter release exist at any stage of the secretory process, including the synthesis of transmitter, the synthesis and recycling of synaptic vesicles, the translocation of vesicles to release sites and the final stages of vesicle fusion with plasma membrane and exocytosis (see Sections 2.1–2.4 below). It is reasonable to assume that all components of release are modulated in concert to maintain neurotransmission at varying levels of nerve activity. Increasing the rate of vesicle fusion and exocytosis would be of little consequence if, for example, the delivery of replacement vesicles to the plasma membrane for subsequent rounds of exocytosis was rate limiting. Similarly, high levels of neurotransmitter release could not be maintained for any period of time without a concomitant increase in transmitter synthesis.

### 2.1 Synthesis of neurotransmitter

The intimate coupling of transmitter synthesis to release was proposed by von Euler and colleagues in the 1950s, when they found that prolonged stimulation of catecholamine secretion from cat adrenal medulla did not reduce the catecholamine content of the gland. It is now known that a variety of physiological and pharmacological stimuli that increase neurotransmitter release also stimulate the catecholamine synthetic pathway. For example, the catalytic activity of tyrosine hydroxylase (the rate-limiting enzyme for catecholamine synthesis) is regulated by $Ca^{2+}$-independent protein kinases, in addition to $Ca^{2+}$-dependent kinases[9]. Cyclic AMP plays a prominent role in the $Ca^{2+}$-independent activation of tyrosine hydroxylase, by a mechanism that is described in detail in Section 11.3.3. The synthesis of catecholamines is also enhanced by elevated transcription of mRNA for tyrosine hydroxylase. Stimulation-coupled gene expression is regulated by the neuronal immediate–early genes, c-*fos* and c-*jun*[20]. The proteins, FOS and JUN, encoded by these two genes, form a heterodimeric transcription factor that regulates the expression of target genes. The expression of c-*fos* is induced by many of the same stimuli that increase both neurotransmitter release and tyrosine hydroxylase mRNA levels[6]. Therefore, it is likely that the tyrosine hydroxylase gene is a target of c-*fos* regulation. Although elevated intracellular $Ca^{2+}$ plays an important role here also, it is only one component in gene activation and may act primarily as a trigger.

The regulatory proteins that control transcription are also modulated by $Ca^{2+}$-independent mechanisms. Multiple second messenger systems are involved in the posttranslational modification of the FOS protein by phosphorylation. Changes in phosphorylation affect the binding of the FOS protein to regulatory sequences on DNA. Hence receptor-mediated changes in second messenger levels could affect mRNA levels by controlling, independent of changes in $Ca^{2+}$, the phosphorylation state of proteins like FOS. In general then, the presence of multiple transmitters and receptors coupled to various second messengers at central and peripheral synapses could recruit $Ca^{2+}$-independent kinases to modulate transmitter synthesis by their action on transcription factors.

### 2.2   Synthesis and recycling of storage vesicles

The secretion of neurotransmitters involves fusion of the exocytotic vesicle with the plasma membrane and a consequent increase in plasma membrane area. Recycling of synaptic vesicles avoids unlimited growth of the plasma membrane and energy expenditure to synthesise new vesicles. Evidence for the reuse of secretory vesicles has been obtained for a variety of cells including chromaffin cells, and sympathetic neurones[28].

Recycling may occur either by simple endocytosis of the vesicle and reuse or by complex processing involving formation of coated pits and large-sized intermediate vesicles. These alternative routes of recycling are determined by the rate of exocytosis and thus also, either directly or indirectly, by the level of $Ca^{2+}$ entry. The more complex processing occurs at high rates of exocytosis and offers more possibilities for $Ca^{2+}$-independent regulation. Although the mechanism of synaptic vesicle cycling is only now beginning to be understood, recent studies offer support for $Ca^{2+}$-independent processes. The elegant work of Hess, Doroshenko and Augustine[13] showed that, in the squid giant synapse, G-proteins control synaptic vesicle cycling and neurotransmitter release independent of $Ca^{2+}$. Injection of GTPγS (a non-hydrolysable GTP analogue) inhibited transmitter release but without affecting the stimulated increase in $[Ca^{2+}]_i$. Furthermore, the number of vesicles docked at the plasma membrane was unchanged, while the number of vesicles near the active zones of the terminals was greatly reduced. This implies that GTPγS locks synaptic vesicles in the docked state, blocking release, and also prevents vesicle cycling into the active zones. Large, heterotrimeric G-proteins act catalytically and non-hydrolysable analogues of GTP and GDP have opposite effects on them. However, Hess and colleagues[13] found that injection of GDPβS (a non-hydrolysable analogue of GDP) also inhibited release without affecting the stimulated increase in $[Ca^{2+}]_i$. This implies that small-molecular-weight, monomeric G-proteins, thought to act cyclically in GDP–GTP exchange, are also regulating transmitter release independent of $Ca^{2+}$. The hypothetical model proposed to explain these findings is reproduced in Fig. 11.2. The physiological implication of the findings is that any manoeuvre that changes intraneuronal GTP levels may modulate neurotransmitter release by this mechanism.

### 2.3   Translocation of vesicles to release sites

Regardless of the mechanisms regulating synaptic vesicle biogenesis and recycling, the

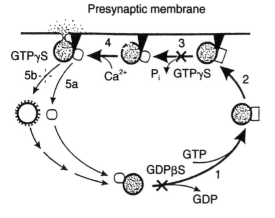

Presynaptic membrane

⊙ Synaptic vesicle  □ GTP-bound protein
▼ Docking site  ○ GDP-bound protein

Fig. 11.2. Hypothetical model proposed by Hess, Doroshenko and Augustine showing the possible involvement of G-proteins in exocytosis. The model can accomodate the block of exocytosis by non-hydrolysable analogues of both GTP and GDP. GDP–GTP exchange (1) precedes docking and is blocked by GDPβS resulting in decreased exocytosis. The GTP bound form of a G-protein regulates docking (2) and hydrolysis of the GTP (release of inorganic phosphorus, $P_i$, in step 3) is necessary for exocytosis (4) to proceed. GTPγS blocks exocytosis by preventing GTP hydrolysis and holding vesicles in the docked position. G-proteins involved in the endocytotic recycling of vesicles (5b) are also blocked by GTPγS. The modulation of exocytosis by regulatory G-proteins occurs without any change in voltage-clamped $Ca^{2+}$ current or $[Ca^{2+}]_i$ measured by fura-2. (From ref. 13, with permission; copyright 1993 by the AAAS.)

availability of vesicles at release sites is dependent on their directed movement through the mesh of cytoplasmic filaments comprising the neuronal cytoskeleton (see Chapter 1). There is considerable evidence that the translocation of synaptic vesicles to release sites is controlled by specific, phosphorylation-dependent interactions between vesicular and cytoskeletal proteins. Synapsin I is a prominent nerve terminal phosphoprotein specifically associated with the cyto-plasmic surface of synaptic vesicles. Synapsin I is also a major substrate for cAMP-dependent and $Ca^{2+}$-calmodulin-dependent protein kinases, which phosphorylate the protein at three distinct sites. Site 1 is located on the globular head region of synapsin I and is the target for cAMP-dependent phosphorylation. Sites 2 and 3 are located on the tail region of the molecule and are phosphorylated by $Ca^{2+}$-calmodulin-dependent protein kinase II. Phosphorylation of synapsin I decreases its binding to fodrin (brain spectrin), to cytoskeletal filaments (F-actin, neurofilaments and microtubules) and to synaptic vesicles. The binding of synapsin I to synaptic vesicles appears to be specifically regulated by $Ca^{2+}$-calmodulin-dependent phosphorylation of the two tail sites. It is suggested that synaptic vesicles held in the cytoskeletal network are released for exocytosis by elevated $[Ca^{2+}]_i$, via its effects on $Ca^{2+}$-calmodulin-dependent protein kinase II. But while $Ca^{2+}$-dependent phosphorylation of synapsin I at sites 2 and 3 controls its binding to synaptic vesicles, it is cAMP-dependent phosphorylation of site 1 that regulates its binding to cytoskeletal actin. Actin is abundant in nerve terminals and F-actin is thought to be linked by fodrin to the presynaptic plasma membrane[7]. Dephosphorylated synapsin I interacts strongly with F-actin and this interaction is greatly reduced by cAMP-dependent phosphorylation of synapsin[4]. Thus, $Ca^{2+}$-independent elevation of intracellular cAMP levels (see Section 3.3 below) might alter transmitter availability adjacent to the cell membrane by phosphorylation of synapsin I at site 1 and consequent reduction of its binding to F-actin. Therefore, it is possible that the interaction between vesicle-associated synapsin I, F-actin and fodrin is concerned closely with regulating the availability of vesicles at presynaptic release sites[7]. In this context, $Ca^{2+}$-independent modulation of release by synapsin has been directly demonstrated in the squid giant synapse, where injection of phosphorylated synapsin I enhanced transmitter release without altering voltage-clamped $Ca^{2+}$ currents[17].

In addition to controlling the interaction of synaptic vesicles with cytoskeletal elements, second messengers may regulate the structure of the cytoskeleton itself[8]. In chromaffin cells, nicotinic stimulation of exocytosis is accompanied by depolymerisation of cortical actin filaments. Like the events described above for neurones, this change in the cytoskeleton is thought to promote the movement of exocytotic vesicles to the sites of release. Also like the events in neurones, $Ca^{2+}$-dependent and $Ca^{2+}$-independent mechanisms are involved. Stimulation with the secretagogue nicotine caused a decrease in actin associated with triton-insoluble cytoskeletal elements in chromaffin cells[8]. The reduction of cytoskeletal actin during nicotinic stimulation was not changed in $Ca^{2+}$-free medium, and was mimicked by phorbol ester activation of protein kinase C. Although $Ca^{2+}$-dependent exocytosis is also accompanied by reduced amounts of cytoskeletal actin, the above findings imply a $Ca^{2+}$-independent modulation of vesicle availability that may involve protein kinase C-dependent phosphorylation.

## 2.4   Vesicle fusion and exocytosis

Protein kinases and G-proteins can provide a means of $Ca^{2+}$-independent modulation of transmitter release by controlling vesicle movement through the cytoskeleton and docking at the sites of release. There is also evidence that exocytosis itself may be subject to $Ca^{2+}$-independent modulation.

The final step in neurotransmitter release involves fusion of the vesicle membrane with the plasma membrane, formation of a fusion pore and exocytotic release of the vesicle contents. The ability of chromaffin granules to undergo fusion with primed plasma membrane vesicles in $Ca^{2+}$-free medium supports the existence of $Ca^{2+}$-independent processes at the final stages of release[14]. In these experiments, isolated adrenal chromaffin granules were labelled with a fluorescent lipid marker at a concentration sufficiently high to quench the fluorescence signal. The labelled chro-

maffin granules were then added to isolated plasma membrane vesicles and fusion was measured by increased fluorescence as the granule membrane is diluted into the plasma membrane. Priming of the target plasma membrane involves $Ca^{2+}$-dependent activation of phospholipase $A_2$ and consequent liberation of fatty acids from membrane phospholipids. However, after priming, phospholipase $A_2$ and $Ca^{2+}$ can be completely removed by repeated washing of the plasma membranes in $Ca^{2+}$-free buffer containing EGTA to chelate residual $Ca^{2+}$. Under these conditions, addition of chromaffin granules allowed vesicle–plasma membrane fusion to the same extent, and with the same kinetics, as the fully reconstituted system. If synaptic vesicles can undergo $Ca^{2+}$-independent fusion with the plasma membrane, then the possibility of $Ca^{2+}$-independent modulatory control may exist at the final step of neurotransmitter release.

Fusion of synaptic vesicles with the plasma membrane is likely to involve the interaction of several vesicular and plasma-membrane-associated factors (see Chapter 1). The experiments described above indicate that plasma membrane substrates of phospholipase $A_2$ may be involved in vesicle fusion. Another factor that is thought to participate in the final stages of exocytosis is synaptophysin (also called p38). Synaptophysin is a major integral membrane protein of synaptic vesicles, has structural similarity to gap-junction proteins, forms channels in lipid bilayers and is required for transmitter secretion reconstituted in *Xenopus* oocytes[1,2] (see also Chapter 1). These properties suggest that synaptophysin plays a major role in transmitter release at the site of exocytosis and may be involved in fusion pore formation.

Important to the subject of this chapter, the synaptophysin step could be part of a $Ca^{2+}$-independent release-modulating mechanism. Synaptophysin is a major substrate for tyrosine kinases in the brain. Relatively high concentrations of the tyrosine kinase (c-*src* product) are present with synaptophysin in synaptic vesicle membranes[7]. Since tyrosine kinase activity can be regulated in a $Ca^{2+}$-independent manner, a possible mechanism for $Ca^{2+}$-independent release modulation by synaptophysin action could be proposed. However, at present the function of synaptophysin in exocytosis and how phosphorylation might alter this function are unknown.

# 3   Factors involved in $Ca^{2+}$-independent modulation of transmitter release

From the above discussion of phosphoprotein involvement in exocytosis, it is possible that some of the messengers likely to be involved in $Ca^{2+}$-independent modulation of transmitter release are protein kinases. It would follow that any phosphoprotein whose activity is regulated by a protein kinase will be regulated in the opposite direction by protein phosphatases. Although the effects of some $Ca^{2+}$-dependent phosphatases (calcineurin, for example) have been examined in the context of transmitter release, there is little information on effects of $Ca^{2+}$-independent phosphatases on release. For this reason, only protein kinases are included in the following discussion. The strongest evidence exists for modulation of transmitter release by cAMP-dependent protein kinase, but other possibilities will be considered first.

## 3.1   Protein kinase C

Protein kinase C is activated by diacylglycerol, a product of membrane phospholipid metabolism, and low levels of $[Ca^{2+}]_i$. Protein kinase C is also activated by the tumour-promoting phorbol esters. In non-neuronal cells, both diacylglycerol and phorbol esters facilitate secretion, and this may occur without changes in $[Ca^{2+}]_i$[15,22]. These findings led to the conclusion that protein kinase C increases the $Ca^{2+}$ sensitivity of the secretory process and, therefore, represents a means for $Ca^{2+}$-independent modulation of release. A specific $Ca^{2+}$-independent action of protein kinase C has not been identified but could

conceivably involve any phosphoprotein-regulated process triggering or modulating exocytosis. For example, $Ca^{2+}$-independent protein kinase C effects on the cytoskeleton may modulate vesicle translocation (see Section 2.3, and ref. 8).

Note that there are studies of protein kinase C effects in neuronal and adrenal chromaffin cells that do not support a totally $Ca^{2+}$-independent mechanism of action on the release process. Facilitation of transmitter release by phorbol esters in neurones is blocked when the presynaptic terminal is voltage clamped[3]. This indicates that voltage-sensitive $Ca^{2+}$ entry plays a part in the protein kinase C enhancement of release. Furthermore, in studies using perfused adrenal glands, the increased catecholamine secretion following protein kinase C activation was associated with an increase in agonist-stimulated $Ca^{2+}$ uptake[18]. On balance, protein kinase C appears to enhance exocytosis mainly by increasing stimulated $Ca^{2+}$ influx. However, $Ca^{2+}$-independent actions of protein kinase C may act positively in concert with the increased $Ca^{2+}$ influx.

## 3.2   Guanine nucleotides

The role of guanine nucleotides in exocytosis is most clearly established in mast cells where GTP analogues are sufficient on their own to stimulate degranulation[16]. GTP analogues also cause secretion from permeabilised chromaffin cells independent of external $Ca^{2+}$ levels[5]. However, $Ca^{2+}$-induced exocytosis in chromaffin cells is inhibited by guanine nucleotides[5,16]. Guanine nucleotide regulation of release implies the involvement of a G-protein in one of the steps in exocytosis: a G-protein provides a physical site at which $Ca^{2+}$-independent modulation could occur. A hypothetical model of G-protein action in modulating exocytosis is presented in Fig. 11.2.

Guanine nucleotides may also be involved in $Ca^{2+}$-independent regulation of neurotransmitter release through the action of cGMP. Cyclic GMP-dependent protein kinase has been identified in nervous tissue and this may regulate exocytotic phosphoproteins. While there is no strong evidence that cGMP is involved in exocytosis *per se*, cGMP-dependent protein kinase may play a role, for example, in synaptic vesicle transport or in transmitter synthesis. In this regard, cGMP-dependent protein kinase may regulate transmitter synthesis by altering the phosphorylation state of transcription factors and/or tyrosine hydroxylase[26].

## 3.3    Adenylyl cyclase and cAMP

The strongest candidate for a $Ca^{2+}$-independent modulator of transmitter release is cAMP acting through cAMP-dependent phosphorylation of proteins associated with transmitter synthesis and synaptic vesicles. Because protein substrates for cAMP-dependent kinases are involved in several stages of neurotransmitter synthesis and release, they provide a variety of possible targets for modulation independent of changes in $[Ca^{2+}]_i$. Certainly, in many neurones, agents that elevate cAMP levels also facilitate transmitter release (see Chapter 9) and in both chick and rat sympathetic neurones, cAMP has been shown to modulate transmitter release independent of $Ca^{2+}$ (see below).

### 3.3.1    Modulation of neurotransmitter release in the cerebral cortex by cAMP

Rat brain slices (neocortex) have been loaded with [³H]-noradrenaline and depolarisation-evoked transmitter release quantified radiometrically. Veratrine, a plant alkaloid that promotes depolarisation by inhibiting $Na^+$-channel inactivation, was then used to evoke [³H]-noradrenaline release. Application of membrane permeable analogues of cAMP, 8-Bromo-cAMP or dibutyryl-cAMP, was found to enhance veratrine-induced [³H]-noradrenaline release in $Ca^{2+}$-free medium[27]. Interestingly, $\alpha_2$-adrenoceptor stimulation with clonidine inhibited and $\alpha_2$-adrenoceptor block with phentolamine enhanced the evoked release in $Ca^{2+}$-free medium. It

has been postulated that $\alpha_2$-adrenoceptors are linked to inhibition of adenylyl cyclase through $G_i$, which, if proved, would give further support for the involvement of cAMP (but see Chapter 9).

The above findings suggest clearly that transmitter release from central adrenergic synapses can be modulated by cAMP-dependent mechanisms apparently independent of external $Ca^{2+}$.

### 3.3.2    Modulation of release in the adrenal medulla by cAMP

A dissociation from $Ca^{2+}$ influx has also been shown for the cAMP-induced facilitation of secretion from the perfused adrenal gland of the rat[18]. In the rat adrenal medullary synapse, VIP is a co-transmitter with acetylcholine in stimulating catecholamine secretion. VIP acts by causing a substantial increase in cAMP content of the postsynaptic chromaffin cells: perfusion of isolated adrenal glands with VIP causes up to an 8-fold increase in the cAMP content of the gland. However, acetylcholine stimulates $^{45}Ca$ uptake and catecholamine secretion but does not stimulate cAMP production. Pretreatment of adrenal glands with VIP caused up to a 3-fold facilitation of acetylcholine-evoked secretion, even at the maximum effective concentrations of acetylcholine. However, there was no change in stimulated $^{45}Ca$ uptake. Forskolin, which increases cAMP content to a degree comparable to VIP treatment, caused a similar increase in acetylcholine-evoked secretion with no change in $^{45}Ca$ uptake. These results strongly suggest that cAMP facilitates catecholamine secretion at a site downstream from $Ca^{2+}$ entry.

### 3.3.3    Modulation of release in sympathetic neurones by cAMP

Further support for $Ca^{2+}$-independent modulation of transmitter release by cAMP has been obtained in studies of (chick) peripheral sympathetic neurones maintained in tissue

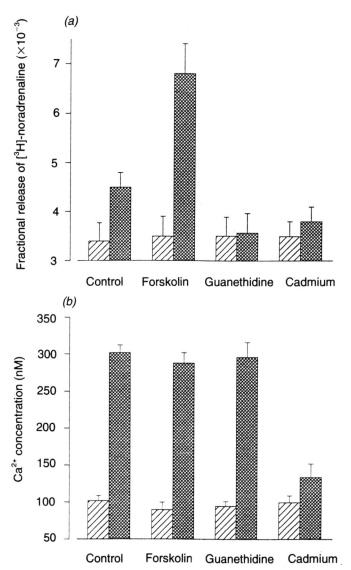

Fig. 11.3. Agents that augment or block transmitter release do not necessarily do so by changing $[Ca^{2+}]_i$. Release of $[^3H]$-noradrenaline (*a*) and stimulated increase in intracellular $Ca^{2+}$ (*b*) during exposure of embryonic chick cultured sympathetic neurones to the compounds indicated. Unstimulated background measurements are shown by the light hatched columns. Measurements following 1 Hz (10 s) electrical field stimulation are shown by the dark shaded columns. Forskolin (10 μM), guanethidine (3 μM) and cadmium (60 μM) were present for 10 min prior to stimulation. None of the agents affected unstimulated background release. However, forskolin enhanced and guanethidine blocked evoked transmitter release with no effect on the increase in $Ca^{2+}$ concentration (measured by indo-1 fluorescence) upon stimulation. Block of voltage-sensitive $Ca^{2+}$ channels by cadmium inhibited transmitter release and the stimulated increase in $Ca^{2+}$ concentration as expected.

culture[23]. Cultured neurones permit the use of patch-clamp and fluorescence-imaging techniques for direct measurement of $Ca^{2+}$ entry and $[Ca^{2+}]_i$ alongside biochemical and transmitter-release studies. Transmitter release can be measured in cultures loaded with [$^3$H]-noradrenaline and stimulated by electrical depolarisation. Whereas cAMP levels are not affected by electrical stimulation, they are significantly increased by activation of membrane receptors coupled to adenylyl cyclase or by treatment with the adenylyl cyclase activator forskolin. Likewise, VIP stimulates cAMP production in cultured sympathetic neurones[23] and in sympathetic ganglia[30] through adenylyl cyclase-coupled receptors. When cultured sympathetic neurones are treated with exogenous VIP or forskolin, cAMP levels are elevated approximately 5- and 10-fold, respectively. Elevated cAMP levels are accompanied by a pronounced enhancement of electrically evoked [$^3$H]-noradrenaline release (2- and 4-fold, respectively, for VIP and forskolin). Furthermore, the cAMP analogue 8-bromo-cAMP also enhanced the evoked release, while the inactive dideoxy forskolin was without effect. These findings show that adenylyl cyclase–cAMP is responsible for the enhanced release caused by forskolin and VIP.

The data summarised in Fig. 11.3 show how transmitter release from cultured sympathetic neurones can be enhanced or suppressed in a cAMP-dependent manner without changing the stimulated increase in $[Ca^{2+}]_i$. The effects of three pharmacological agents on the electrically evoked release of [$^3$H]-noradrenaline are given in Fig. 11.3a. Forskolin enhanced the evoked [$^3$H]-noradrenaline release by the cAMP-dependent mechanism noted above. Guanethidine, a well-known inhibitor of sympathetic neurotransmitter release *in vivo*, effectively blocked the stimulated release of [$^3$H]-noradrenaline in cultured neurones. Cadmium, a non-specific blocker of VSCC, reduced evoked release by about 70%. The bar graphs in Fig. 11.3b show that neither forskolin nor guanethidine altered the stimulated increase in $[Ca^{2+}]_i$. The positive results with cadmium indicate that when an agent affects transmitter release by altering $Ca^{2+}$ entry $[Ca^{2+}]_i$ appropriately reflects the change.

Voltage-sensitive $Ca^{2+}$ entry can be measured directly by monitoring voltage-clamped $Ca^{2+}$ current. Consistent with Fig. 11.3, Fig. 11.4 shows that agents which enhance (forskolin, VIP) or decrease (guanethidine) [$^3$H]-noradrenaline release have no effect on $Ca^{2+}$ current in sympathetic neurones. Cadmium, as expected, is an effective inhibitor of $Ca^{2+}$ current.

Whether guanethidine inhibits transmitter release by a cAMP-dependent mechanism is not known. However, the above observations still offer strong support for cAMP enhancement of transmitter release independent of altered $Ca^{2+}$ entry or mobilisation of internal $Ca^{2+}$. Facilitation of exocytosis by cAMP has also been found to be independent of altered $Ca^{2+}$ entry in a prolactin-secreting tumour cell line[10] and in bovine adrenal chromaffin cells[21].

In conclusion, although some investigators have cast doubt on whether cAMP-dependent modulation of secretion occurs in bovine chromaffin cells[16], data from the other neuronal and non-neuronal preparations described above support the idea that, in general, cAMP facilitates exocytosis by a $Ca^{2+}$-independent mechanism.

### 3.3.4  Targets for cAMP-dependent protein kinase phosphorylation

There are two stages of the secretory process at which cAMP-dependent protein kinases can facilitate transmitter release independent of changes in $[Ca^{2+}]_i$. One is by the phosphorylation of synapsin I with consequent increased availability of synaptic vesicles (see Section 2.3 above). The other is by increased catecholamine synthesis regulated by phosphorylation of tyrosine hydroxylase. With respect to the latter, stimulation of splanchnic nerves, which releases

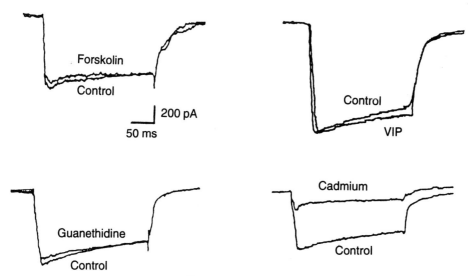

Fig. 11.4. Whole-cell, voltage-clamped $Ca^{2+}$ currents in chick sympathetic neurones. Currents recorded from the same cell during control and the indicated drug treatment are shown superimposed. Treatments that facilitated transmitter release (upper traces) were forskolin (10 $\mu$M) or VIP (10 $\mu$M) for 10 min. Treatments that blocked release (lower traces) were guanethidine (1 $\mu$M) for 15 min and cadmium (30 $\mu$M) for 5 min. Note that only cadmium blocked $Ca^{2+}$ current. Currents were evoked by 200 ms depolarisations from a holding potential of −70 mV. Tetrodotoxin and tetraethylammonium in the bath and caesium in the patch pipette were used to suppress other voltage-sensitive currents.

acetylcholine and VIP, or adrenal perfusion with VIP increases radiolabelled phosphate incorporation into tyrosine hydroxylase[11]. The phosphorylation is associated with increased catalytic activity of the enzyme. Tyrosine hydroxylase can be phosphorylated at four distinct serine residues, serine 8, 19, 31 and 40. The function of Ser-8 phosphorylation is not known. VIP causes up to an 8-fold increase in Ser-40 phosphorylation with no change at the other three sites. Importantly, Ser-40 is the substrate for cAMP-dependent protein kinase and phosphorylation of Ser-40 is specifically associated with increased tyrosine hydroxylase activity[11]. Protein kinase C-dependent and $Ca^{2+}$-calmodulin-dependent kinases (which target Ser-31 and Ser-19, respectively) do not increase enzymatic activity. Likewise, the nicotinic and muscarinic receptors for acetylcholine stimulate phosphorylation of Ser-19 and Ser-31, respectively, and do not increase

tyrosine hydroxylase activity[11]. (It was proposed that the function of Ser-19 and Ser-31 phosphorylation by acetylcholine is to regulate the extent of enzyme activation produced by Ser-40 phosphorylation. However, the interactions between the different sites in regulating enzymatic activity has not yet been investigated.) Thus, in rat adrenal gland, the catalytic activity of tyrosine hydroxylase is controlled by the $Ca^{2+}$-independent action of VIP via cAMP dependent phosphorylation of Ser-40.

In sympathetic ganglia, cAMP-dependent activation of tyrosine hydroxylase is a result of VIP released from presynaptic nerve endings[30]. Therefore, here as well, cAMP appears to play an important part in maintaining transmitter release by stimulating transmitter synthesis.

The fact that processes maintaining both vesicle availability (synapsin I) and transmitter synthesis (tyrosine hydroxylase activity)

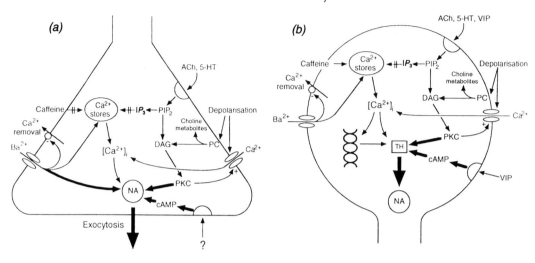

Fig. 11.5. Interacting cellular messengers control transmitter release through $Ca^{2+}$-dependent and $Ca^{2+}$-independent mechanisms. Thicker arrows show the pathways thought to be involved in $Ca^{2+}$-independent modulation of release, but do not necessarily reflect the relative importance of the different pathways in controlling release. (a) In sympathetic nerve terminals, acetylcholine (ACh) and 5-HT, for example, acting via their respective receptors stimulate phosphatidylinositol bisphosphate ($PIP_2$) metabolism. This produces Ins(1,4,5)$P_3$ and diacylglycerol (DAG), which activates protein kinase C (PKC). Protein kinase C may facilitate exocytosis by stimulating $Ca^{2+}$ entry or by increasing the sensitivity of the release process to $Ca^{2+}$. In these terminals, intracellular pools of $Ca^{2+}$ are sensitive to $Ba^{2+}$ but apparently not to Ins(1,4,5)$P_3$ or caffeine. Barium can enter through $Ca^{2+}$ channels and, in addition to possible direct effects on release, displaces internal $Ca^{2+}$ and blocks $Ca^{2+}$ removal. cAMP has no effect on $[Ca^{2+}]_i$ but facilitates evoked release of noradrenaline (NA) by affecting vesicle transport or fusion. The endogenous ligand responsible for stimulating cAMP production in nerve terminals has, however, not been identified. Depolarisation of the nerve terminal stimulates the phosphatidylcholine (PC) pathway in addition to voltage-dependent $Ca^{2+}$ entry. (b) In the neuronal cell body, receptor-coupled second messenger systems parallel those in the terminal. However, $Ca^{2+}$-independent pathways here are also involved in the control of transmitter synthesis, e.g. by affecting the activity of tyrosine hydroxylase (TH). Stores of $Ca^{2+}$ in the cell body appear to be different from those in the terminals in that they are sensitive to both caffeine and $Ba^{2+}$. Metabolism of $PIP_2$ is stimulated by acetylcholine, 5-HT and VIP, acting through their membrane receptors. As in the terminals, Ins(1,4,5)$P_3$ apparently does not affect $[Ca^{2+}]_i$. VIP also stimulates cAMP production, which increases TH activity through phosphorylation. Calcium-independent regulation of transcription factors (not shown) may also affect TH mRNA levels (see refs. 23, 24, 25 and 29).

are targets of cAMP stimulation suggest a compelling scenario for cAMP modulation of transmitter release independent of changes in $[Ca^{2+}]_i$.

## 3.4 Other $Ca^{2+}$-independent modulators of transmitter release

In synapses of cultured invertebrate neurones, the neuropeptide, FMRF-amide causes a reduction of acetylcholine release.

The inhibition of release results partially from the reduction of voltage-sensitive $Ca^{2+}$ entry. However, a significant reduction of acetylcholine release caused by FMRF-amide still occurs in $Ca^{2+}$-free medium. The $Ca^{2+}$-independent target of this peptide is not known, but it was initially proposed to involve dephosphorylation (inhibition) of synapsin I or similar proteins controlling vesicle availability at release sites[19]. More recently, FMRF-amide was found to reduce transmitter release in the presence of constant elevated $[Ca^{2+}]_i$ (produced by photolysis of intracellular caged $Ca^{2+}$), and at low FMRF-amide concentrations ($\leq 10^{-7}$ M) to inhibit transmitter release without changing $[Ca^{2+}]_i$ measured by Fura-2 fluorescence[12]. These results show clearly that FMRF-amide modulates transmitter release without altering $Ca^{2+}$ influx or mobilisation of intracellular $Ca^{2+}$. Furthermore, it has been shown that the $Ca^{2+}$-independent modulation of release requires a pertussis toxin-sensitive G-protein[12]. Because G-proteins play an important role in $Ca^{2+}$-independent synaptic vesicle cycling at the sites of release (see Section 11.2.2 above), it is possible that FMRF-amide acts by reducing the availability of releasable synaptic vesicles.

## 3.5 Interacting signals may modulate release

It is well established that pre- and postsynaptic elements affect each others' characteristics *in vivo*. Accordingly, cultured neurone preparations that contain only one element provide a useful, but not necessarily ideal, model of their counterparts in the body. The model in Fig. 11.5 summarises the interaction of $Ca^{2+}$-dependent and $Ca^{2+}$-independent pathways controlling transmitter release as defined in cultured sympathetic neurones of the chick. The general conclusions are: (i) terminal regions and not cell bodies are the important sites of neurotransmitter release[24;] and (ii) second messengers, including $Ca^{2+}$, regulate different aspects of catecholamine metabolism in different neuronal regions. For example, in nerve terminals, interacting messengers affect vesicle availability and transmitter release whereas in the neuronal cell body interacting messengers affect transmitter synthesis.

Note that $Ca^{2+}$ stores are also different in the two regions. For example, caffeine mobilises internal $Ca^{2+}$ in cell bodies but not in terminals. Barium, however, mobilises $Ca^{2+}$ in both regions and, unlike caffeine, stimulates transmitter release[25] (but see

Chapter 1). Interestingly, agonist-stimulated $Ins(1,4,5)P_3$ generation appears to have no effect on $[Ca^{2+}]_i$ in either region in cultured sympathetic neurones[29].

It is clear that facilitation of $Ca^{2+}$-dependent transmitter release by cAMP occurs without further changes in $Ca^{2+}$ influx or $[Ca^{2+}]_i$. However, the concerted actions of elevated $[Ca^{2+}]_i$ and cAMP may produce greater or additional effects, which are, moreover, different in different cellular regions. In the cell body of sympathetic neurones, $Ca^{2+}$ stimulates gene transcription while both $Ca^{2+}$ and cAMP stimulate tyrosine hydroxylase activity and the synthesis of neurotransmitter. VIP released from preganglionic neurones is the likely physiologic agonist that elevates cAMP in chromaffin cells and neuronal cell bodies in sympathetic ganglia. In nerve terminals, $Ca^{2+}$-independent facilitation of exocytosis may be related to phosphorylation of synapsin I by cAMP-dependent protein kinase. Elevation of cAMP in nerve terminals *in vitro* can be produced by forskolin or application of VIP. However, the important question that remains unanswered is what is the physiological stimulus for cAMP production in sympathetic nerve terminals *in vivo*?

## 4 Summary

Calcium ions play an important role in triggering neurotransmitter release by their action at the site of exocytosis. They also either directly or indirectly, regulate most processes involved in the synthesis of transmitter and the translocation of synaptic vesicles to the site of release. These $Ca^{2+}$-sensitive processes distant from the sites of release are the probable targets for intracellular $Ca^{2+}$ mobilised by second messengers (see also Chapter 1). There is a growing body of evidence that neurotransmitter release can also be modulated independent of altered $Ca^{2+}$ levels. Many of the $Ca^{2+}$-dependent components of exocytosis can be modulated by phosphorylation via $Ca^{2+}$-independent protein kinases. Although specific sites for $Ca^{2+}$-independent modulation are not well defined, possible targets include transcription factors, cytosolic and vesicular proteins regulating the synthesis and packaging of transmitter, and proteins involved in vesicle docking and fusion with the plasma membrane. The strongest evidence for $Ca^{2+}$-independent modulation of neurotransmitter release comes from studies of cAMP-facilitated exocytosis in a variety of secretory cells and sympathetic neurones. New evidence for $Ca^{2+}$-independent control of exocytosis at the sites of release is emerging from studies on the role of G-proteins in vesicle cycling.

The $Ca^{2+}$ hypothesis predicted that elevated $[Ca^{2+}]_i$ was responsible for stimulating transmitter release. However, direct measurement of $[Ca^{2+}]_i$ was not possible in the perfused neuro-effector organs used to develop this hypothesis. The more recent use of cultured cells and $Ca^{2+}$-sensitive fluorescent dyes has led to important new ideas concerning $[Ca^{2+}]_i$ and the release of neurotransmitters. One of these ideas, which continues to gain support, is that concerning $Ca^{2+}$-independent modulation of release.

## References

1. Alder J, Lu B, Valtorta F, Greengard P and Poo M-m (1992) Calcium-dependent transmitter secretion reconstituted in *Xenopus* oocytes: requirement for synaptophysin. *Science* **257**: 657–661
2. Almers W (1990) Exocytosis. *Annual Reviews of Physiology* **52**: 607–624
3. Augustine GJ, Charlton MP and Smith SJ (1987) Calcium action in synaptic transmitter release. *Annual Reviews of Neuroscience* **10**: 633–693
4. Bähler M and Greengard P (1987) Synapsin I bundles F-actin in a phosphorylation dependent manner. *Nature* **326**: 704–707
5. Bittner M, Holtz RW and Neubig RR (1986) Guanine nucleotide effects on catecholamine secretion from digitonin-permeabilized adrenal chromaffin cells. *Journal of Biological Chemistry* **261**: 10182–10188
6. Black IB, Chikaraishi DM and Lewis EJ (1985) Trans-synaptic increase in RNA coding for tyrosine hydroxylase in a rat sympathetic ganglion. *Brain Research* **339**: 151–153
7. Burgoyne RD and Cheek TR (1987) Role of fodrin in secretion. *Nature* **326**: 448
8. Burgoyne RD, Morgan A and O'Sullivan AJ (1989) The control of cytoskeletal actin and exocytosis in intact and permeabilized adrenal chromaffin cells: role of calcium and protein kinase C. *Cellular Signalling* **1**: 323–334
9. Cahall AL and Perlman RL (1987) Preganglionic stimulation increases the phosphorylation of tyrosine hydroxylase in the superior cervical ganglion by both cAMP-dependent and $Ca^{2+}$-dependent protein kinases. *Biochimica et Biophysica Acta* **930**: 454–462
10. Frey EA, Kebabian JW and Guild S (1986). Forskolin enhances calcium-evoked prolactin release from 7315c tumor cells without increasing the cytosolic calcium concentration. *Journal of Pharmacology and Experimental Therapeutics* **29**: 461–466
11. Haycock JW and Wakade AR (1992) Activation and multiple-site phosphorylation of tyrosine hydroxylase in perfused rat adrenal glands. *Journal of Neurochemistry* **58**: 57–64
12. Haydon PG, Man-Son-Hing H, Doyle RT and Zoran M (1991) FMRFamide modulation of secretory machinery underlying presynaptic inhibition of synaptic transmission requires a pertussis toxin-sensitive G-protein. *Journal of Neuroscience* **11**: 3851–3860
13. Hess SD, Doroshenko PA and Augustine GJ (1993) A functional role for GTP-binding proteins in synaptic vesicle cycling. *Science* **259**: 1169–1172
14. Karli UO, Schäfer T and Burger MM (1990) Fusion of neurotransmitter vesicles with target membrane is calcium independent in a cell-free system. *Proceedings of the National Academy of Sciences USA* **87**: 5912–5915
15. Knight DE and Baker PF (1983) The phorbol ester TPA increases the affinity of exocytosis for calcium in 'leaky' adrenal medullary cells. *FEBS Letters* **160**: 98–100
16. Knight DE, von Grafenstein H and Athayde CM (1989) Calcium-dependent and calcium-independent exocytosis. *Trends in Neurosciences* **12**: 451–458
17. Llinas RR, McGuiness TL, Leonard C, Sugimori M and Greengard P (1985) Intraterminal injection of synapsin I or

calcium-calmodulin-dependent protein kinase II alters neurotransmitter release at the squid giant synapse. *Proceedings of the National Academy of Sciences USA* **82:** 3035–3039

18. Malhotra RK, Wakade TD and Wakade AR (1989) Cross-communication between acetylcholine and VIP in controlling catecholamine secretion by affecting cAMP, inositol triphosphate, protein kinase C and calcium in rat adrenal medulla. *Journal of Neuroscience* **9:** 4150–4157

19. Man-Son-Hing H, Zoran MJ, Lukowiak K and Haydon PG (1989) A neuromodulator of synaptic transmission acts on the secretory apparatus as well as on ion channels. *Nature* **341:** 237–239

20. Morgan JI and Curran T (1986) Role of ion flux in the control of c-*fos* expression. *Nature* **322:** 552–555

21. Morita K, Dohi T, Kitayama S, Koyama Y and Tsujimoto A (1987) Enhancement of stimulation-evoked catecholamine release from cultured bovine adrenal chromaffin cells by forskolin. *Journal of Neurochemistry* **48:** 243–247

22. Pozzan T, Gatti G, Dozio N, Vicentini LM and Meldolesi J (1984) $Ca^{2+}$-dependent and -independent release of neurotransmitters from PC12 cells: a role for protein kinase C activation. *Journal of Cell Biology* **99:** 628–638

23. Przywara DA, Bhave SV, Bhave A, Wakade TD and Wakade AR (1991) Dissociation between intracellular $Ca^{2+}$ and modulation of [$^3$H]-noradrenaline release in chick sympathetic neurons. *Journal of Physiology* **437:** 201–220

24. Przywara DA, Bhave SV, Chowdhury PS, Wakade TD and Wakade AR (1993) Sites of transmitter release and relation to intracellular $Ca^{2+}$ in cultured sympathetic neurons. *Neuroscience* **52:** 973–986

25. Przywara DA, Chowdhury PS, Bhave SV, Wakade TD and Wakade AR (1993) Barium-induced exocytosis is due to internal calcium release and block of calcium efflux. *Proceedings of the National Academy of Sciences USA* **90:** 557–561

26. Roskoski R Jr, Vulliet PR and Glass DB (1987) Phosphorylation of tyrosine hydroxylase by cyclic GMP-dependent protein kinase. *Journal of Neurochemistry* **48:** 840–845

27. Schoffelmeer AN and Mulder AH (1983) $^3$H-noradrenaline release from rat neocortical slices in the absence of extracellular $Ca^{2+}$ and its presynaptic alpha$_2$-adrenergic modulation. *Naunyn-Schmiedeberg's Archives of Pharmacology* **323:** 188–192

28. Wakade AR (1979) Recycling of noradrenergic storage vesicles of isolated rat vas deferens. *Nature* **281:** 374–376

29. Wakade TD, Bhave SV, Bhave A, Przywara DA and Wakade AR (1990) $Ca^{2+}$ mobilized by caffeine from the inositol 1,4,5-trisphosphate-insensitive pool of $Ca^{2+}$ in somatic regions of sympathetic neurons does not evoke [$^3$H] norepinephrine release. *Journal of Neurochemistry* **55:** 1806–1809

30. Zigmond RE, Schwarzschild MA and Rittenhouse AR (1989) Acute regulation of tyrosine hydroxylase by nerve activity and by neurotransmitters via phosphorylation. *Annual Reviews of Neuroscience* **12:** 415–461

# 4 Modulation of neurotransmitter release: physiological function

# 12 *In vivo* evidence for presynaptic modulation of neurotransmitter release

Ben H. C. Westerink

Most of the data on which our views of the process of modulation of neurotransmitter release are based have been obtained from *in vitro* experimentation. Often somewhat extreme manoeuvres have had to be employed in order to demonstrate modulatory phenomena in these *ex situ* preparations. Therefore, it is relevant to ask the questions: do these modulatory mechanisms occur *in vivo* and, furthermore, do they have physiological relevance? More recently, investigators have begun to try to answer these questions by devising experimental paradigms to demonstrate whether neurotransmitter release is indeed modulated under normal physiological conditions by the receptor-mediated mechanisms described in the earlier parts of this book. In this chapter, Ben Westerink describes some of the experimental techniques that have been employed in the attempt to measure what actually happens in the physiological situation. From the experimental data he describes, it appears that neurotransmitter-release modulation probably does occur *in vivo*.

## 1 Introduction

To study presynaptic transmitter modulation *in vivo*, it is necessary to monitor the 'release' of neurotransmitters in the brain of living experimental animals. For this purpose, cannulae or chemical electrodes need to be implanted in brain areas. These record the content of neurotransmitters and related metabolites in the extracellular fluid, which is in direct contact with the implanted device. Based upon the assumption that the transmitter concentration in the extracellular fluid is directly related to its concentration in the synaptic cleft, the calculated neurotransmitter concentration is often referred to as 'release'. Various authors have questioned this assumption; for example, the release of neurotransmitters might be modified by uptake into nerves or glial cells or by

metabolism before it reaches the cannula or electrode. Therefore, the sampled transmitter content might better be expressed as 'overflow' or 'extracellular content'. Although aware of its limitation, the word 'release' is used here in its broad sense.

In this chapter, the *in vivo* evidence for presynaptic modulation of neurotransmitter release is briefly reviewed, but first a characterisation of the various methods that are currently used to study neurotransmitter release *in vivo* is given.

## 2 *In vivo* measurement of transmitter release

During the early period of neurochemical research, analysis of neural tissue content of neurotransmitters and their metabolites

217

served as an important source of knowledge of the biochemical aspects of neurotransmission. However, such analyses represent a determination of content in homogenised tissue taken from a killed animal and its significance as an index of release of neurotransmitters is very doubtful for the following reason. Neurotransmitters are stored in nerve terminals and large concentration gradients (1000–10 000-fold) between the intra- and extracellular compartments are typical. It is the (much lower) extracellular concentration of neurotransmitters that is of significance for communication between neurones, but it is the (much higher) concentration that would be measured experimentally. Therefore, various attempts have been made to sample the extracellular compartment of nervous tissue in living animals to obtain a better indication of the amounts of neurotransmitter released.

The first attempts to analyse extracellular fluid were achieved in the late 1960s by the development of the cup- and push-pull-techniques. In 1973, Adams and colleagues reported on the use of carbon paste electrodes for the detection of oxidisable molecules in the extracellular fluid of the brain[16]. This formed the basis for development of *in vivo* voltammetry for measuring neurotransmitters and related metabolites. The microdialysis technique was introduced in 1984 by Ungerstedt[21] and can be considered as a refinement of the push-pull method.

## 2.1   Push-pull perfusion

For a push-pull perfusion experiment, two concentric tubes are stereotactically implanted into a precise localised brain area. Fluid is introduced through the inner tube by a perfusion pump and removed through the outer tube by a second pump. The perfusion fluid comes into direct contact with brain tissue that surrounds the tip of the cannula. Endogenous substances are taken up by the perfusion fluid, which is removed to the exterior for analysis. Push-pull perfusion has been used to measure the release from various discrete brain areas of a variety of compounds, such as catecholamines and their related metabolites, amino acids, peptides and acetylcholine.

Technically push-pull perfusion is somewhat more complicated than the microdialysis method that was developed later. Two exactly calibrated pumps are necessary to transport both the pushed and pulled fluids. Relatively high flow rates are used during push-pull perfusions (10–30 μl/min); thus build up of back-pressure may occur. Clogging of cannulae is also a potential problem, especially when smaller cannulae (< 0.5 mm outside diameter) are used.

It is clear that most push-pull perfusions are carried out during anaesthesia and with artificial respiration, although studies in conscious animals have been reported. Push-pull perfusions are, therefore, generally unsuitable for behavioural studies. In addition, the use of anaesthesia may be disadvantageous for pharmacological studies, as certain drug effects are masked.

## 2.2   Microdialysis

Microdialysis, like push-pull methods, involves the implantation of a pair of fine tubes into the brain. The difference between a push-pull cannula and a microdialysis probe is that to make the latter the inlet and outlet tubing of the former are covered by a (semipermeable) dialysis membrane. The presence of the membrane has several advantages. First, the dialysis membrane is a mechanical barrier and acts to reduce turbulence in the fluid flow. Turbulent, high-velocity fluid flow causes damage when it is directed at brain tissue. Turbulence is a problem in the push-pull perfusion method, which uses concentric tubes that are completely open to the extracellular fluid and high flow rates (see above). Damage to tissue is greatly reduced when the fluid flow is contained inside the probe and is of a low rate, as occurs in microdialysis. Typical flow rates used in microdialysis experiments are between 0.5 and 3 μl/min. These flow rates result in small and concentrated samples.

A second advantage of the dialysis membrane is that it acts as a filter to prevent entry into the probe of the large molecules, for example enzymes, present in the extracellular fluid. Enzymatic degradation of the sample is eliminated once the material has crossed the membrane into the probe. This property is especially advantageous when acetylcholine is sampled, as the extracellularly located acetylcholine esterase normally causes rapid hydrolysis of the transmitter. The filtration has beneficial consequences for the surrounding tissue as well. By preventing their removal, the large molecules, enzymes and other species such as neurotransmitter peptides are kept *in situ* in the brain, thus minimising this aspect of perturbation of the neural environment. However, the fact remains that other neurotransmitters, small molecules and ions are still being removed and may disturb the homeostatic balance of the extracellular environment; such effects are less pronounced in microdialysis than in push-pull methods.

Nevertheless, microdialysis has certain disadvantages compared with push-pull perfusion. The presence of a membrane barrier means that a lower amount of the transmitter of interest will become available to be measured. When such compounds hardly penetrate through the dialysis membrane, e.g. neuropeptides, use of the alternative push-pull cannula is clearly necessary.

Since 1985, microdialysis in conscious animals has become firmly established as a versatile and reliable *in vivo* method to monitor neurotransmitter release. For example, by using flexible tubing the probe in the brain of a freely moving experimental animal can be directly connected to the analytical equipment. With the help of electronically controlled valves, a completely automated on-line microdialysis system can be achieved. The impact of microdialysis on neuropharmacology is illustrated by the fact that more than 1000 articles reporting use of the method have already appeared.

## 2.3 *In vivo* voltammetry

Voltammetry is based on the application of a potential to an electrode in a conducting solution. At potentials sufficient to cause oxidation of the molecules of interest, a current is generated as molecules are oxidised at the electrode surface. Different molecules have different oxidation potentials, depending on the structure of the molecule and the functional groups present. The recorded oxidation current, usually in the nanoampere to picoampere range, is amplified and can be related directly to the concentration of the oxidised molecule. Voltammetry in the brain is carried out with stereotaxically implanted carbon-fibres (diameter 5–30 μm).

Voltammetric measurements are made in the extracellular fluid of the brain and, thus, provide information about the same environment as that of push-pull or microdialysis studies. The method is limited to the measurement of electroactive molecules. However, this includes the catecholamines and indoleamines and, therefore, is applicable to many neurochemically significant classes of molecule. Voltammetry has some unique capabilities that permit observations not possible otherwise. In particular, voltammetry is much faster than perfusion techniques: the ability to monitor rapidly changing concentrations of neurochemicals at a high sampling frequency is one of the most attractive features of *in vivo* voltammetry. However, separating the signal of interest from interfering signals has had to be the focus of a major effort in voltammetric research. This is because many compounds besides the neurotransmitter of interest, e.g. catecholamine metabolites, ascorbic acid and uric acid, are easily oxidised. In addition, the molecules of most interest, the neurotransmitters, are usually present in significantly lower concentrations than are their metabolites or other interfering compounds. Currently, separation of the signals is based on differences in the oxidation potentials of the electroactive molecules. Also, chemical modifications of the electrode surface have been made to increase the sensitivity to certain neurotransmitters[1].

## 2.4 Selection of techniques

The microdialysis technique is, in general, more sensitive than the voltammetric technique. However, the ultimate sensitivity of the microdialysis method depends on the species measured and the method of analysis. For catecholamines and related electroactive molecules, HPLC with electrochemical detection provides a very sensitive analytical method that is convenient to use with dialysates. Since microdialysis does not allow proteins and other large molecules into the perfusate, the sample is automatically cleaned up and can be injected without further purification into a HPLC system. Detection limits of 0.5–2 pg (10–30 fmol) transmitter, present in a few microlitres of dialysate, are routinely reached.

There is a significant difference in spatial resolution between voltammetry and microdialysis. The small size of microelectrodes for voltammetry allows a much more localised region to be sampled than is possible with microdialysis. Diameters of carbon-fibres are typically between 5 μm and 30 μm, with lengths of 100–500 μm. Sampling is thought to occur within 20 μm of the surface. The volume sampled by dialysis probes is considerably larger. Probes are usually 200–300 μm in diameter and several millimetres long. However, because of the continuous removal of material by the probe, concentration gradients are created that may extend as much as several millimetres radially into the tissue.

*In vivo* voltammetry has a temporal resolution of the order of seconds and is, therefore, much faster than microdialysis. Voltammetry can be used to study processes associated with stimulated neurotransmitter release that take place over a few seconds, such as analysing the impulse-dependency of autoreceptors. Microdialysis measurements, however, typically take from 5 to 20 min. In addition, in microdialysis the signal is integrated over the period to produce an average value for the sampling period. Microdialysis is the procedure of choice for analysing the neurochemistry of behaviours that change in the order of minutes (e.g. sexual behaviour, sleep–wake patterns) rather than seconds.

An important advantage of the microdialysis technique (and also of the push-pull method) is that the probe can be used to deliver compounds to local brain regions while simultaneously monitoring the neurochemical response to the infused drug. Used in this way, tetrodotoxin sensitivity and $Ca^{2+}$ dependency of the recorded transmitter release can be established (see below). The microdialysis procedure can be used to stimulate certain neuronal pathways to evoke behavioural changes if neurochemicals are added to the perfusing medium. Likewise, the modulation of the 'naturally' evoked transmitter release can be studied by infusion of neuronal receptor-specific compounds. Direct infusion of compounds into nerve terminal areas is an important tool to characterise presynaptic receptors *in vivo*.

In a nutshell, the differences between voltammetry and microdialysis are that voltammetry is much faster and samples from a smaller region, but it is not as sensitive as microdialysis. While microdialysis is very sensitive and records from a wider field, it is relatively slow.

## 3 Criteria for *in vivo* neurotransmitter release

It is evident that sampling methods cannot be used to study physiological changes without first giving careful consideration to the alterations introduced by the technique itself. *In vivo* sampling techniques are invasive and will always cause damage to nervous tissue. Acute, as well as chronic, use of implanted cannulae will cause artefacts resulting from mechanical damage and consequent gliosis and decrease of oxygen availability to the surrounding nervous tissue. It is particularly important to establish whether the neurotransmitter found in the sample was derived

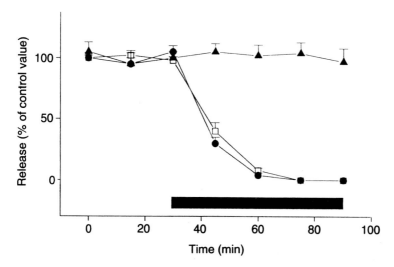

Fig. 12.1.  Effect of tetrodotoxin infusion (60 min, 1 μM; black bar) on the spontaneous release of dopamine (□), acetylcholine (●) and glutamate (▲), recorded with a microdialysis cannula.

from neurotransmission or whether it resulted from mechanically disrupted nerve terminals. The following criteria should be considered.

## 3.1   Recovery from the surgical procedures

Various authors have emphasised that after the surgical implantation of a cannula a certain period of time must be allowed for recovery of the nervous tissue. In the case of dopamine sampled by microdialysis, for example, it has been shown that during the first hours after implantation a considerable proportion of the dialysate content of dopamine is derived from damaged terminals; 8 h after implantation of the probe, virtually all sampled transmitter originated from neuronal activity. Others have emphasised that a period of 24–48 h after implantation of the cannula is necessary for the recovery of nervous tissue from surgical damage.

## 3.2   Tetrodotoxin dependency

A classical feature of neuronal activity is membrane depolarisation caused by the opening of (fast) $Na^+$ channels to allow $Na^+$ influx. Infusion of the $Na^+$-channel blocker tetrodotoxin through the dialysis probe or push-pull cannula can be used to investigate the neuronal origin and release by exocytosis of the sampled neurotransmitter[24]. However, it is emphasised that the interpretation of tetrodotoxin dependency in microdialysis studies differs from that in *in vitro* studies. For example, in (*in vitro*) experiments with brain slices, tetrodotoxin is often used to exclude indirect effects that are caused by excitation of interneuronal connections. This means of discriminating direct from indirect effects cannot be made in microdialysis studies. However in microdialysis studies, tetrodotoxin can be used to discriminate the voltage dependence or independence of drug-induced release. An example of tetrodotoxin-independent (and, therefore, voltage (depolarisation)-independent) neurotransmitter release is the increase in dopamine content of dialysate after administration of amphetamine or certain neurotoxins. Another example is shown in Fig. 12.1: 24 h after implantation of microdialysis probes, the release of neurotransmitters, such as dopamine and acetylcholine, is virtually abolished by tetrodotoxin infusion, judged by its absence from the dialysate samples. In the case of 5-HT and noradrenaline, however, a certain fraction (about 20%) of the transmitter output is often resistant to tetrodotoxin. It is uncertain at this time how to explain the origin of this residual amount of monoamines.

Again, it is difficult to interpret the origin of extracellular GABA recorded by microdialysis or push-pull cannulae. Although it has been reported that drug-induced changes in GABA are often moderate and difficult to quantify, various authors have reported little, if any, effect of tetrodotoxin infusion on GABA levels, whereas others have observed a moderate decrease to 80–60% of control levels[2]. Taking the data together, it can probably be concluded that an important part of the extracellular GABA does not result from neuronal depolarisation. In this respect, it is known that extracellular GABA is compartmentalised in both neuronal and nonneuronal pools.

Extracellular concentrations of neurotransmitter amino acids, such as aspartate and glutamate, are not sensitive to tetrodotoxin infusion (Fig. 12.1). The probable reason is that the appearance of these amino acids in the extracellular fluid are more the result of metabolic processes, such as protein metabolism, than of neurotransmission. Whether measured extracellular levels of glutamate and aspartate have any relation to neurotransmission is unknown at the present time.

### 3.3   $Ca^{2+}$ dependency

Exocytotic transmitter release is $Ca^{2+}$ dependent. The influx of $Ca^{2+}$ during depolarisation of the neurone is an important modulator of transmitter release. Presynaptic receptors are believed to act principally via modulation of the $Ca^{2+}$ influx (see Chapters 9 and 10, but see also Chapter 11). The $Ca^{2+}$ dependency of neurotransmitter release can be investigated by omitting $Ca^{2+}$ from the perfusion fluid. The microdialysis probe does not, however,

remove endogenous $Ca^{2+}$ from its surrounding extracellular fluid, so complete inhibition of neurotransmitter release is difficult to achieve. A better method to evaluate $Ca^{2+}$ dependency is to use relatively high concentrations (12.5–40 mM) of the $Ca^{2+}$ antagonist $Mg^{2+}$ in the perfusing medium. Alternatively since the $Ca^{2+}$ channels that are involved in the neurotransmitter release process are of the N-type, low concentrations of $Cd^{2+}$ (0.3 mM) can be used[23].

The extracellular $Ca^{2+}$ concentration of the brain is about 1.1 mM. When the extracellular $Ca^{2+}$ is elevated by infusion via the microdialysis probe of fluids containing high $Ca^{2+}$ levels, a pronounced increase in the release of transmitters such as dopamine, noradrenaline and serotonin has been observed[24]. Initially, microdialysis studies were carried using classical Ringer solutions that had $Ca^{2+}$ concentrations of 2.4–3.4 mM. With hindsight, it is clear that these studies were carried out under conditions where artificially high levels of neurotransmitter release would have prevailed: the data from these studies should be evaluated with caution.

The $Ca^{2+}$ dependency of the extracellular neurotransmitter content has been investigated in many microdialysis studies. It is a general observation that neurotransmitter release that is sensitive to tetrodotoxin also responds to $Ca^{2+}$ depletion. Omitting $Ca^{2+}$ from the perfusion fluid usually removes 70–80% of the extracellular content of dopamine, noradrenaline, 5-HT or acetylcholine. An almost total depletion of these transmitters in the sampled perfusate is achieved when high $Mg^{2+}$ concentrations or $Cd^{2+}$ are infused. The appearance of GABA in the perfusate is not, or only partly, affected by $Ca^{2+}$ depletion. Likewise, the appearance of the neurotransmitter amino acids glutamate and aspartate is not reduced or may even increase during $Ca^{2+}$ antagonism[23].

It would be of interest to compare the tetrodotoxin and $Ca^{2+}$ sensitivity of push-pull and microdialysis methods. Because of the intimate contact with nervous tissue, push-pull perfusions cause more cell damage than the microdialysis method. Moreover push-pull perfusions are usually carried out in acute experiments. Unfortunately, the relative degree of the damage in push-pull experiments is largely unknown, as data on the tetrodotoxin and $Ca^{2+}$ dependency are scarce in the push-pull literature.

In cats, infusion of tetrodotoxin only partly inhibited the release of [$^3$H]-dopamine from the striatum, whereas the release of the transmitter from the substantia nigra was even stimulated[18].

## 4 *In vivo* evidence for presynaptic autoreceptors

In a recent impressive review on presynaptic autoreceptors Starke *et al.*[19] summarised more than 700 papers on the subject. The authors concluded that release-modulating autoreceptors are widely distributed, although they may not occur on every neurone. The great majority of the studies cited in the review by Starke used *in vitro* methods. In this section, the discussion focuses on the consideration of whether the *in vitro* evidence is supported by *in vivo* studies.

Glowinski and co-workers[4–7,12,13,15,18] were pioneers in the 1970s and early 1980s in investigating the properties of autoreceptors *in vivo*. They used anaesthetised cats, the brains of which were perfused with one or several push-pull cannulae. Neurotransmitter release was measured as radiolabelled compounds after prior administration of radioactive precursors. These studies provided the first *in vivo* support for the existence of various presynaptic auto- and heteroreceptors on cholinergic, dopaminergic, noradrenergic and serotonergic neurones.

### 4.1 *In vivo* criteria for presynaptic receptors

Presynaptic receptors are localised – by definition – on nerve terminals (but see Chapter 15 and also below). To determine the relationship between presynaptic mechanisms and neurotransmitter release, it is important that experimental drugs are infused to that part of a neuronal system where only nerve terminals are localised. The monoaminergic systems are very useful in this respect. The cell bodies of dopaminergic, noradrenergic and serotonergic neurones arc clustered in nuclei in the brain stem and the nerve terminal fields are found in several cortical and subcortical areas. But even infusion of receptor-specific compounds onto nerve terminals does not absolutely guarantee that the recorded changes in neurotransmitter release were caused by presynaptic processes. Interneuronal connections may indirectly contribute in the observed drug effect. Tetrodotoxin infusions cannot be used to exclude possible indirect effects (see Section 12.3.2) as it will abolish direct effects as well. It is necessary, therefore, to remove postsynaptic neurones by pretreatment of the perfused brain area with cytotoxins (such as ibotenic acid) that destroy cell bodies but spare axons.

### 4.2 Dopamine receptors

In the early 1970s, it was observed that dopamine receptor agonists decrease the impulse activity of dopaminergic neurones and inhibit the release and synthesis rate of dopamine; the reverse is true for dopamine antagonists. Initially these changes were interpreted by assuming the presence of a striatonigral interneuronal loop, which was believed to be inhibitory towards nigral dopaminergic cells. However, the use of neurotoxins that destroy postsynaptic neurones, and further electrophysiological investigations, provided evidence that there are autoreceptors localised also at soma-dendritic sites that are able to modify the impulse activity of dopaminergic neurones. The situation then became more complex. Hemisection experiments (in which the dopaminergic cell bodies were separated from the nerve terminals) indicated that when dopaminergic terminals were separated from their cell bodies dopamine release

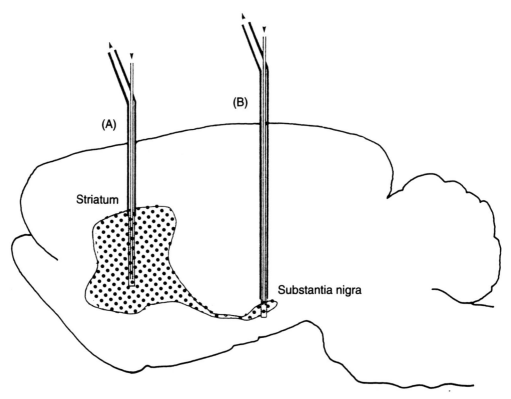

(B)

(A)

Striatum

Substantia nigra

Fig. 12.2. Two microdialysis probes are implanted here into the dopaminergic neurones of the nigrostriatal system. Probe A is located in the nerve terminal area (striatum) and probe B is inserted into the cell body area (substantia nigra).

(from the terminals) could still be modulated as could dopamine synthesis (by the cell bodies). It was concluded that autoreceptors were localised both on presynaptic dopaminergic terminals and at soma-dendritic sites, both contributing to the control of dopamine release. In fact, dopaminergic receptors on nigrostriatal neurones were among the first autoreceptors described.

Microdialysis studies in which dopamine agonists and antagonists were infused into the caudate nucleus provided direct *in vivo* evidence for the presence of presynaptic autoreceptors[14,22]. Pretreatment with cell body neurotoxins excluded a postsynaptic involvement in the measured effects. The autoreceptor was defined pharmacologically as the $D_2$ subtype. The contribution of the

recently discovered $D_3$ and $D_4$ subtypes needs further investigation.

The relative contribution of the autoreceptors on cell bodies and nerve terminals was estimated by simultaneous implantation of two microdialysis probes. Such an experiment is shown in Figs. 12.2 and 12.3. One probe is implanted into the cell body area (in the substantia nigra) and the second probe is implanted into the nerve terminal area (in the striatum). Infusion of a $D_2$ receptor agonist or antagonist into one cannula or the other reveals the response of the cell bodies/dendrites and nerve terminals, respectively. An alternative experiment, by which the relative contribution of autoreceptors on cell bodies and nerve terminals can be readily estimated, is shown in Fig. 12.4. In this

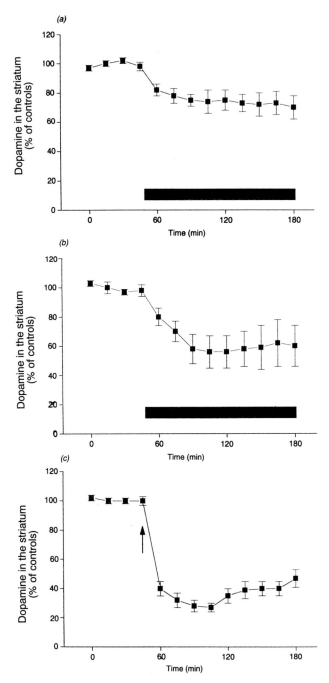

Fig. 12.3. A dopamine $D_2$ agonist $((-)$N-0437) was administered by three different routes to the brain using a push-pull cannula. (a) The agonist (10 μM, black bar) is infused into the soma-dendritic area (substantia nigra) of nigrostriatal dopaminergic neurones (see Fig. 12.2). Dopamine release in the ipsilateral striatum decreased to about 75% of controls. (b) The agonist (1 μM, black bar) was infused into the nerve-terminal area (striatum) and, as a consequence, striatal dopamine release decreased to about 55% of controls. (c) When the agonist was administered systemically (1 μM/kg, intraperitoneally; arrow), dopamine release in the striatum decreased to about 30% of controls. The last effect can be interpreted as a summation of the effects shown in (a) and (b).

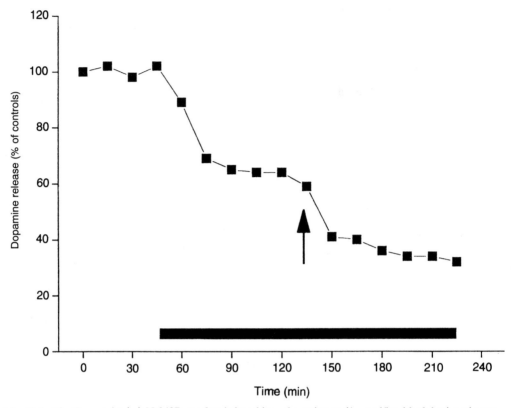

Fig. 12.4. The D$_2$ agonist $(-)$-N-0437 was first infused into the striatum (1 μmol/kg, black bar) and next administered systemically (1 μmol/kg, intraperitoneally, arrow). The decrease in the release of dopamine that was observed in the striatum derives from stimulation of both autoreceptors localised on nerve terminals (first decrease) and also those at soma-dendritic sites (second decrease).

experiment, an intrastriatal infusion of a D$_2$ receptor agonist (to stimulate nerve terminal receptors alone) is followed by a peripheral injection of the same compound (to stimulate both sets of receptors). The results clearly show that release-controlling autoreceptors on nerve terminals and impulse-flow-controlling autoreceptors on cell bodies both contribute to the decrease of striatal dopamine release that is observed when a maximal effective dose of a D$_2$ receptor agonist is systemically administered.

### 4.3   Adrenoceptors

The presence of presynaptic α$_2$-adrenoceptors modulating noradrenaline release was clearly demonstrated by microdialysis studies on rat frontal cortex[11]. As expected, the autoreceptor stimulated a negative feedback mechanism. Systemic administration of the α$_2$-adrenoceptor agonist clonidine reduced, whereas the α$_2$-adrenoceptor antagonists yohimbine and idazoxan increased, the basal release of noradrenaline. When the drugs were infused locally into the nerve-terminal field, similar effects were seen. These effects were unaltered when postsynaptic neurones were destroyed by pretreatment with the cell body neurotoxin ibotenic acid, indicating that the α$_2$-adrenoceptors were, indeed, presynaptically localised.

## 4.4    Presynaptic 5-HT receptors

The first *in vivo* evidence that 5-HT release is modulated by presynaptic autoreceptors came from a push-pull study in which lysergide, infused into the cat, caudate nucleus, was shown to decrease the release of radiolabelled 5-HT[13]. Since then several voltammetric studies have confirmed and extended these observations.

At present, several groups are using microdialysis for the subtyping of 5-HT autoreceptors *in vivo* using the new, selective agonists and antagonists that have been synthesised. In general, 5-HT$_1$ agonists decrease the release of 5-HT in the brain. The reverse is true for 5-HT$_3$ agonists. The subtypes of the 5-HT$_1$ receptor, divided into 5-HT$_{1A}$ and 5-HT$_{1B}$, are of particular interest. It was demonstrated that the soma-dendritic autoreceptor behaves like the 1A type (for which 8-hydroxy-(di-*n*-propylaminotetralin (8-OH-DPAT) is a selective agonist). However, serotonergic terminals probably do not possess 5-HT$_{1A}$ receptors as they do not respond to 8-OH-DPAT infusion. In contrast, nerve terminals are believed to use 5-HT$_{1B}$ receptors to modulate serotonin release. This conclusion is based on experiments in which a decreased release of serotonin was observed when the compound RU24969 (an agonist for 5-HT$_{1A}$ as well as 5-HT$_{1B}$) was infused into the nerve-terminal fields.

## 4.5    Cholinergic receptors

Push-pull and microdialysis studies of the *in vivo* release of acetylcholine revealed that certain anticholinergic drugs increase and cholinomimetics decrease the release of the transmitter when infused into the caudate nucleus[12]. These observations support the presence of muscarinic release-modulating autoreceptors. Strictly speaking, the presynaptic location of these autoreceptors is not yet proved, as potential autoreceptors present on cell bodies were not excluded in these experiments.

Studies on endogenous acetylcholine release usually require the presence of an esterase inhibitor (added to the perfusion fluid) to prevent hydrolysis and thereby allow the analytical chemical detection of the transmitter. However, the presence of an esterase inhibitor had other, unexpected effects on the result in some experiments using the microdialysis technique[10]. In the absence of the inhibitor, the muscarinic antagonist atropine was unable to enhance the release of acetylcholine. However, in the presence of an esterase inhibitor, atropine markedly stimulated the output of acetylcholine. The reverse was true for the cholinomimetic oxotremorine, which decreased the release of acetylcholine only in the absence of esterase inhibition. These observations have implications for presynaptic modulation theory. They indicate that cholinergic autoreceptors are not occupied under normal *in vivo* conditions; i.e. during resting conditions acetylcholine exerts no tonic feedback inhibition on its own release. It is of note that several *in vitro* studies have reached similar conclusions.

## 4.6    Amino acid receptors

A few push-pull studies have provided *in vivo* evidence for the existence of presynaptic GABA$_A$ as well as GABA$_B$ autoreceptors on GABAergic neurones[15]. Only one microdialysis study has reached similar conclusions[2], whereas others have reported an inability to detect such GABAergic presynaptic receptors. The difficulties in interpreting data concerning extracellular levels of GABA (discussed above) may be contributing to the controversy.

## 4.7    The frequency dependence of autoreceptors

Consideration of the phenomenon of presynaptic inhibition mediated by autoreceptors suggests that it is impulse-frequency dependent. The criteria that can be applied experimentally are as follows. First, because of competition between endogenous neurotransmitter and exogenous agonist at presynaptic autoreceptors, the effectiveness of the latter should decrease as the impulse frequency increases. Second, the enhancement of neurotransmitter release by antagonists should increase as the impulse frequency increases. Fulfilment of these criteria proving impulse-frequency dependence has been widely documented by *in vitro* studies. *In vivo* observations, using differential pulse amperometry, are consistent. It has been shown[20] that inhibition of dopamine release by a dopamine receptor agonist declined when the stimulation frequency was increased. Furthermore, it has been shown that, in the presence of antagonists, the stimulation of transmitter release was more pronounced when higher frequencies were applied.

# 5  *In vivo* evidence for presynaptic heteroreceptors

Studies with *in vitro* preparations have described numerous heteroreceptors in various neuronal systems. Direct *in vivo* evidence for presynaptic heteroreceptors is now beginning to accumulate. The monoaminergic neuronal systems have received much attention in this respect. As an example of this research, the presynaptic heteroreceptors found on dopaminergic neurones are discussed below in some detail.

## 5.1  Heteroreceptors on dopaminergic neurones

### 5.1.1  Cholinergic receptors

Various *in vitro* studies using striatal slices and synaptosomes have produced evidence for the presence of presynaptic muscarinic (cholinergic) receptors on dopaminergic terminals. Similar conclusions were drawn by workers using push-pull studies in cats[12]. However, microdialysis studies have been controversial so far. Damsma *et al.*[9] adminis-

tered muscarinic receptor agonists and antagonists systemically to rats and found no effect on the levels of extracellular dopamine in the striatum. Carter *et al.*[3] infused various concentrations of carbachol and atropine into the striatum and likewise found no effect on the release of dopamine. The balance of opinion is that cholinergic modulation of dopamine release is probably not localised at the level of presynaptic heteroreceptors.

### 5.1.2  GABA receptors

*In vitro* studies have provided evidence for the localisation of $GABA_A$ as well as $GABA_B$ receptors on nerve terminals of dopaminergic neurones. Push-pull studies in cats have confirmed that there are interactions between GABA receptors and dopamine release in the striatum, but these effects were interpreted as indirect, acting through interneuronal processes[4]. A microdialysis study found no evidence for the presence of GABA heteroreceptors on dopaminergic nerve terminals (see Fig. 12.5).

### 5.1.3  Excitatory amino acid receptors

Several *in vivo* studies have demonstrated that dopaminergic terminals in the striatum possess receptors for excitatory amino acids. Some controversy exists about the subtypes (NMDA or non-NMDA) of receptors involved. *In vitro* evidence has indicated that NMDA receptors are directly localised on dopaminergic nerve terminals. However, microdialysis studies have concluded that NMDA-modulated release of striatal dopamine is an indirect effect that is mediated probably by cholinergic (inter) neurones[3,25]. There is general agreement that non-NMDA receptors are located on dopaminergic neurones. Microdialysis studies have provided evidence that non-NMDA receptor agonists (AMPA and kainate) were much more potent than NMDA with respect to stimulation of dopamine release in the striatum.

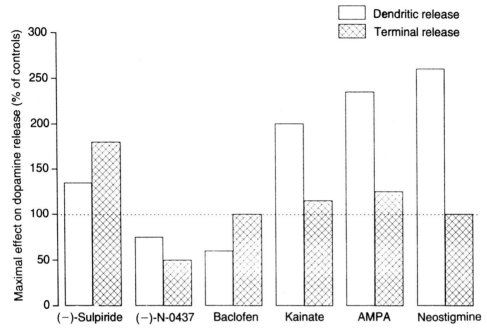

Fig. 12.5. Six different receptor-specific drugs were infused (in separate experiments) into the striatum and substantia nigra (see Fig. 12.2): the $D_2$ antagonist (−)-sulpiride (1 μM), the $D_2$ agonist (−)-N-0437 (1 μM), the $GABA_B$ agonist baclofen (10 μM), the non-NMDA agonists kainate (30 μM) and AMPA (100 μM) and the cholinomimetic agent neostigmine (1 μM). Extracellular dopamine was measured via the same probe. Dopamine release in the striatum (terminal release) responded to (−)-sulpiride, (−)-N-0437, AMPA and kainate. The response was weak to the last two. Dopamine release in the substantia nigra (soma-dendritic release) responded to all six infused drugs. The results indicate that functional receptors are not homogeneously distributed over the dopaminergic neurone.

### 5.1.4 Peptide receptors

The presence of least 12 peptidergic receptors localised on dopaminergic neurones has been reported in *in vitro* studies[5]. Many of these putative heteroreceptors have not yet been confirmed by *in vivo* studies. However, microdialysis studies in which cholecystokinin analogues and neurotensin were directly administered to nerve-terminal fields have provided evidence for localisation of presynaptic peptidergic receptors on dopaminergic nerve terminals. It is of interest to note that cholecystokinin and neurotensin co-exist with dopamine in a subpopulation of ventral tegmental dopaminergic neurones. Presynaptic inhibition by co-localised trans-mitters (co-transmitters) offers an alternative way to modulate neurotransmission (see Chapter 2).

### 5.1.5 Opiates and opioid peptides

The classical observation on opiates was made by Chesselet *et al.*[7] who showed, with a push-pull cannula, that local administration of the μ-opiate agonist morphine and δ-opiate agonists stimulated *in vivo* the spontaneous release of dopamine in the caudate nucleus of the cat. Since then, many studies on the effect of opiates on the *in vivo* release of dopamine have appeared, most of these being concerned with peripheral administration of the opiates (see Chapter 16). Agonists of μ- and δ-opiates stimulated the spontaneous release of dopamine, whereas κ-agonists decreased the release of the transmitter. Infusion of inhibitors of enkephalin-degrading enzymes by microdialysis strongly indicated that local enkephalins may tonically modulate the release of dopamine *in vivo*.

The possible presynaptic localisation of opiate receptors has been studied by infusion of opioid peptides[17]. Administered during microdialysis, δ-agonists stimulated the spontaneous release of dopamine. The effect was seen in the nucleus accumbens but not in the striatum. However, μ-agonists were without effect when infused into either the striatum or nucleus accumbens.

### 5.1.6 Cellular location of heteroreceptors on dopaminergic neurones

For our understanding of heteroreceptors, it is of interest to know whether receptors are always evenly distributed over the whole neurone or whether certain receptors are restricted to either soma-dendritic sites or to nerve terminals. For example, as noted above, $5-HT_{1A}$ receptors are thought to be exclusively localised on cell bodies whereas $5-HT_{1B}$ receptors are found on nerve terminals. What is known about dopaminergic neurones in this respect? The most direct way to study this question is to use an *in vivo* model in which the release of dopamine is sampled by cannulae at different locations along the nigrostriatal bundle. The nigrostriatal dopaminergic system is of particular value in such studies because the soma-dendritic sites and nerve terminals are anatomically well separated. Moreover, soma-dendritic and nerve-terminal receptors are both directly involved in the local release of dopamine (called respectively dendritic and terminal release; see also Chapter 15). This has been investigated with the microdialysis technique (see Fig.12.5). Five different receptors ($D_2$, $GABA_B$, NMDA, non-NMDA (kainate, AMPA) and muscarinic), each

believed to be involved in the regulation of dopaminergic neurotransmission, were studied. Prototypic drugs of these receptors expected to produce marked effects were infused into the brain in separated experiments. In one set of experiments, drugs were infused into the substantia nigra, where the soma-dendritic part of the dopaminergic bundle is localised. The dopamine release that is recorded at this site is, therefore, considered to be dendritic release. In separate experiments, the drugs were infused into the striatum, where the nerve endings of the dopaminergic bundle are localised, and the terminal release of dopamine was recorded.

The results in Fig. 12.5 show that certain functionally active receptors ($D_2$, non-NMDA) are found both on soma-dendritic and terminal sites of dopaminergic neurones. Other receptors (cholinergic receptors, $GABA_B$ receptors) were found to be active on soma-dendritic sites only. It is concluded that an even distribution of functional release-controlling receptors over the cell membrane is not a general feature of neurones.

## 5.2 Heteroreceptors on cholinergic neurones

Detailed anatomical knowledge of neuronal systems has facilitated the detection of heteroreceptors. One heteroreceptor that has, as a consequence of such knowledge, received much attention in neuropharmacology is the $D_2$ receptor that modulates the release of acetylcholine in the striatum. *In vitro* studies have indicated that the $D_2$ receptor is associated with axon–axon contacts and it can, therefore, be considered as a presynaptic heteroreceptor of cholinergic neurones. Microdialysis studies have showed that infusion of $D_2$ antagonists increases the release of acetylcholine whereas $D_2$ agonists decrease the transmitter output[8]. These observations demonstrate that $D_2$ receptors are able to modulate the release of acetylcholine in an inhibitory manner.

## 6   Summary

*In vivo* models that sample the release of neurotransmitters have improved our insight into presynaptic mechanisms. Although many conditions still have to be investigated, it can be concluded that *in vivo* methods have generally confirmed the existence of presynaptic receptors as proposed from *in vitro* experiments. It has become apparent that certain receptor (sub)types are not homogeneously distributed. Some of them are found only on a subpopulation of neurones in a system; even on a single neurone some receptors are restricted to soma-dendritic sites, others to nerve terminals.

Among the various *in vivo* techniques that have been used, microdialysis is of great potential. To date, microdialysis has been used to study receptors in the CNS. Future microdialysis studies no doubt will provide detailed information about properties of receptors *in vivo,* such as receptor reserve, receptor occupancy and up- and down-regulation. It is also probable that microdialysis will be applied to the study of presynaptic receptors on peripheral nerves *in vivo.* Selective presynaptic agonists and antagonists are continually being developed for the many subtypes of receptors that are now being discovered. Microdialysis will be of great value in the evaluation of these new drugs and in determining how they might affect the activity of the nervous system in intact organisms.

In the future, microdialysis might be combined with specific detection methods, perhaps using immobilised enzymes to construct biosensors, such as glutamate sensors. New possibilities to investigate presynaptic processes will appear when microdialysis probes and related biosensors are combined with electrophysiological recording techniques such as single-unit recording in conscious subjects.

## References

1. Blaha CD and Lane RF (1984) Chemically modified electrode for *in vivo* monitoring of brain catecholamines. *Brain Research Bulletin* **10:** 861–864
2. Bourdelais AJ and Kalivas PW (1992) Modulation of extracellular γ-aminobutyric acid in the ventral pallidum using in vivo microdialysis. *Journal of Neurochemistry* **58:** 2311–2320
3. Carter CJ, l'Heureux R and Scatton B (1988) Differential control by *N*-methyl-D-aspartate and kainate of striatal dopamine release *in vivo*: a trans-striatal study. *Journal of Neurochemistry* **51:** 462–468
4. Chéramy A, Nieoullon A and Glowinski J (1978) GABA-ergic process involved in the control of dopamine release from nigrostriatal dopaminergic neurons in the cat. *European Journal of Pharmacology* **48:** 281–295
5. Chéramy A, Barbeito L, Godeheu G *et al.* (1990) Respective contributions of neuronal activity and presynaptic mechanisms in the control of the *in vivo* release of dopamine. *Journal of Neural Transmission* **29:** 183–193
6. Chéramy A, Leviel V, and Glowinski J (1981) Dendritic release of dopamine in the substantia nigra. *Nature* **289:** 537–542
7. Chesselet MF, Chéramy A, Reisine TD and Glowinski J (1981) Morphine and δ-opiate agonists locally stimulate *in vivo* dopamine release in cat caudate nucleus. *Nature* **291:** 320–322
8. Damsma G, de Bocr P, Westerink BHC and Fibiger HC (1990) Dopaminergic regulation of striatal cholinergic interneurons: an in vivo microdialysis study. *Naunyn-Schmiedeberg's Archives of Pharmacology* **342:** 523–527
9. Damsma G, Westerink BHC, de Vries JB and Horn AS (1988) The effect of systemically applied cholinergic drugs on the striatal release of dopamine, as determined by automated brain dialysis in conscious rats. *Neuroscience Letters* **89:** 349–354
10. de Boer P, Westerink BHC and Horn AS (1990) The effect of acetylcholinesterase inhibition on the release of acetylcholine from the striatum *in vivo*: interaction with autoreceptor responses. *Neuroscience Letters* **116:** 357–360
11. Dennis T, l'Heureux R, Carter C and Scatton B (1986) Presynaptic alpha-2 adrenoreceptors play a major role in the effects of idazoxan on

cortical noradrenaline release (as measured by *in vivo* dialysis) in the rat. *Journal of Pharmacology and Experimental Therapeutics* **241:** 642–649

12. Giorguieff M-F, Le Floc'h ML, Glowinski J and Besson M-J (1977) Involvement of cholinergic presynaptic receptors in the control of the spontaneous release of dopamine from striatal dopaminergic terminals in the rat. *Journal of Pharmacology and Experimental Therapeutics* **200:** 535–544

13. Hery F, Simonnet G, Bourgoin S *et al.* (1979) Effect of nerve activity on the *in vivo* release of [$^3$H] serotonin continuously formed from L-[$^3$H] tryptophan in the caudate nucleus of the cat. *Brain Research* **169:** 317–334

14. Imperato A and Di Chiara G (1988) Effects of locally applied $D_1$ and $D_2$ receptor agonists and antagonists studied with brain dialysis. *European Journal of Pharmacology* **156:** 385–393

15. Kemel ML, Gauchy C, Glowinski J and Besson M-J (1983) *In vivo* release of [$^3$H]GABA in cat caudate nucleus and substantia nigra. I. Bilateral changes induced by a unilateral application of muscimol. *Brain Research* **272:** 331–340

16. Kissinger PT, Hart JB and Adams RN (1973) Voltammetry in brain tissue – a new neurophysiological measurement. *Brain Research* **55:** 209–213

17. Longoni R, Spina L, Mulas A *et al.* (1991) (D-Ala)Deltorhin II: $D_1$-dependent stereotypes and stimulation of dopamine release in the nucleus accumbens. *Journal of Neuroscience* **11:** 1565–1576

18. Nieoullon A, Chéramy A and Glowinski J (1977) Release of dopamine *in vivo* from cat substantia nigra. *Nature* **266:** 375–377

19. Starke K, Göthert M and Kilbinger H (1989) Modulation of neurotransmitter release by presynaptic autoreceptors. *Physiological Reviews* **69:** 864–989

20. Suaud-Chagny MF, Ponec J and Gonon F (1991) Presynaptic autoinhibition of the electrically evoked dopamine release studied in the rat olfactory tubercle by *in vivo* electrochemistry. *Neuroscience* **45:** 641–652

21. Ungerstedt U (1984) Measurement of neurotransmitter release by intracranial dialysis. In: Marsden CA (ed), *Measurement of Neurotransmitter Release* in vivo, pp 81–107 John Wiley, New York

22. Westerink BHC and de Vries JB (1989) On the mechanism of neuroleptic increase in striatal dopamine release: brain dialysis provides direct evidence for mediation by autoreceptors localized on nerve terminals. *Neuroscience Letters* **99:** 197–202

23. Westerink BHC, Hofsteede HM, Damsma G and de Vries JB (1988) The significance of extracellular $Ca^{2+}$ for the release of dopamine, acetylcholine and amino acids in conscious rats, evaluated by brain microdialysis. *Naunyn-Schmiedeberg's Archives of Pharmacology* **337:** 373–378

24. Westerink BHC, Hofsteede RM, Tuntler J and de Vries JB (1989) The use of $Ca^{2+}$ antagonism for the characterization of drug-evoked dopamine release from the brain of conscious rats determined by microdialysis, *Journal of Neurochemistry* **52:** 705–712

25. Westerink BHC, Santiago M and de Vries JB (1992) The release of dopamine from nerve terminals and dendrites of nigrostriatal neurons induced by excitatory amino acids in the conscious rat. *Naunyn-Schmiedeberg's Archives of Pharmacology* **345:** 523–529

# 13 Modulation of secretion from neurosecretory cells

Michael R. Boarder

Modulation of release appears to be a ubiquitous phenomenon in the nervous system and has been demonstrated in a very large number of types of synapse in a wide range of animal species. The phenomenon appears to be even more widespread: the general concept of modulation of release applies also to neurosecretion at the interface of the nervous and the endocrine systems. In this chapter, Michael Boarder considers two illustrative examples of neurosecretion where the products of specialised neurones or neuronally derived cells are released into the bloodstream (rather than into a synaptic cleft), but whose release is clearly modulated at, or close to, the site of release.

## 1 Introduction

A commonly recognised characteristic of neurones is that they communicate with other cells by release of a transmitter that is delivered directly to, or close to, the surface of the target cell. This target cell is usually thought of as a neurone, a muscle cell or a secretory (e.g. exocrine) cell, but it may also be one of a variety of other cell types (e.g. glial, endothelial and epithelial cells). This form of cell–cell communication (neurotransmission) is distinct from endocrine secretion, where the released agent (the hormone) reaches the target cell via the bloodstream. However, there are a number of other situations in which neurones or related cells (neurone-like cells such as adrenal chromaffin cells) release substances that reach their target cells by way of their blood supply (see also Chapter 7). This release of a hormone by a neurone or neurone-like cell is called neurosecretion. Beyond the obvious and defining characteristic of the ontogenic equivalent of neurosecretory cells and neurones, the process of neurosecretion has much in common with that of neurotransmission. The aim of this chapter is to describe the process of neurosecretion and to show that neurosecretion may be modulated in much the same way as is neurotransmission in neurones. First, the general nature of neurosecretion is described and compared with neurotransmission and hormone release. Then specific examples of release from neurosecretory cells of the hypothalamus and the adrenal medulla will be given to illustrate central and peripheral neurosecretion, respectively, and the modulatory mechanisms that pertain.

### 1.1 Neurosecretion compared with neurotransmission

One aspect of neurosecretion that places it in close relationship with neurotransmission is the nature of the communicating molecules:

233

hormones and neurotransmitters (see also Chapter 7). Neurotransmitters are lipophobic compounds that do not readily pass biological membranes and that, prior to their release by exocytosis, are stored in a reservoir comprising vesicles. After release, neurotransmitters exert their biological effects by combining with specific cell-surface receptors that transduce the stimulation into an intracellular signal[†] The presence of a neurotransmitter reservoir means that the rate of release can be dissociated from the rate of synthesis. The neurosecretory hormones conform to this pattern and, therefore, the modulation of secretion of the neurohormones might be expected to have much in common with the release of neurotransmitters. Hormones released from other endocrine sites, i.e. non-neuronal sites, display a greater diversity in form and function. For example, the lipophobic hormones from the adrenal cortex are not stored, are released as they are synthesised and enter their target cells to exert their biological effects after combining with an intracellular receptor, rather than via an interaction with cell surface receptors (but see Chapter 8).

## 1.2  Biochemical nature of neurohormones

With respect to their biochemical nature, the neurosecretory hormones are principally biogenic amines and peptides, although other substances are certainly involved.

### 1.2.1  Biogenic amines

Two examples of biogenic amines as neurohormones are given here. Hypothalamic dopamine neurones provide for both neuro-

transmitter release and for neurohormone release, the latter from terminals in the median eminence releasing into the hypthalamo–pituitary portal system (see below). The target cells of this dopamine are the lactotrophs of the anterior pituitary, and here dopamine acts as a prolactin release-inhibiting hormone. This is probably the only instance of a 'classical' neurotransmitter acting directly on secretory cells of the anterior pituitary. The second example is release of noradrenaline and adrenaline from the chromaffin cells of the adrenal medulla. Some aspects of the modulation of release of these catecholamines from chromaffin cells will be detailed below. These two examples illustrate the principle that biogenic amines in the role of neurohormones are the same compounds as those acting as neurotransmitters in the central and peripheral nervous systems.

### 1.2.2  Peptides

Many neurones in the brain and periphery are known to secrete peptides as well as classical neurotransmitters, such as biogenic amines[2] (see Chapter 2). Neurones store classical transmitters in small translucent vesicles of 40–50 nm diameter, while peptide neurotransmitters are stored in a smaller population of large dense-cored vesicles, which may, in addition, contain classical neurotransmitters (see Chapter 4). In neurosecretion, the peptides are strongly represented. Some aspects of the processes associated with peptide neurotransmission are poorly understood. Studies of the synthesis, storage and release of neurosecretory peptides have played a very important role in providing an understanding of how neurones function.

### 1.2.3  Common transmitters that are not neurohormones

By contrast with the catecholamines, acetylcholine is a classical neurotransmitter that does not behave as a neurohormone. Acetylcholine is not found in the circulation because it is effectively removed by

---

[†] An interesting exception to this rule is nitric oxide, which plays an important neuromodulatory (neurotransmitter?) role in the brain (see also Chapter 7). It is a compound that does readily pass through biological membranes, it is not stored in a reservoir, it is released at the rate at which it is synthesised, it is not released by exocytosis and its 'receptor' is an intracellular enzyme.

cholinesterases following release into the extracellular compartment. This illustrates a simple principle: a compound which is unstable or rapidly degraded cannot function as a hormone, although these may be very desirable attributes in a neurotransmitter (but see Section 3.3.1 below concerning ATP release from the adrenal medulla).

In central neurones, the excitatory (e.g. glutamate) and inhibitory (e.g. GABA and glycine) amino acid transmitters are ubiquitous but do not appear to act as neurohormones.

## 1.3 Modulation of neurosecretion: special considerations for neuropeptides

As mentioned above, peptides play a dominant role in neurosecretion. The differences between biogenic amine and peptide biosynthesis in neurones, the relationship to vesicular supply and the consequences for supply of neurotransmitters for release have been described previously[2]. In this section the consequences for presynaptic modulation of different modes of supply and release of neurohormones are considered.

In a 'conventional' neurone, the principal sites of release (terminals) are physically remote from the cell body where proteins are synthesised. Therefore, proteins involved in the functioning of the nerve terminals have to be transported down the axon. This is a relatively slow process, which may take up to several days. With catecholamines, for example, the enzymes for biosynthesis are transported to the terminals from the cell body. Therefore, an adaptive response of a neurone, which involves increased or decreased biosynthesis of enzymes, will take hours or days before it can have an effect on the capacity to synthesise neurotransmitter at the nerve terminal. However, biosynthesis of the neurotransmitter is principally at the site of release and so local changes in demand can be accommodated by rapid changes in supply. Presynaptic receptors play a central role in this rapid adapative process, modulating not only release itself but also changes in

biosynthesis. This is best illustrated in the brain by the dopaminergic terminals of the basal ganglia. Here, the consequences of changes in membrane polarity and activation of presynaptic receptors by released dopamine jointly control the activity of tyrosine hydroxylase. Together they rapidly link supply to demand.

The situation as it applies to peptide neurotransmitters is quite different. Here the peptide sequence is synthesised *de novo* as part of a longer precursor (the pro-peptide) in the cell body. This is then packaged in the Golgi apparatus and processed by partial proteolysis and covalent modification to form the mature peptide contained within the vesicles. In this case, the supply of peptides for release is delivered down the axon to the terminals. Membrane polarity changes and activation of presynaptic receptors cannot rapidly modulate supply in response to demand (Fig. 13.1).

There is, however, a reservoir of peptide stored in the vesicles. The presence of a reservoir of neurotransmitters enables rate of release to be dissociated from rate of synthesis. This is of particular importance for the neuropeptides, since it means that presynaptic events can modulate release even though, in the short term, they cannot modulate supply (biosynthesis).

It is known that this situation pertains to neurohormone release: indeed, early work on neurohypophysial peptides contributed to the development of this picture of peptide neurochemistry[9]. For example, vasopressin and oxytocin, along with their neurophysins, are synthesised by neurones in the supraoptic and paraventricular nuclei of the hypothalamus and transported down the axons to the nerve terminals in the posterior pituitary, from where they are released into the blood supply. Studies labelling the hypothalamic nuclei *in vivo* with [$^{35}$S]-cysteine established that *de novo* synthesis of the peptide chains occurs in the hypothalamic cell bodies in the form of a precursor containing the respective neurophysin sequence. Processing to the mature peptides occurs intragranularly

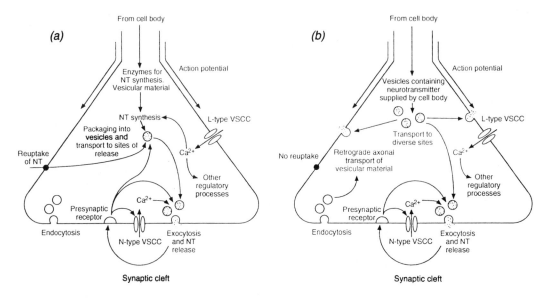

Fig. 13.1. Autonomy of the nerve terminal: comparison between biogenic amines and peptides. (a) A biogenic amine neurotransmitter or neurohormone (NT) terminal. Recycling of vesicles, local biosynthesis and packaging into vesicles and reuptake of released NT all contribute to local control. Presynaptic receptors modulate both supply and release of NT. Release is shown to be localised to hot-spots adjacent to N-type (ω-conotoxin-sensitive) VSCC. (b) Peptide neurotransmitter or neurohormone biosynthesis does not occur in the terminals. As a result, local autonomy is lost. There is no reuptake. Endocytosis of vesicles does occur, but these cannot be refilled. Modulation by presynaptic receptors is limited to regulating release, which can occur at diverse sites at the nerve-terminal plasma membrane. A situation such as this exists with the vasopressin and oxytocin terminals of the posterior pituitary.

during transport to the terminals, where the [$^{35}$S]-labelled peptide is released[25]. These studies also showed that rates of biosynthesis and processing could be modulated by changes in salt intake.

This understanding of the relationship between cell body and terminals and the inability of the neurohypophysial neurones to regulate synthesis in response to presynaptic factors is important for our understanding of physiological and pathophysiological processes such as diabetes insipidus[†].

† While the hypothalamic vasopressin- and oxytocin-containing nuclei are usually considered from the point of view of the neurosecretory function of their posterior pituitary projections, magnocellular cell bodies from these nuclei also project direct into the brain, where they make axosomatic and axodendritic contacts[11]. This shows that the lessons learnt from neurosecretory cells also apply to true neurotransmission.

## 1.4 Exocytosis and endocytosis in neurosecretion

One of the pieces of evidence that supports the notion that neurohypophysial hormones are released by exocytosis is the concurrent increase in membrane capacitance[11]. A capacitance increase is a consequence of the incorporation of the vesicular membrane into the terminal plasmalemma and the ability to make measurements of small capacitance changes has facilitated the study of exocytosis in single neurohypophysial nerve terminals. The neurohypophysial nerve endings have been the subject of a number of studies on retrieval of membrane into vesicles from the synaptic plasma membrane. These include a recent report that adds considerably to the view that following exocytosis the vesicle membrane rapidly undergoes endocytosis, selectively retrieving this membrane unconta- minated by plasma membrane to provide a population of terminal vacuoles[17]. This pro- vides an important addition to our understanding of secretion from neurones: the vesicle appears to fuse with the terminal plasma membrane, opens to the extracellular spaces and releases its contents, then rapidly recloses in an endocytotic phase returning it to the terminal interior. As a result of the exocytosis/endocytosis model, the synaptic vesicle pathway has been described as a 'local, autonomous pathway independent of organelles, such as the Golgi complex'[27]. However, in the hypothalamic posterior pitu- itary nerve terminals where vasopressin and oxytocin synthesis or reuptake does not occur, it is clear that this is not the case (Fig. 13.1). New vesicles for release are dependent on a Golgi-derived supply of pep- tide sequences from the cell bodies. The rapid retrieval of vesicular material has no effect on short-term kinetics of release, which is predictably transient despite sustained depolarisation[12].

It is likely that, in most cases, neurotrans- mission involves co-release of peptides and 'classical' neurotransmitters. It is doubtful, therefore, whether local autonomy (of termi- nals) is generally the case. This limits the role that presynaptic receptors can have on the functioning of nerve terminals, particularly with respect to synthesis and release of peptides.

## 2 Modulation of hypophysiotrophic hormone secretion

The process of hypophysiotrophic hormone release involves secretion directly from ter- minals of hypothalamic nerves into the portal blood supply, which connects the hypothala- mus and terminals in the pituitary stalk to the secretory cells of the anterior pituitary (Fig. 13.2). Neurones with cell bodies located in the periventricular regions of the hypothal- amus and with terminal fields in the median eminence secrete hormones controlling endocrine cells of the anterior pituitary. The question of regulation of these hypothalamic neuroendocrine secretions by cell surface receptors is clearly important for the orches- tration of the endocrine system. An interest- ing example is the reciprocal regulation of growth hormone (GH) secretion from the somatotrophs of the anterior pituitary by the hypophysial neurohormones that stimulate (GH-releasing hormone: GHRH) or inhibit (somatotrophin release-inhibiting factor: SRIF, synonymous with somatostatin) the release of GH.

### 2.1 Modulation of growth hormone release

#### 2.1.1 Mechanisms acting at the cell body

There is an inverse relationship between release of GHRH and SRIF into the portal system, such that when GHRH is high then SRIF is low and vice-versa. This has a cycle time of about 4 h and underlies the regula- tion of pulsatile GH secretion[22]. Multiple inputs regulate this system and a hypothesis for the maintenance of the relationship of GHRH release to SRIF release is that SRIF terminals form direct inhibitory synapses with GHRH-releasing cells and are them- selves under the negative control of GHRH (Fig. 13.3). The majority of GHRH-releasing terminals in the median eminence have their cell bodies in the ventrolateral part of the arcuate nucleus of the hypothalamus.

Information currently available concern- ing the regulation of GHRH synthesis and release from these cells by SRIF receptors is as follows.

1. Neutralisation of SRIF influence by pas- sive immunisation leads to an increase in GHRH secretion and consequently of pituitary GH secretion[22].
2. Injection of cysteamine selectively depletes hypothalamic SRIF and causes an increase in GHRH immunoreactivity and GHRH mRNA-positive neurones in the arcuate nucleus[23].

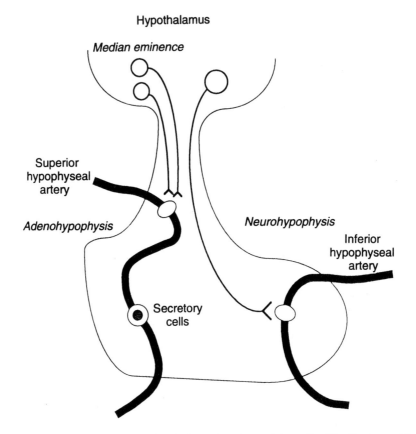

**Hypothalamus**

*Median eminence*

Superior
hypophyseal
artery

*Adenohypophysis*

*Neurohypophysis*

Inferior
hypophyseal
artery

Secretory
cells

Fig. 13.2. Delivery of neurohormones to the pituitary. Neurones with small cell bodies located in periventricular and paraventricular regions of the hypothalamus release their neurohormones into the descending portal system of the pituitary stalk. They are carried through this to the anterior pituitary (adenohypophysis) where they interact with endocrine target cells. In addition, magnocellular neurones of the hypothalamus project via long axons to the posterior pituitary (neurohypophysis) where they directly release their hormones into the bloodstream.

3. Physical disruption of SRIF projections to the arcuate nucleus increases GHRH immunoreactivity and GHRH release.
4. The arcuate nucleus contains a network of SRIF-containing axons originating from cell bodies located both within the arcuate nucleus itself and in other hypothalamic sites[29].
5. Cells showing SRIF receptor binding within the arcuate nucleus are concentrated in the ventrolateral portion and show considerable

co-localisation with both GHRH immunoreactive cells and those positive for GHRH mRNA[1].

These physiological and anatomical observations have established that the release of GHRH is negatively correlated with the release of SRIF, so that release of GHRH is at a peak when that of SRIF is minimal. This negative correlation is maintained, at least in part, by the inhibitory influence of local SRIF

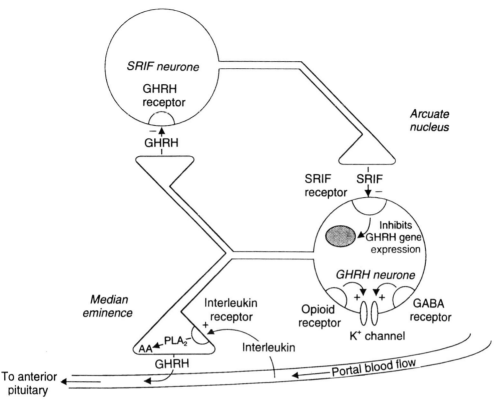

Fig. 13.3. Modulation of GHRH secretion from terminals in the median eminence of the hypothalamus by receptors on these nerve terminals and by receptors on their cell bodies in the arcuate nucleus. The figure shows a two-way interaction between SRIF release-inhibiting GHRH neurones and GHRH release-inhibiting SRIF neurones. In addition, GHRH is shown as being released into the portal blood by which it is carried to the adenohypophysis. GHRH release may be under the inhibitory control of interleukins, acting at the nerve terminals and stimulating phospholipase $A_2$ ($PLA_2$) activity and formation of modulatory metabolites of arachidonic acid (AA).

neurones exerted directly on the GHRH cell bodies (Fig. 13.3). The immunohistochemical and *in situ* hybridisation (GHRH mRNA) studies listed above suggest that the occupation of SRIF receptors on the GHRH cell bodies reduces the expression of the gene for GHRH and, thus, its synthesis, as shown in Fig. 13.3. Therefore, these studies point to regulation of GHRH release and synthesis by cell-surface SRIF receptors; however, the biochemical mechanisms underlying this regulation remain unclear.

It is interesting to note that the reciprocally inverse relationship between release of GHRH and SRIF provides for a flexibility in response to the major inhibitory central neurotransmitter, GABA, which explains both the GABA-mediated enhancement (GABA receptors on SRIF neurones) and the GABA-mediated inhibition (GABA receptors on GHRH neurones) reported in the literature. It is apparent that the perikarya of the arcuate nucleus contain both $GABA_B$ and $\mu$-opioid receptors (Fig. 13.3), both linked to a single population of inwardly rectifying ligand-gated $K^+$ channels[14]. These studies have provided insight into the biochemical events underlying control of neurohormone release and should lead to advances in providing a molecular model for the modulation of release by inputs at the levels of the perikarya.

### 2.1.2 Mechanisms acting at secretory terminals

Various indications suggest the presence of receptors on the terminals of the neurones in the median eminence. There is also an ascending component to the hypothalamic pituitary vascular system, which would allow hormones from the pituitary to be delivered directly to the nerve terminals of the median eminence. The presence of these components allows for the possibility that pituitary hormones modulate the production and secretion into the descending portal blood flow of their own releasing hormones by an action at presynaptic sites. There is evidence that this takes place.

Another example of regulation of hormone release by receptors at the terminals within the median eminence concerns the interleukins. Interleukin-1 (IL-1) and interleukin-6 (IL-6) have emerged as principal mediators between the immune system and the endocrine system. Evidence suggests that the main site of action is at the level of the hypothalamic neuroendocrine system. Although interleukins and other cytokines do not cross the blood–brain barrier, one point at which the barrier is necessarily weak within the hypothalamus is at the sites of neuroendocrine release in the median eminence. There is evidence that it is here that interleukins act, regulating release of GHRH as well as CRH[20,26]. While it is likely that this is a direct action at presynaptic receptors on the nerve-terminal plasmalemma, the characteristics and mechanisms involved are, once again, not well understood. However, there is evidence to suggest that IL-6 stimulation of CRH release involves the products of arachidonic acid metabolism resulting from the activation of phospholipase $A_2$ (see also Chapter 7 and 9). This is the enzyme that cleaves arachidonic acid, normally a rate-limiting intermediate in the synthesis of prostaglandins and related compounds, from its readily available phospholipid precursor. It has previously been described as an effector mechanism for certain cell surface receptors (see Chapter 9). Dexamethasone, which acts as an indirect inhibitor of $PLA_2$ activity, and inhibitors of enzymes responsible for converting arachidonic acid to its varied active products attenuate the IL-6 stimulated release of CRH[15]. This is in accord with the observations that some products of arachidonic acid metabolism (e.g. leukotriene $B_4$ and prostaglandins) regulate CRH release. These various observations suggest that the release of the hypothalamic hypophysial-releasing hormones is regulated by presynaptic receptors within the median eminence that utilise phospholipase $A_2$ and arachidonic acid metabolites as their effector mechanisms. This is illustrated in Fig. 13.4 for CRH release from nerve terminals of paraventricular neurones, but is also shown in Fig. 13.3 for GHRH release.

It seems likely that presynaptic modulation of hypothalamic hormones at their site of release in the median eminence is widespread. Other examples include instances of neurohormone release by neurotransmitters derived from the neural network of the brain. Specifically, a recent report suggests that the hypophysiotrophic hormone LHRH is regulated by dopaminergic terminals making direct synaptic contacts with LHRH-containing terminals in the median eminence[7].

From the foregoing, it is apparent that the site of neurohormone release in the median eminence is one of the principal points of integration of the endocrine system. The weakness of the blood–brain barrier, the blood supply both into the portal system and perhaps from the ascending component of the portal system, the input of information from the immune system via, for example, the cytokines, and the direct input from the brain neurones all converge and are integrated at the median eminence. Presynaptic receptors clearly play a key role in neurohormone release modulation. Despite this little

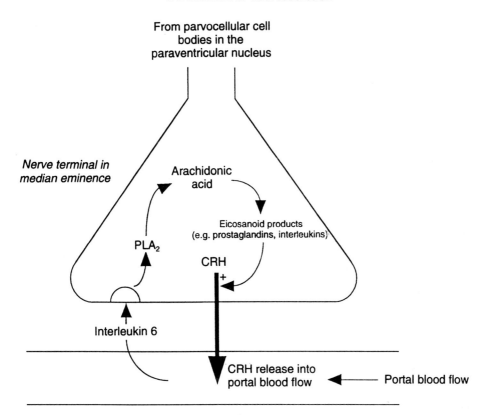

Fig. 13.4. Modulation of CRH release by presynaptic interleukin receptors. The figure is a cartoon of an axon in the median eminence (originating from a hypothalamic CRH-containing cell body) with its nerve terminal adjacent to the capillary plexus of the portal system which passes to the anterior pituitary. Interleukin-6 modulates release by activation of phospholipase $A_2$ ($PLA_2$).

is known about the receptors and the effector mechanisms that are responsible for this presynaptic integration.

## 3    Modulation of secretion from the adrenal medulla

The neurosecretory cells of the adrenal medulla, the chromaffin cells, are conveniently considered as postganglionic sympathetic neurones which have no axon: release occurs from the cell body[6,13]. They are neuroendocrine cells because their secretory products, mainly catecholamines, reach target cells via the circulation. The functioning of the chromaffin cells is modulated by a wide variety of substances of diverse origin (see Fig. 13.5). Like true postganglionic neurones, they are subject to regulation by neurotransmitter released from their preganglionic innervation. In the case of adrenal chromaffin cells, this is a branch of the splanchnic nerve. Also in common with other peripheral neurones, the chromaffin cells, are influenced by blood-borne agents. However, specific to the adrenal medulla is the influence of steroids produced by the adjacent adrenal cortex and delivered in high concentration by the intra-adrenal blood supply. In addition, the highly vascularised adrenal medulla, with dense secretory cells interspersed with small blood vessels, means that the chromaffin cells may also be subject to the influence of

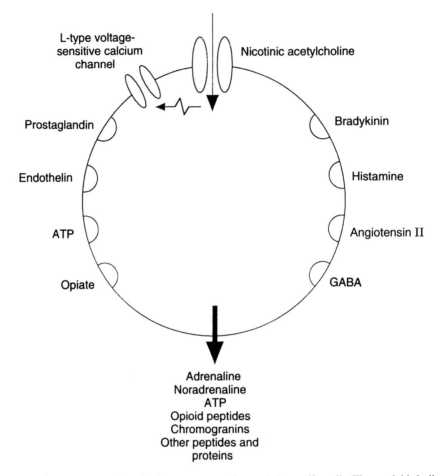

Fig. 13.5. Multiple receptors and multiple secretory products of chromaffin cells. The model is built principally from data from bovine chromaffin cells. The nicotinic acetylcholine receptor elicits the largest secretory response, mediated by $Na^+$ (and $Ca^{2+}$) influx through the receptor channel causing local depolarisation. This depolarisation opens (mainly) L-type voltage-sensitive $Ca^{2+}$ channels, allowing $Ca^{2+}$ influx that is independent of voltage-sensitive $Na^+$ channels. Activation of their respective receptor(s) by the other agents indicated stimulates secretion, or positively or negatively modulates acetylcholine-evoked secretion. In all cases, stimulation of secretion requires $Ca^{2+}$ influx. This may again be via L-type voltage-sensitive channels (e.g. with stimulation by prostaglandins[21]), or by another route (e.g. with stimulation by bradykinin[19]). Other receptors (e.g. muscarinic acetylcholine receptors) are present on these cells and may play a role in both short-term and long-term modulation of release elicited by activation of receptors by other agonists shown. For example, the effects evoked by bradykinin and histamine are subject to modulation by other agonists that stimulate protein kinase C[3].

substances released by the microvascular endothelium (see Fig. 13.6).

Chromaffin cells have certain basic characteristics by which they are distinguished from true neurones. Some salient examples are:

1. There is no spatial separation between the protein synthetic and packaging (Golgi)

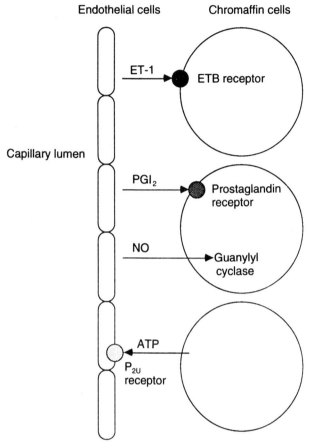

Fig. 13.6. The relationship between microvascular endothelial cells and chromaffin cells in the adrenal medulla. The figure shows the release of two substances from the endothelium that act on chromaffin cell-surface receptors, endothelin-1 (ET-1) and prostacyclin (PGI$_2$), and one, nitric oxide (NO), that acts at an intracellular site. Among the vasoactive substances released from the chromaffin cells is ATP, released in large amounts and which acts on 'nucleotide' (P$_{2U}$) receptors on the endothelial cells. In this way, the adrenal medulla can be seen as a model for the (mutual modulatory) interaction of elements of the nervous system with the local vasculature.

machinery and the site of 'neurotransmitter' storage and release. This will affect some aspects of the supply of both amines and peptides (see Section 1.3 above).

2. Most neurones studied have a characteristic distribution of voltage-sensitive Ca$^{2+}$ channels, such that the L-type (dihydropyridine-sensitive) channels are widely distributed but others, such as the N-type ($\omega$-conotoxin-sensitive) channels, are located adjacent to the sites of release. The result is that release from most neurones in response to depolarisation is not inhibited by dihydropyridines such as nitrendipine[4] (see Chapter 10). In the chromaffin cell, the high density and widespread distribution of L-type channels ensures that the major part of the depolarisation-evoked release is dihydropyridine sensitive. However, this release is insensitive to

blockers of other $Ca^{2+}$ channels, such as ω-conotoxin[18], despite the presence of ω-conotoxin-sensitive channels in chromaffin cells.

3. In neurones, cell-body depolarisation reaches the terminals via fast $Na^+$ channel-dependent and, therefore, tetrodotoxin-sensitive action potentials. While $Na^+$ channel-based action potential firing is induced in chromaffin cells in response to nicotinic stimulation, release is not inhibited by tetrodotoxin.

Other differences between chromaffin cells and true neurones relate to their function: the time course of a neuroendocrine response, for example, is much longer than that of responses in neurones, both central and peripheral. In this sense, the chromaffin cells resemble other neuroendocrine cells. Only some aspects of the large literature on this subject are introduced here.

### 3.1 Cholinergic regulation of adrenomedullary secretion

*In vivo*, the adrenal medullary chromaffin cells are innervated by the splanchnic nerve. This releases acetylcholine, which stimulates adrenal medullary secretion by acting at nicotinic acetylcholine receptors located on the chromaffin cell plasmalemma. In bovine adrenal chromaffin cells maintained in tissue culture, a number of receptors are linked to exocytosis, but stimulation of the nicotinic receptor elicits the largest response (Fig. 13.5). This observation is a reflection of the dominant role of acetylcholine released from the splanchnic nerve in stimulating adrenal medullary secretion *in vivo*. There are two types of receptor for acetylcholine: nicotinic and muscarinic. There is some species difference in the linkage to the secretion pathway of the two types of cholinergic receptor: bovine cells possess muscarinic receptors but do not secrete in response to selective muscarinic agonists. On the other hand guinea-pig and rat chromaffin cells

exhibit a substantial secretory response to both nicotinic and muscarinic stimulation.

The nicotinic response is mediated by a receptor-linked channel permeable to cations. The channel is relatively selective for $Na^+$ but has appreciable permeability for $Ca^{2+}$. In bovine tissue, the number, distribution and total conductivity of these channels for cation entry is sufficient to dominate release, i.e. release is independent of voltage-sensitive $Na^+$ and $Ca^{2+}$ channels, and of $Na^+$ entry, and presumably reflects $Ca^{2+}$ entry direct through the nicotinic channel[4]. In bovine chromaffin cells, muscarinic receptors are linked to adenylyl cyclase, phospholipase C and inhibit $K^+$ channels, all of which may modulate nicotinic receptor-evoked secretion (see Chapters 9 and 10).

### 3.2 Non-cholinergic modulation of adrenomedullary secretion

#### 3.2.1 Neurally released modulators

The splanchnic nerve releases a number of co-transmitters in addition to acetylcholine. These include peptides (such as the tachykinins and VIP) and other substances which may play a role in modulation of acetylcholine-stimulated release. Substance P is a tachykinin that inhibits nicotinic receptor-evoked release from bovine chromaffin cells (thereby reducing the amplitude of the secretion) but simultaneously protects against desensitisation of the acetylcholine response (thereby prolonging secretion). While desensitisation is known to occur at many levels in chromaffin cells[16], it seems likely it is mainly the nicotinic receptor itself that is involved: desensitisation being regulated by the phosphorylation state of the δ-subunit.

#### 3.2.2 Blood-borne modulators

The blood supply is a source of several agents that modulate adrenal medullary secretion. Histamine, bradykinin and angiotensin II, for example, all stimulate release from bovine chromaffin cells by triggering mechanisms that result in the influx of extracellular $Ca^{2+}$. These substances also trigger the phospholipase C-mediated breakdown of inositol phospholipids and the generation of $Ins(1,4,5)P_3$ and diacylglycerol; these too might be involved in secretion–modulation mechanisms (see Chapters 1 and 9). The physiological significance of this release is not documented. However, it is possible to speculate, for example, that in cases of anaphylactic shock, enhanced adrenaline and noradrenaline output stimulated by histamine would present some protection against cardiovascular collapse and respiratory insufficiency.

The supply to the adrenal medulla of blood directly from the adrenal cortex ensures that the chromaffin cells are bathed in high concentrations of steroids. It is interesting to speculate on possible mechanisms by which steroids may influence adrenal medullary secretion. It may be that the principal influence of the steroids is phenotypic modification via regulation of gene expression (see Chapter 8). There are well-documented effects of glucocorticoids upon expression of genes relating to the biosynthesis of both catecholamines and opioid peptides released from chromaffin cells. Alternatively, or additionally, steroid-induced inhibition of phospholipase $A_2$ and eicosanoid production may play a release-modulating role (see Section 2.1.2).

### 3.2.3 Locally released modulators

Adrenal medullary chromaffin cells have intimate contact with a dense capillary network and this juxtaposition provides interesting possibilities for modulatory interactions between vascular endothelial cells and the chromaffin cells. Endothelial cells produce substances that regulate associated vascular smooth muscle. Among these substances are nitric oxide, prostaglandins and endothelins, which also have been shown to modulate the secretion of chromaffin cells. Nitric oxide activates soluble guanylyl cyclase inside the cells, while prostaglandins and endothelins

act on cell surface receptors. In turn, chromaffin cells release substances that act on the local endothelial cells. The best example of the latter is ATP, which is stored in chromaffin granules and released with catecholamines. Furthermore, receptors with the pharmacology of $P_{2U}$ receptors, linked to phospholipase C, are found on the endothelial cells. There is a maintained gradient of ATP from the chromaffin cells that results from the rapid degradation of ATP by $5'$-ectonucleotidases. Therefore, each component that is necessary for a two-way (mutually modulatory) communication between local endothelial cells and chromaffin cells has been described (Fig. 13.6).

## 3.3 Autocrine modulation of adrenal medullary secretion

Catecholamines are not the only substances released from chromaffin cells in response to stimulation. The diversity is too great to be described here but some are indicated in Fig. 13.5. However, in terms of their potential importance as modulators of adrenal medullary secretion, ATP, opioid peptides and chromogranins are briefly considered. Each of these have been proposed to modulate the release from the cell from which they are released, or adjacent chromaffin cells, by acting on specific cell surface receptors. Unlike in postganglionic sympathetic neurones, catecholamines do not modulate their own release from chromaffin cells: there appears to be no functional α- or β-adrenoceptors on the chromaffin cell membrane[24,28].

### 3.3.1 Modulation by ATP

The chromaffin cell membrane contains receptors for ATP ($P_2$ receptors) that are linked to phospholipase C, increased activity of which may augment secretion (see Chapter 9). The presence of $P_2$ purinoceptors on the plasmalemma of neurones is quite common, as is the release of ATP as a cotransmitter, so this short positive feedback loop may be widespread. It has also been reported, however, that prolonged exposure to ATP may inhibit release from chromaffin cells. This negative feedback loop may act to regulate the time course of secretion[8] (see also discussion of the modulatory role of substance P above).

### 3.3.2 Opioid peptides

Opioid peptides of great diversity are also co-stored and released from adrenal chromaffin cells. These include the products of the proenkephalin A and the dynorphin/neoendorphin genes in most animals, and also of the ACTH/β-lipotrophin gene in man. The presence of multiple opioid receptors in the adrenal medulla has been reported[5], and while there are reports of lack of effects of many opioids, it does appear that adrenal medullary secretion can be inhibited by certain peptides from the opioid families, effecting a local negative feedback.

### 3.3.3 Chromogranins

An interesting example of peptide autoregulation of adrenal medullary secretion derives from studies of chromogranin A. Chromogranin A is a glycoprotein with widespread distribution and great abundance in the nervous and endocrine systems. In the chromaffin cell, chromogranin A is concentrated within the (secretory) granules, where it accounts for about 40% of the soluble protein. Shortly after it was sequenced, it was recognised that it contained a segment with considerable homology to pancreostatin, a peptide which inhibits insulin secretion. Further studies have shown that proteolytic cleavage of chromogranin A generates a peptide fragment, known as chromostatin. This was found to inhibit cholinergic and $K^+$ depolarisation-stimulated secretion from chromaffin cells[10]. Chromostatin was potent in the nanomolar concentration range, with almost complete inhibition at 1 μM, an effect apparently mediated by blocking stimulus-evoked $Ca^{2+}$ entry. It appears that chromostatin can be generated from chromogranin A in the extracellular compartment of chromaffin cell experimental preparations. The very high concentration of chromogranin A at the site of release from granules suggests that this system could function as a short feedback loop to modulate adrenal medullary secretion. However, given that chromogranin A is also found in the circulation, it is possible that its conversion to chromostatin may occur at distant sites. In this way, neurosecretion elsewhere in the body may be regulated by chromogranin released from the adrenal medulla.

## 4 Summary

This brief overview of some aspects of chromaffin cell function reveals that these cells form a point at which a wide range of inputs, of diverse origins and chemical nature, are integrated and an output, the modulated release of chromaffin granule contents, is computed. The intracellular 'wiring' of this computational process consists of signals generated mostly, but not exclusively, at cell surface receptors. These produce a complex variety of biochemical changes, which may include alterations in ion flux, phospholipid, inositol (poly)phosphate and cyclic nucleotide generation, and in protein kinase and phosphatase activity. These converge on the exocytotic machinery of the cell to produce short-term changes in release and longer-term responses (e.g. gene expression) that comprise the long-term memory of the cell and modulate the potential for future release.

## References

1. Bertherat J, Dournaud P, Berod A *et al.* (1992) Growth hormone releasing hormone synthesising neurons are a subpopulation of somatostatin receptor-labelled cells in the rat arcuate nucleus: a combined in situ hybridisation and receptor light-microscopic radioautographic study. *Neuroendocrinology* **56:** 25–31

2. Boarder MR (1989) Presynaptic aspects of cotransmission: relationship between vesicles and neurotansmitters. *Journal of Neurochemistry* **53**: 1–11

3. Boarder MR and Challiss RAJ (1992) Role of protein kinase C in the regulation of histamine and bradykinin stimulated inositol polyphosphate turnover in adrenal chromaffin cells. *British Journal of Pharmacology* **107**: 1140–1145

4. Boarder MR, Marriott DB and Adams M (1987) Stimulus secretion coupling in cultured chromaffin cells: dependency on external $Na^+$ and on dihydropyridine sensitive $Ca^{2+}$ channels. *Biochemical Pharmacology* **36**: 163–167

5. Bunn SJ, Marley PD and Livett BG (1988) The distribution of opioid binding subtypes in the bovine adrenal medulla. *Neuroscience* **27**: 1081–1094

6. Burgoyne RD (1991) Control of exocytosis in adrenal chromaffin cells. *Biochimica et Biophysica Acta* **1071**: 174–202

7. Contijoch AM, Gonzalez C, Singh HN, Malamed S, Trancoso S and Advis J-P (1992) Dopaminergic regulation of luteinizing hormone-releasing hormone release at the median eminence level: immunocytochemical and physiological evidence in hens. *Neuroendocrinology* **55**: 290–300

8. Diverse-Pierluissi M, Dunlop K and Westhead EW (1991) Multiple actions of extracellular ATP on $Ca^{2+}$ currents in cultured bovine chromaffin cells. *Proceedings of the National Academy of Sciences USA* **88**: 1261–1265

9. Gainer H, Sarne Y and Brownstein MJ (1977) Biosynthesis and axonal transport of rat neurophyseal proteins and peptides. *Journal of Cell Biology* **73**: 366–381

10. Galindo E, Rill A, Bader M-F and Aunis D (1991) Chromostatin, a 20-amino acid peptide derived from chromogranin A, inhibits chromaffin cell secretion. *Proceedings of the National Academy of Sciences USA* **88**: 1426–1430

11. Lim NF, Nowycky MC and Bookman RJ (1990) Direct measurement of exocytosis and $Ca^{2+}$ currents in single vertebrate nerve terminals. *Nature* **344**: 449–451

12. Lindau M, Stuenkel EL and Nordmann JJ (1992) Depolarisations, intracellular $Ca^{2+}$ and exocytosis in single nerve terminals. *Biophysics Journal* **61**: 19–30

13. Livett BG (1984) Adrenal medullary chromaffin cells *in vitro*. *Physiological Reviews* **64**: 1102–1161

14. Loose MD, Ronnekleiv OK and Kelly MJ (1991) Neurons in the rat arcuate nucleus are hyperpolarised by $GABA_B$ and μ-opioid receptor antagonists: evidence for convergence at a ligand gated potassium conductance. *Neuroendocrinology* **54**: 517–544

15. Lyson K and McCann SM (1992) Involvement of arachidonic acid cascade pathways in interleukin-6-stimulated corticotropin releasing factor release *in vitro*. *Neuroendocrinology* **50**: 708–715

16. Marley PD (1988) Desensitization of the nicotinic secretory response of adrenal chromaffin cells. *Trends in Pharmacological Sciences* **9**: 102–107

17. Nordmann JJ and Artault J-C (1992) Membrane retrieval following exocytosis in isolated neurosecretory nerve endings. *Neuroscience* **49**: 201–207

18. Owen PJ, Marriott DB and Boarder MR (1989) Evidence for dihydropyridine sensitive and conotoxin insensitive release of noradrenaline and uptake of $Ca^{2+}$ with adrenal chromaffin cells. *British Journal of Pharmacology* **97**: 133–138

19. Owen PJ, Plevin R and Boarder MR (1989) Characterisation of bradykinin stimulated release of noradrenaline from cultured bovine adrenal chromaffin cells. *Journal of Pharmacology and Experimental Therapeutics* **248**: 1231–1236

20. Paynes LC, Obal F, Opp MR and Krueger JM (1992) Stimulation and inhibition of growth hormone secretion by interleukin-1β: the involvement of growth hormone releasing hormone. *Neuroendocrinology* **56**: 118–123

21. Plevin R, Owen PJ, Marriott DB and Boarder MR (1990) Role of phosphoinositide turnover and cyclic AMP accumulation in prostaglandin stimulated noradrenaline release from cultured adrenal chromaffin cells. *Journal of Pharmacology and Experimental Therapeutics* **252**: 1296–1303

22. Plotsky PM and Vale W (1985) Patterns of growth hormone releasing factor and somatostatin secretion into hypophysical portal circulation of the rat. *Science* **230**: 461–463

23. Polkovits M, Brownstein MJ, Eiden LE *et al.* (1982) Selective depletion of somatostatin in rat brain by cysteamine. *Brain Research* **240**: 178–180

24. Powis DA and Baker PF (1986) $\alpha_2$-
    Adrenoceptors do not regulate catecholamine
    secretion by bovine adrenal medullary cells: a
    study with clonidine. *Molecular Pharmacology*
    **29:** 134–141
25. Russell JT, Brownstein MJ and Gainer H
    (1981) Time course of appearance and release
    of [$^{35}$S]cysteine labelled neurophysins and
    peptides in the neurohypophysis. *Brain
    Research* **205:** 299–311
26. Spinedi E, Hadid R, Daneva T and Gaillard
    RC (1992) Cytokins stimulate the CRH but
    not vasopressin neuronal system: evidence for
    a median eminence site of interleukin-6 action.
    *Neuroendocrinology* **56:** 46–53

27. Sudhof TC and Jahn R (1991) Proteins of
    synaptic vesicles involved in exocytosis and
    membrane recycling. *Neuron* **6:** 665–677
28. Wan DC-C, Powis DA, Marley PD and Livett
    BG (1988) Effects of $\alpha$- and $\beta$-adrenoceptor
    agonists and antagonists on ATP and
    catecholamine release and desensitization of
    the nicotinic response in bovine adrenal
    chromaffin cells. *Biochemical Pharmacology*
    **37:** 725–736
29. Willoughby JO, Brogan M and Kapoor R
    (1989) Hypothalamic interconnections of
    somatostatin and growth hormone releasing
    factor neurons. *Neuroendocrinology* **50:**
    584–591

# 5 Modulation of neurotransmitter release: clinical relevance

# 14 Possible role of presynaptic receptors in hypertension

Kazimierz R. Borkowski

There are thought to be many chronic human afflictions that arise as a consequence of pathophysiological changes in body neurochemistry. It is possible that some are caused in part by untoward changes in neurotransmitter release-modulating mechanisms. Such changes could result in an augmentation or a diminution in the degree to which release-regulating control is manifested and thence to a reduction or an increase, respectively, in the amount of neurotransmitter in a synapse. In this chapter, Kazimierz Borkowski considers the condition of essential hypertension and evaluates the suggestions and hypotheses that have been made with respect to the part played by neurotransmitter release-modulating mechanisms in the natural history of the disease.

## 1 Hypertension, vascular smooth muscle tone and sympathetic activity

Sir George Pickering, arguably the father of modern 'hypertensionology', considered that there was no upper limit of normal blood pressure[19]. Nevertheless, it is acknowledged that elevated blood pressures are associated with increased rates of morbidity and mortality[22] and normotension is commonly defined, and is generally accepted, as pressures at or below 140/90 mmHg. It is worth noting, however, that increased rates of cardiovascular morbidity and mortality are also associated with abdominal obesity, hyperlipidaemia and hyperinsulinaemia, and that these conditions and hypertension often co-exist. This association of conditions may be one reason why successful control of blood pressure alone has not achieved the expected improvement in rates of morbidity and mortality in hypertensive populations.

Primary hypertension is a progressive disorder, the aetiology of which is not yet fully understood and, whilst current antihypertensive drugs reduce blood pressure, there is no cure. Therefore, therapeutic intervention to reduce blood pressure to acceptable levels is, at present, a life-long prospect. However, 70% of individuals with elevated blood pressure have hypertension that is considered mild and, being essentially asymptomatic, often do not feel better when taking antihypertensive drugs, particularly as these agents are not devoid of unwanted side effects. Hence, the search for antihypertensive drugs with novel mechanisms of action, and the possibility of improved efficacy and achieving a more acceptable side-effect profile continues unabated. Parallel studies focus on identifying the underlying cause of hypertension, in the hope that this may lead to the development of therapies effective in preventing hypertension, rather than reducing an already elevated blood pressure, and, perhaps, the development of a cure.

Multiple factors are involved in modulating blood pressure and maintaining cardiovascular homeostasis[10] and a dysfunction in any one may result in undesirable blood pressure elevation. Of these factors, an altered control of vascular smooth muscle tone, leading to narrowed blood vessels and an increased peripheral vascular resistance, is probably the major underlying cause of high blood pressure. Indeed, a relationship between vascular smooth muscle tone and blood pressure in the general population is indicated by observations that peripheral vascular resistance increases with the progression of hypertension, that it also increases with ageing, and that the incidence of hypertension increases with ageing.

Samuel Schaarschmidt, professor of medicine in Berlin until 1747, was the first to describe a condition, now known as hypertension, the symptoms of which were a bounding pulse and a high occurrence of vascular accidents. He considered that these symptoms were caused by a 'spastic constriction of the vascular bed'. Vascular smooth muscle tone is affected by a variety of constrictor and dilator influences, including physical, humoral and neurogenic stimuli[10]. From a systemic perspective, the sympathetic nervous system is, perhaps, the most important regulator of vascular smooth muscle tone, and an increase in sympathetic nervous activity leads to vasoconstriction in many parts of the circulation. Noradrenaline is the major neurotransmitter of postganglionic sympathetic nerves in the periphery and, when released in response to nerve activation, elicits vascular smooth muscle contraction with a consequent increase in peripheral resistance and a rise in blood pressure. The constrictor effects of noradrenaline are mediated by postsynaptic (i.e. located on the effector cell) $\alpha$-adrenoceptors. Vascular smooth muscle cells, especially those in skeletal muscle beds, the coronary circulation and the liver, also contain $\beta$-adrenoceptors, which mediate vasodilatation. These postsynaptic receptors are of the $\beta_2$-subtype, at which adrenaline (from the adrenal medulla) is the natural agonist.

Given the cardiovascular effects of noradrenaline (vasoconstriction and increased cardiac contractility and rhythmicity, all of which contribute to an increase in blood pressure), many of the early antihypertensive drugs were intended to interfere with the sympathetic nervous system itself (e.g. guanethidine, a neuronal 'blocking' agent) or with the postsynaptic effects of noradrenaline once released (e.g. phentolamine, a non-selective $\alpha$-adrenoceptor antagonist). However, it is now recognised that, whilst the activity of sympathetic nerves measured in terms of frequency of recorded action potentials is governed within the CNS, the actual release of noradrenaline from sympathetic nerve terminals (varicosities) in response to action potentials is modulated in a quantitatively important manner by receptors located on the nerve terminals themselves. Therefore, the pharmacological manipulation of these presynaptic receptors also represents a possible means of regulating blood pressure. The development of antihypertensive drugs that modulate the amount of noradrenaline released (as opposed to drugs that either block release altogether or prevent its postsynaptic effects once released) is a further option that may have significant advantages over traditional antihypertensive drugs in terms of its focus and specificity.

## 2  Presynaptic receptors on sympathetic nerves

The history of presynaptic receptors, their identification and their effects on neurotransmitter release and end-organ responses have been the subject of a number of excellent reviews (see refs. 11, 12, 23, 25 and also other Chapters in this book). Functional presynaptic receptors can be allocated into one or other of two categories. The majority of presynaptic receptor types exert an inhibitory influence on neurotransmitter release (i.e. the receptors mediate a negative feedback, reducing the per-pulse release of neurotransmitter). Pharmacological stimulation of these receptors on sympathetic varicosities would attenuate noradrenaline release and thereby exert antihypertensive effects. A minority of presynaptic receptor types exert a facilitatory influence on neurotransmitter release (these receptors mediate a positive feedback, increasing the per-pulse release of neurotransmitter and, on sympathetic nerve terminals, would augment noradrenaline release). Pharmacological blockade of these receptors on sympathetic varicosities would be expected to exert antihypertensive effects.

Whether noradrenaline release from a single sympathetic varicosity affects subsequent noradrenaline release from the same varicosity (a true autoreceptor feedback mechanism) by an action at presynaptic receptors remains subject to debate (Chapter 5, see also ref. 1). The release of neurotransmitter from a single varicosity is very intermittent; the probability that an action potential passing through a varicosity will release a packet of noradrenaline is in the order of 0.01 (see Chapters 3 and 4). Moreover, recent experiments indicate that noradrenaline release from one varicosity does not affect subsequent release from the same varicosity but appears rather to affect the probability of the release of noradrenaline in response to an action potential in spatially close varicosities[24]. Nevertheless, under *in vivo* conditions and also in isolated perfused tissues, pharmacological manipulation of presynaptic receptors certainly modulates the per-pulse release of sympathetic neurotransmitter. Observations of the effects of drugs on neurogenic transmitter efflux and end-organ responses have lead to the identification of a host of functional presynaptic receptor populations (Fig. 14.1).

## 2.1 Presynaptic α-adrenoceptors

The first observations that α-adrenoceptor antagonists increased stimulation-evoked noradrenaline efflux were made in the late 1950s. The phenomenon was explained as being a consequence not so much of altered neurotransmitter release but rather of the

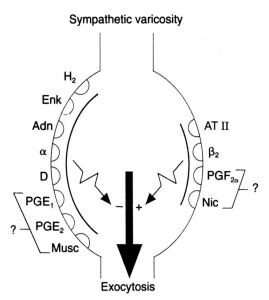

Sympathetic varicosity

Exocytosis

Fig. 14.1. Presynaptic receptor subtypes that have been putatively identified on sympathetic nerve varicosities: α- and $\beta_2$-adrenoceptors, dopamine receptors (D), nicotinic (Nic) and muscarinic (Musc) cholinergic receptors, angiotensin II receptors (ATII), histamine receptors ($H_2$), opioid receptors (Enk), adenine nucleotide receptors (Adn) and prostaglandin receptors ($PGE_1$, $PGE_2$ and $PGF_{2\alpha}$). An inhibitory effect on neurotransmitter release and a facilitatory effect is shown by arrow (+) and by arrow (−). Question marks indicate that the experimental data available are not unequivocal.

inhibition of its neuronal and extraneuronal uptake. It was not until the early 1970s that the concept of presynaptic receptors (i.e. receptors on nerve endings, as opposed to postsynaptic receptors on effector cells) was proposed and the hypothesis advanced that presynaptic receptor mechanisms were involved in the modulation of neuronal noradrenaline release.

When the presence of distinct pre- and postsynaptic α-adrenoceptors was acknowledged, the terminology postsynaptic $\alpha_1$-adrenoceptors and presynaptic $\alpha_2$-adrenoceptors was proposed; the latter mediating an inhibition of stimulation-evoked noradrena-

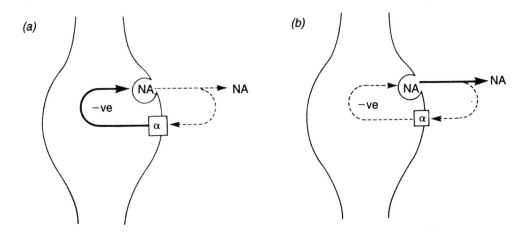

Fig. 14.2. Inhibition of sympathetic neurotransmitter release mediated by α-adrenoceptors. Under normal conditions (*a*), the released noradrenaline (NA) activates presynaptic α-adrenoceptors, which mediate a strong inhibitory influence to limit further noradrenaline release. In the presence of dysfunctional presynaptic α-adrenoceptors (*b*), their inhibitory influence is attenuated and noradrenaline release increases (but see Chapters 4 and 5).

line release. The continued development and use of selective agonists and antagonists has, however, led to the conclusion that both subtypes are present in both sites, but that $\alpha_1$-adrenoceptors are predominant postsynaptically, while presynaptically $\alpha_2$-adrenoceptors are predominant. Both postsynaptic α-adrenoceptor subtypes mediate vascular smooth muscle contraction, and both presynaptic α-adrenoceptor subtypes appear to inhibit neuronal noradrenaline release (but see Chapters 5 and 7). Noradrenaline, whether exogenously applied or released from sympathetic nerve varicosities, is a full agonist at $\alpha_1$- and $\alpha_2$-adrenoceptors and there is evidence of increasing feedback inhibition of neuronal noradrenaline efflux with increasing frequency of nerve stimulation. This can be envisaged as an attempt to limit the release of excessive amounts of noradrenaline in order to keep end-organ responses within the physiological range. An impairment of inhibitory presynaptic $\alpha_2$-adrenoceptor function would be predicted to result in the release of inappropriate amounts of nor-

adrenaline (Fig. 14.2) and augmented end-organ responses that might play a role in hypertension.

Since postsynaptically mediated pressor responses to $\alpha_2$-adrenoceptor agonists are relatively small (see above), the pharmacological stimulation of $\alpha_2$-adrenoceptors *in vivo* would be expected to elicit a reduction in peripheral resistance and blood pressure as a result of the attenuation of noradrenaline release via stimulation of (the predominant) inhibitory presynaptic $\alpha_2$-adrenoceptors.

## 2.2   Presynaptic β-adrenoceptors

During the 1970s and early 1980s, there was also an accumulation of evidence supporting the existence of presynaptic β-adrenoceptors, which mediate a facilitation of stimulation-evoked noradrenaline release. Whilst there is some pharmacological evidence for facilitatory presynaptic $\beta_1$-adrenoceptors and that facilitatory $\beta_1$- and $\beta_2$-adrenoceptors may coexist, the weight of evidence indicates that the receptors are of the $\beta_2$-subtype, at which adrenaline appears to be the natural agonist and at which noradrenaline is only a weak agonist. Circulating plasma adrenaline, from the adrenal medulla, would, therefore, be expected to facilitate neuronal noradrenaline release directly via stimulation of presynaptic $\beta_2$-adrenoceptors. However, adrenaline is also a substrate for uptake$_1$ and, when present in the circulation, would be taken up along with noradrenaline and co-sequestered in storage vesicles in sympathetic varicosities. Upon subsequent nerve activity, it would be released as a co-transmitter with noradrenaline and stimulate facilitatory presynaptic $\beta_2$-adrenoceptors and thereby augment noradrenaline release. This effect would be particularly pronounced at lower frequencies of nerve discharge, when intrasynaptic levels of noradrenaline would not be expected to be sufficient to activate inhibitory presynaptic $\alpha_2$-adrenoceptors (Fig. 14.3).

A sensitisation of presynaptic $\beta_2$-adrenoceptors also might be expected to result in an inappropriate augmentation of neuronal noradrenaline release (Fig. 14.3) and, thus, to increased peripheral resistance and blood pressure.

Despite the blockade of postsynaptic vasodilator $\beta$-adrenoceptors, which theoretically should increase peripheral resistance and elevate blood pressure, at least in the short term, $\beta$-adrenoceptor antagonists are effective antihypertensive drugs. Whilst this is primarily a result of their lowering of cardiac output, the antihypertensive effects of $\beta$-adrenoceptor antagonists may, in part, be also the result of the attenuation of noradrenaline release via the blockade of presynaptic $\beta$-adrenoceptors.

The facilitatory effect of presynaptic $\beta$-adrenoceptors on noradrenaline release is, however, small compared with the inhibitory effect of presynaptic $\alpha$-adrenoceptors: blockade of presynaptic $\alpha$-adrenoceptors increases stimulation-evoked noradrenaline efflux by up to 300%; stimulation of presynaptic $\beta$-adrenoceptors increases noradrenaline efflux by only 30–60% (but see Section 4).

## 2.3  Angiotensin II receptors

Angiotensin II is a powerful vasoconstrictor, causing an increase in blood pressure by increasing total peripheral vascular resistance. It also stimulates aldosterone release from the adrenal cortex, causing sodium retention by the kidney and a resultant increase in plasma volume. Angiotensin II, an octapeptide, is generated by the action of angiotensin converting enzyme (ACE), from a decapeptide precursor (angiotensin I) that, in turn, is generated by the action of renin upon the inactive precursor angiotensinogen, a plasma protein. Renin is released from juxtaglomerular cells in the kidney in response to increased sympathetic activity or to a local fall in renal afferent arteriolar pressure. This activation of the renin–angiotensin–aldosterone system, and consequent generation of angiotensin II, leads to a redistribution of the blood volume and an increase in blood pressure in an attempt to maintain renal perfusion pressure and kidney function.

ACE inhibitors are proving to be effective antihypertensive drugs and are enjoying widespread use. By preventing the conversion of angiotensin I into angiotensin II, inhibitors of ACE are thought to cause lowering of blood pressure by decreasing formation of a potent vascular smooth muscle constrictor. Although the antihypertensive efficacy of ACE inhibitors may be largely the result of this reduction of angiotensin II-mediated vasoconstriction, there is evidence that blood-borne angiotensin II, and also that synthesised locally by endothelial cells in blood vessel walls (see also Chapter 7), facilitates the per-pulse release of sympathetic neurotransmitter by an action at presynaptic angiotensin II receptors. Thus, decreased presynaptic angiotensin II receptor-mediated facilitation of sympathetic activity, following ACE inhibition, may also contribute to the blood pressure-lowering effects of these drugs.

Since the $\beta$-adrenoceptor agonist isoprenaline enhances neurogenic pressor responses and the release of locally generated

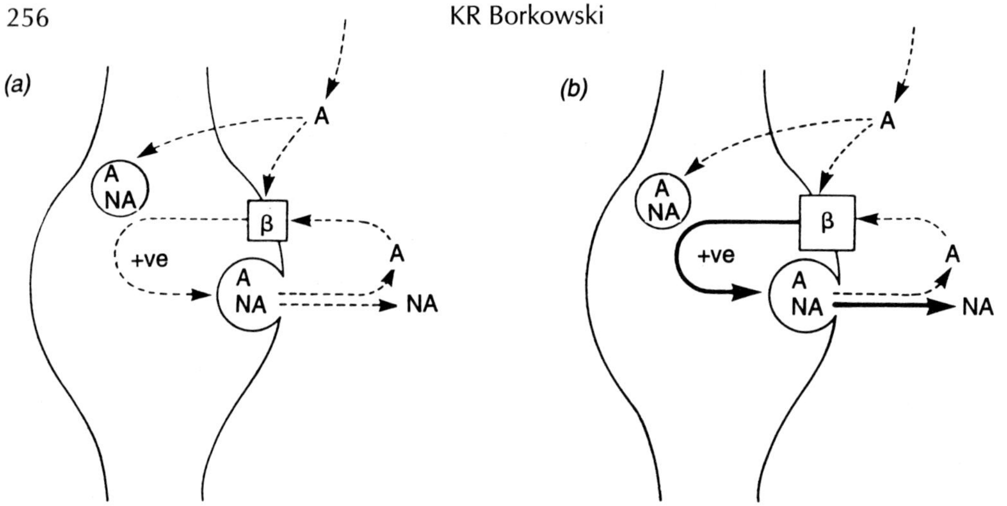

Fig. 14.3. Facilitation of sympathetic neurotransmitter release mediated by β-adrenoceptors. Under normal conditions (*a*), adrenaline (A) present in the bloodstream and that released as a co-transmitter from sympathetic nerve vesicles activates presynaptic β-adrenoceptors, which mediate a facilitatory influence on evoked-noradrenaline (NA) release. This facilitatory influence is more readily observed at lower frequencies of nerve activity, when synaptic concentrations of noradrenaline are low and less likely to activate adjacent presynaptic α-adrenoceptors. In the presence of 'sensitised' presynaptic β-adrenoceptors (*b*), the facilitatory influence is augmented and noradrenaline release increases.

angiotensin II in isolated perfused mesenteric arteries, it has been suggested that presynaptic β-adrenoceptors mediate their facilitatory effects through the activation of a local renin–angiotensin system. An inhibition of the isoprenaline-induced effects in the presence of the β-adrenoceptor antagonist propranolol or the ACE-inhibitor captopril, and an inhibition of isoprenaline-induced angiotensin II release by the $\beta_2$-adrenoceptor antagonist ICI 118,551 but not by the $\beta_1$-adrenoceptor antagonist atenolol has also been demonstrated. This suggests an involvement of $\beta_2$-adrenoceptors in the release of locally generated angiotensin II, in some situations at least[16,17].

Whether or not locally generated and released angiotensin II is involved always in presynaptic β-adrenoceptor-mediated facilitation of sympathetic neurogenic responses, angiotensin II does facilitate neuronal noradrenaline release. However, this facilitatory effect approximates that of presynaptic β-adrenoceptor stimulation. Therefore, the antihypertensive efficacy of ACE inhibitors is unlikely to be predominantly caused by the attenuation of sympathetic neurotransmitter release resulting from the prevention of angiotensin II formation and the consequent reduction in stimulation of facilitatory presynaptic angiotensin II receptors. Moreover, interpreting the effects of ACE inhibitors solely on the basis of their effect on angiotensin II generation is inadequate since they also inhibit kininase II, the enzyme involved in bradykinin degradation. The potentiation of the vasodilator effects of bradykinin may, therefore, also contribute to the effects of ACE inhibitors.

A better quantitative appreciation of the facilitating role of release-modulating presynaptic angiotensin II receptors is likely to result from experiments using novel agents such as losartan, a selective antagonist of angiotensin II receptors.

## 2.4   Dopamine receptors

In a number of tissues, exogenous dopamine has been shown to stimulate postsynaptic α-adrenoceptors but with a potency between 10- and 100-fold less than that of noradrenaline. However, with respect to its presynaptic effect in attenuating stimulation-evoked neuronal noradrenaline release, dopamine was found to be approximately equipotent with noradrenaline. Initially, it was believed that noradrenaline and dopamine acted on a single presynaptic receptor system that differed from postsynaptic α-adrenoceptors in that it was particularly sensitive to dopamine. It now appears that a discrete population of presynaptic dopamine receptors exists. It is, however, evident that presynaptic dopamine receptors are less common and less widely distributed than inhibitory presynaptic α-adrenoceptors.

Agonists of dopamine receptors inhibit stimulation-evoked noradrenaline release in the rabbit ear artery, an effect blocked by dopamine receptor antagonists. However, these antagonists alone do not appear to enhance stimulation-evoked noradrenaline release, as would be expected if endogenous dopamine activated inhibitory presynaptic dopamine receptors to suppress noradrenaline release. Indeed, while dopamine and the enzymes responsible for its synthesis and degradation are found in vascular tissues, the release of endogenous vascular dopamine appears not to occur in amounts sufficient to inhibit neuronal noradrenaline release. Nor have the dopamine receptor antagonists haloperidol and metoclopramide been widely reported to raise blood pressure. Therefore, there is little evidence that endogenous dopamine plays a role in the presynaptic modulation of neuronal noradrenaline release *in vivo*.

With the exception of the CNS, in which there is an abundance of nerves that secrete dopamine as their neurotransmitter (see, for example, Chapter 15), the concentration of dopamine in tissues is small and more consistent with a role for dopamine as a precursor rather than as a neurotransmitter. Dopamine can be converted to noradrenaline by dopamine-β-hydroxylase and, subsequently, in the adrenal medulla and a very small number of nerves in the CNS, noradrenaline is converted to adrenaline by phenylethanolamine-*N*-methyltransferase.

## 2.5   Cholinergic receptors

Nicotinic receptor agonists cause release of noradrenaline from sympathetic nerve terminals. There is some evidence that such agonists also increase nerve stimulation-induced transmitter efflux, suggesting the presence of (facilitatory) presynaptic nicotinic receptors. Conversely, the activation of presynaptic muscarinic receptors attenuates nerve stimulation-induced noradrenaline efflux. It should be noted that not all investigators have been successful in demonstrating facilitatory nicotinic and inhibitory muscarinic receptors, and the issue of presynaptic cholinergic modulation of sympathetic neurotransmitter release is not finally established. The story is further complicated by reports that the enhancement of noradrenaline release by very low concentrations of acetylcholine is resistant to both antinicotinic and antimuscarinic agents.

## 2.6   Prostaglandin receptors

Many sympathetic nerve terminals appear to be endowed with prostaglandin receptors. Vascular endothelial cells are capable of synthesising some prostaglandins, e.g. $PGI_2$. Testing the hypothesis that endothelium-derived and circulating prostaglandins may modulate sympathetic neurotransmitter release, it has been shown that activation of presynaptic receptors by exogenous $PGE_1$ and $PGE_2$ attenuates the per-pulse release of noradrenaline in some, but not all, tissues. This inhibitory effect is much smaller than that mediated by presynaptic α-adrenoceptors. There are also some reports that $PGF_{2\alpha}$ enhances noradrenaline efflux. However, the effects of prostaglandins on sympathetic neurotransmission have not been tested extensively and the physiological role, if any, of presynaptic prostaglandin receptors is unclear.

## 2.7  Histamine receptors

Histamine has been shown to decrease neurogenic (sympathetic) venoconstriction and the efflux of radiolabelled noradrenaline from innervated tissues *in vitro*. Similar effects have been obtained with $H_2$ agonists, and these effects of histamine and $H_2$ receptor agonists were reversed by $H_2$ receptor antagonists. Assuming for the moment that release of radiolabelled noradrenaline accurately reflects release of endogenous sympathetic neurotransmitter, these results suggest the presence of inhibitory presynaptic $H_2$ receptors. However, sympathetic nerve stimulation-induced vasoconstriction in feline cerebral vessels has been shown to be reduced in the presence of the $H_1$ receptor agonist pyridylethylamine or the $H_2$ receptor agonist impromidine, which suggests the presence of both inhibitory presynaptic $H_1$ and $H_2$ receptors. The source of endogenous histamine that could act upon presynaptic receptors and the physiological significance of such an action is unclear. Furthermore, there has not yet been a clear demonstration of a dis-inhibition of sympathetic neurotransmission in the presence of histamine receptor antagonists alone.

## 2.8  Opioid receptors

There are a few reports that morphine and the naturally occurring enkephalins reduce the per-pulse release of radiolabelled noradrenaline, indicating the presence of inhibitory presynaptic opioid receptors. Under certain conditions, for example in haemorrhagic shock, the non-selective opioid receptor antagonist naloxone can induce an increase in blood pressure. It can be speculated that antagonism of the inhibition of sympathetic activity, by naloxone's blockade of inhibitory presynaptic opioid receptors, may contribute to this effect. However, as is the case with many other presynaptic receptor populations, the physiological significance of this release-modulating effect mediated by opioid receptors remains obscure.

## 2.9  Adenine nucleotide receptors

Transmitter storage vesicles in sympathetic varicosities contain high concentrations of the nucleotides ATP and ADP and of adenosine, in addition to noradrenaline. ATP is clearly released as a co-transmitter, and exogenous ATP, ADP and adenosine have all been shown to attenuate stimulation-evoked release of noradrenaline from sympathetic nerve terminals (see Chapter 6). Moreover, it is interesting to note that adenosine is released during sympathetic nerve stimulation in amounts that are similar to those which, when applied exogenously, have been shown to inhibit neuronal noradrenaline release. This clearly suggests the presence of presynaptic receptors for adenine compounds, which inhibit sympathetic activity. It can be speculated that the dephosphorylation of ATP, associated with elevated levels of nerve activity, may lead to the appearance of high concentrations of adenosine, which would act presynaptically in an attempt to minimise further neurotransmitter release and limit end-organ responses. Nonetheless, the physiological importance of these receptors has not yet been established conclusively (see also Chapters 7 and 9).

## 3  Presynaptic α-adrenoceptors and hypertension

### 3.1  Presynaptic modulation of sympathetic activity

There have been many reports, published since the early 1970s, concluding that presynaptic $\alpha_2$-adrenoceptors mediate inhibition and presynaptic $\beta_2$-adrenoceptors mediate facilitation of noradrenaline release. This will then reduce or enhance, respectively, sympathetic neurogenic responses. However, it must be noted that in the absence of pharmacological manipulation to optimise conditions, the demonstration of inhibition and facilitation has often been equivocal[1]. Notwithstanding, a dysfunction in either one or both of these presynaptic receptor systems could be envisaged to have pathophysiological consequences. Thus, a decrease in inhibitory presynaptic $\alpha_2$-adrenoceptor responsiveness (Fig. 14.2) or an increase in facilitatory presynaptic $\beta_2$-adrenoceptor responsiveness (Fig. 14.3) would be expected to augment the per-pulse release of noradrenaline. As a consequence peripheral vascular resistance would increase causing an elevation of blood pressure. Conversely, the appropriate pharmacological manipulation of these presynaptic receptors would be expected to lower blood pressure by reducing noradrenaline release and, thus, enabling a decrease in peripheral vascular resistance.

To ascribe a role to presynaptic receptors in the aetiology of hypertension is clearly dependent not only upon demonstrating the presence of these receptors but also upon demonstrating the appropriate dysfunction in their responsiveness which would result in an enhancement of sympathetic neurogenic responses. Presynaptic $\alpha$- and $\beta$-adrenoceptors have been studied extensively from this standpoint.

### 3.2 Presynaptic $\alpha$-adrenoceptors: experiments in animals

In testing the hypothesis that presynaptic $\alpha$-adrenoceptor responsiveness is altered in hypertension, it has been shown that nerve stimulation-induced efflux of radiolabelled noradrenaline and vasopressor responses are both greater in perfused kidneys from 7-week-old spontaneously hypertensive rats (SHR), i.e. during the developing phase of genetic hypertension, compared with those from kidneys of age-matched normotensive rats. Similar increases in noradrenaline efflux were observed in kidneys from both normotensive and hypertensive animals in the presence of cocaine to block uptake$_1$ (the

major route of inactivation of sympathetic neurotransmitter by reuptake into the nerve terminals), indicating that the increased noradrenaline efflux in the hypertensive rats was indeed caused by increased neuronal release and not to differences in uptake. Therefore, the increased release of noradrenaline occurring in early hypertension[26] may reflect decreased responsiveness of inhibitory presynaptic $\alpha$-adrenoceptors and play a role in the development of hypertension. However, stimulation-induced release of radiolabelled noradrenaline was lower from kidneys of adult (6-month-old) SHRs with established hypertension compared with that from kidneys of age-matched normotensive rats, suggesting that inhibitory presynaptic $\alpha$-adrenoceptors may be more, rather than less, responsive once hypertension is established.

That presynaptic $\alpha$-adrenoceptor responsiveness is reduced in young SHRs, but increases steadily and later attenuates noradrenaline release as hypertension progresses and becomes established (arguably an adaptive response attempting to decrease sympathetic activity in the face of elevated blood pressure) is not supported by other observations, however. Administration of the $\alpha_2$-adrenoceptor antagonist yohimbine led to similar increases in stimulation-induced efflux of both radiolabelled and endogenous noradrenaline from isolated arteries and veins of age-matched 6- and 10-week-old SHRs and normotensive rats. It also led to smaller increases in efflux from tissues of 28-week-old SHRs with established hypertension compared with those from tissues of age-matched normotensive rats[26]. In contrast to those above, these results suggest that presynaptic $\alpha$-adrenoceptors are less responsive in established hypertension and may contribute to hypertension maintenance rather than to its development.

Despite the use of different tissues and pharmacological agents to stimulate or block presynaptic $\alpha$-adrenoceptors, it is difficult to reconcile the differences in the findings of these studies. The role, if any, of altered presynaptic $\alpha$-adrenoceptor responsiveness in hypertension and its development remains unclear. Indeed, in chronic neurogenic hypertension induced by sinoaortic baroreceptor denervation, the blockade of presynaptic α-adrenoceptors with the antagonist phentolamine caused similar increases in stimulation-induced (radiolabelled) noradrenaline efflux in isolated perfused mesenteric arteries from operated hypertensive and sham-operated normotensive rats. This appears to indicate that, at least in this model of chronic neurogenic hypertension, presynaptic α-adrenoceptor responsiveness is unaffected throughout the phases of development of hypertension.

Whether or not changes in the responsiveness of inhibitory presynaptic α-adrenoceptors occur in hypertension, there is little doubt that these receptors are present in both normotensive and hypertensive animals and their stimulation by appropriate agonists would be expected to reduce sympathetic neurotransmitter release and blood pressure. The $\alpha_2$-adrenoceptor agonist clonidine causes hypotension in experimental animals and is used as an antihypertensive in man. Whilst there is evidence to suggest that a major component of clonidine's blood pressure-lowering effect is caused by stimulation of postsynaptic α-adrenoceptors within the CNS, which leads to reduced central sympathetic outflow, a presynaptic site of action for clonidine in peripheral sympathetic neurones cannot be excluded.

### 3.3 Presynaptic α-adrenoceptors: experiments in humans

Functional inhibitory presynaptic α-adrenoceptors and facilitatory β-adrenoceptors have been demonstrated in isolated human vascular tissues such as the digital and omental arteries *in vitro*. However, the role of presynaptic receptors *in vivo* is more difficult to study in humans than in experimental animals, primarily because of the limitations of using plasma noradrenaline levels as an index of sympathetic nerve activity. Regional noradrenaline spillover (i.e. the noradrenaline measurable in blood draining a given limb or organ) results from not only the level of sympathetic nerve activity in the area but also the variation in noradrenaline reuptake by the nerves and regional blood flow, which affects noradrenaline washout. Nevertheless, a small number of, often quite elegant, studies have been performed to demonstrate the presence of presynaptic receptors that modulate sympathetic neurotransmitter release and end-organ responses in man *in vivo*.

Despite the mechanisms underlying the increase being unclear, plasma noradrenaline levels were found to be elevated in 14 out of 15 studies of young hypertensives. Moreover, direct recordings from multifibre postganglionic sympathetic nerves showed increased activity in young men with borderline hypertension compared with age-matched normotensive controls. In addition, submaximal exercise caused an increase in plasma noradrenaline levels in young (17–26-year-old) prehypertensive offspring of hypertensive parents that was 75–79% greater than that observed in age-matched normotensive controls with normotensive parents[21]. These findings do not, of course, necessarily suggest altered presynaptic modulation of neurotransmitter release, but they do indicate that increased sympathetic activity is not secondary to blood pressure elevation but precedes it and may, therefore, be important in hypertension development in humans.

Intravenous infusion of the $\alpha_2$-adrenoceptor antagonist idazoxan increased both plasma noradrenaline levels and blood pressure in healthy volunteers, as would be expected following blockade of inhibitory presynaptic α-adrenoceptors. Conversely, stimulation of presynaptic $\alpha_2$-adrenoceptors by infusion of the selective agonists clonidine or guanfacine reduced plasma noradrenaline. Therefore, noradrenaline release in humans appears to be attenuated by presynaptic $\alpha_2$-adrenoceptor stimulation. Agonists at these receptors might reasonably be expected to possess antihypertensive efficacy. Though guanfacine infusion reduces plasma noradrenaline levels, it, surprisingly, does not lower blood pressure. However, the $\alpha_2$-adrenoceptor agonist clonidine does both and has proved to be a useful antihypertensive drug in humans. However, as noted in Section 3.2, it is by no means clear what proportion of clonidine's effect is caused by stimulation of presynaptic $\alpha_2$-adrenoceptors in the periphery, which reduces noradrenaline release, and what is caused by stimulation of postsynaptic $\alpha$-adrenoceptors within the CNS, which reduces sympathetic nerve action potential frequency.

It is difficult to determine sympathetic activity from measurements of plasma noradrenaline levels and to construct complete dose–response curves in humans. It must also be acknowledged that pre- and postsynaptic receptors may not exhibit the same pharmacological properties and this will complicate attempts to elucidate the nature and role of presynaptic receptors on the basis of their interactions with agents whose pharmacological properties may have been determined according to their interactions with postsynaptic receptors. As a result, it is not surprising that there have been no systematic studies of potential changes in presynaptic receptor responsiveness and its possible role in human hypertension.

### 3.4  Summary

Presynaptic $\alpha$-adrenoceptors, predominantly of the $\alpha_2$-subtype that mediate an inhibitory influence on sympathetic neurotransmitter release, have been demonstrated in normotensive and hypertensive experimental animals and in humans both *in vivo* and *in vitro*. Agonists of $\alpha_2$-adrenoceptors, such as clonidine, have proved to be effective antihypertensive drugs. However, the role of presynaptic $\alpha$-adrenoceptors in the aetiology of hypertension, whether or not changes in presynaptic $\alpha$-adrenoceptor responsiveness occur with the progression of hypertension and, further, the potential contribution of such changes to the hypertensive disease process remain to be fully elucidated.

## 4  Presynaptic β-adrenoceptors and hypertension

### 4.1  Presynaptic β-adrenoceptors and sympathetic facilitation

Whereas the stimulation of presynaptic $\alpha$-adrenoceptors attenuates (decreases) the per-pulse release of sympathetic neurotransmitter, stimulation of presynaptic β-adrenoceptors facilitates (increases) noradrenaline release. Therefore, increased sympathetic neurotransmitter release and, consequently, blood pressure elevation might be expected to result either from a decreased presynaptic $\alpha$-adrenoceptor responsiveness or an increased presynaptic β-adrenoceptor responsiveness or, indeed, a combination of the two. Attempts to identify changes in facilitatory presynaptic β-adrenoceptor responsiveness in hypertension have proved difficult and not entirely conclusive, largely because the facilitatory effect of presynaptic β-adrenoceptors is relatively small (see above).

While there is some evidence that presynaptic β-adrenoceptors are of the $\beta_1$-subtype and that presynaptic $\beta_1$- and $\beta_2$-adrenoceptors may co-exist in some tissues[15], most studies indicate that presynaptic β-adrenoceptors are of the $\beta_2$-subtype, at which noradrenaline is only a weak agonist. Therefore, presynaptic $\beta_2$-adrenoceptors would not be part of a true feedback loop in which the release of endogenous noradrenaline affects the subsequent release of noradrenaline from the same varicosity (but see Chapters 4 and 5). Adrenaline is the naturally occurring, and full, agonist at $\beta_2$-adrenoceptors and appears to facilitate sympathetic neurotransmitter release and end-organ responses by a direct action at presynaptic $\beta_2$-adrenoceptors (see Section 2.2). In addition, there is evidence that adrenaline also facilitates noradrenaline release by an 'indirect' action, whereby it is taken up into sympathetic nerve varicosities, becomes sequestered in storage vesicles together with noradrenaline and facilitates sympathetic activity by stimulating presynaptic $\beta_2$-adrenoceptors when it is released as a result of subsequent nerve activity. In this fashion, adrenaline undergoes a subtle change in function from that of circulating hormone to that of neurally released co-transmitter.

### 4.2 Presynaptic β-adrenoceptors: experiments in animals

Evidence for functional facilitatory presynaptic β-adrenoceptors comes predominantly from observations (in a variety of vascular tissues including rat portal vein, guinea-pig atria, cat spleen and hind limb, dog heart and coronary sinus) that β-adrenoceptor antagonists decrease neurogenic sympathetic transmitter efflux, that β-adrenoceptor agonists increase efflux and that this effect of β-adrenoceptor agonists is abolished by appropriate antagonists. Other studies of neurogenic sympathetic end-organ responses (in pithed rats, in rat isolated perfused mesenteric arteries and kidneys, and in canine mesenteric arteries) not only indicate that these too are enhanced by stimulation of presynaptic β-adrenoceptors but also suggest that these receptors are of the $\beta_2$-subtype (for reviews see refs. 2, 3 and 13). However, in rat cerebral cortex and rabbit pulmonary artery, β-adrenoceptor antagonists did not reduce stimulation-evoked noradrenaline release and β-adrenoceptor agonists did not cause an increase in evoked release.

That presynaptic β-adrenoceptors can be involved in mediating facilitatory effects is demonstrated conclusively by observations of β-adrenoceptor-mediated modulation of noradrenaline release from axonal sprouts in rat superior cervical ganglia maintained in tissue culture. In this preparation, there are no postsynaptic elements to obscure interpretation. It was found that, while the β-adrenoceptor antagonist propranolol prevented increases in evoked noradrenaline efflux caused by the presence of the β-adrenoceptor agonist isoprenaline, propranolol alone had little or no effect on stimulation-evoked release of noradrenaline. The same was found in experiments of this type with cat

spleen. These observations can be explained on the basis that noradrenaline is only a weak agonist at $\beta_2$-adrenoceptors. As such, (and as noted above) noradrenaline would not be expected to facilitate its own release and, therefore, in the absence of an effective agonist at $\beta_2$-adrenoceptors, one could not expect blockade of presynaptic $\beta_2$-adrenoceptors to reduce neurotransmitter release.

However, the observations that the effective $\beta_{1,2}$-adrenoceptor agonist isoprenaline was either without effect, or even inhibited, stimulation-evoked efflux of noradrenaline from nerve terminals in mouse atria, rat cerebral cortex, rabbit pulmonary artery and cat spleen are not so readily explained.

Together, the results reinforce the impression of variability between tissues and species and are compatible with the view that presynaptic β-adrenoceptors are less ubiquitous than presynaptic α-adrenoceptors and that, even where they do occur, they do not necessarily mediate a facilitation of the neuronal release of noradrenaline[11,23].

Not only is there a degree of uncertainty regarding the presence and functional status of presynaptic β-adrenoceptors, there are also conflicting data regarding potential changes in the responsiveness of these receptors in hypertension. For example, in isolated mesenteric arterial beds from 14–16-week-old SHRs, the enhancement by isoprenaline of neurogenic increases in perfusion pressure and radiolabelled noradrenaline efflux was greater than that observed in arterial beds from age-matched normotensive Wistar Kyoto (WKY) rats. Likewise the $\beta_2$-adrenoceptor agonist salbutamol also caused a greater enhancement of neurogenic pressor responses in SHR compared to WKY mesenteries, and the perfusion pressure effects were attenuated by non-selective β-adrenoceptor antagonists but not by the relatively selective $\beta_1$-adrenoceptor antagonist practolol. These results suggest not only that presynaptic β-adrenoceptors are of the $\beta_2$-subtype but also that presynaptic $\beta_2$-adrenoceptor-mediated facilitation of sympathetic neurotransmitter release and the consequent vascular response is enhanced in SHRs and, therefore, may play a role in hypertension maintenance.

However, in other studies, there was no difference in the facilitation by isoprenaline of neurogenic responses in isolated perfused kidneys from 18-week-old SHRs compared with that observed in kidneys from age-matched WKY rats. Moreover, isoprenaline's facilitation of field stimulation-induced radiolabelled noradrenaline release from isolated superfused spleen strips from 15-week-old SHR and WKY rats was not significantly different. In contrast to the above, these results indicate a similar responsiveness of presynaptic $\beta_2$-adrenoceptors in normotensive rats and in SHRs with elevated blood pressure.

In yet other studies, isoprenaline-induced facilitation of the field stimulation-induced release of radiolabelled noradrenaline was greater in isolated superfused spleen strips from 5-week-old prehypertensive SHRs compared with that observed in tissues from age-matched WKY rats. These data support the hypothesis that facilitatory presynaptic $\beta_2$-adrenoceptors exhibit increased responsiveness early in the time course of the hypertensive disease process and may be involved in hypertension development rather than its maintenance. Here again there is room for doubt, as the magnitude of isoprenaline's facilitation of field stimulation-induced radiolabelled noradrenaline efflux in isolated portal vein from 6–8-week-old SHR and WKY rats was found to be similar.

From these and similar findings, it can be argued that facilitatory presynaptic $\beta_2$-adrenoceptor responsiveness appears to be enhanced only in developing hypertension, and even then only in SHRs younger than 6 weeks of age. On balance the data available indicate the considerable variability between tissues and are also testimony to the difficulties inherent in investigations of presynaptic modulation of sympathetic neurotransmission.

### 4.3 Presynaptic $\beta$-adrenoceptors: experiments in humans

*In vitro,* $\beta$-adrenoceptor agonists have been shown to cause a dose-dependent increase in the nerve stimulation-evoked release of transmitter in human omental arteries and veins, and in digital arteries, suggesting the presence of functional facilitatory presynaptic $\beta$-adrenoceptors. These receptors are of the $\beta_2$-subtype, since only the selective $\beta_2$-adrenoceptor agonists salbutamol and terbutaline, and not the selective $\beta_1$-adrenoceptor agonist tazolol, enhance stimulation-evoked neurotransmitter release. However, while the $\beta_{1,2}$-adrenoceptor antagonist propranolol prevented isoprenaline-induced increases in transmitter efflux, alone it had little or no effect on nerve stimulation-induced release of transmitter in omental blood vessels and in oviduct.

Notwithstanding the limitations associated with such human experiments *in vivo,* plasma catecholamine levels have been studied extensively in normotensive and hypertensive subjects. Although the differences measured have often been small and inconsistent, patients with primary hypertension appear to have elevated plasma adrenaline levels. Since adrenaline is the natural agonist at $\beta_2$-adrenoceptors, adrenaline has been implicated in the pathophysiology of human primary hypertension[7].

Increases in arterial and venous noradrenaline levels, presumably as a result of stimulation of facilitatory presynaptic $\beta_2$-adrenoceptors, have been found during infusions of adrenaline. Moreover, the adrenaline-induced increases in plasma noradrenaline were greater in hypertensive than in normotensive subjects and were prevented by $\beta$-adrenoceptor antagonists. This suggests an increased responsiveness of $\beta_2$-adrenoceptors in hypertensive subjects. Further, the data with the antagonists show that the changes in plasma noradrenaline levels were not simply caused by the displacement of neuronal noradrenaline by adrenaline consequent upon its uptake by noradrenergic nerves. However, the crucial experiments to measure the effects of systemic infusions of β-adrenoceptor agonists (e.g. adrenaline, isoprenaline and salbutamol) on plasma noradrenaline levels have been somewhat inconsistent, and in those experiments in which increases in plasma noradrenaline levels were observed, the increases were similar in normotensive and hypertensive subjects[8].

### 4.3.1   Effect of β-adrenoceptor agonists

Infusions of adrenaline or isoprenaline, in doses too small to have direct effects upon blood pressure, have been shown to induce marked tachycardia. The increase in heart rate subsided quickly following the cessation of isoprenaline infusion, but was sustained for up to an hour following adrenaline infusion even though plasma adrenaline returned to normal levels within minutes of the cessation of its infusion. These results indicate clearly that the tachycardia induced by isoprenaline and adrenaline was not caused solely by the stimulation of postsynaptic β-adrenoceptors on cardiac muscle but must also have involved an enhancement of sympathetic cardio-accelerator drive, most probably via stimulation of facilitatory presynaptic β-adrenoceptors. The long-lasting effect of adrenaline is consistent with the suggestion that adrenaline is taken up into sympathetic nerves and facilitates neurotransmitter release upon subsequent nerve activation (see Sections 2.2 and 4.4). In this regard, note that the half-life of adrenaline in plasma is approximately 1 min, whereas in innervated tissues it is in the order of 4 h.

Further support for the notion that the sustained stimulatory action of adrenaline in these experiments was mediated by facilitatory presynaptic β-adrenoceptors is provided by observations that administration of glucagon, a physiological stimulus for the release of adrenaline from the adrenal medulla, also elicited increases in blood pressure, heart rate and plasma noradrenaline, which were sustained after plasma adrenaline levels had returned to normal (Fig. 14.4). In

the presence of β-adrenoceptor blockade with propranolol, administration of glucagon induced a similar increase in plasma adrenaline, but, despite the initial increase in pressure being greater than that observed in the absence of propranolol, there was no longer a sustained increase in plasma noradrenaline, heart rate or even blood pressure. This result is to be expected from the combined blockade of release-facilitating presynaptic β-adrenoceptors and vasodilator postsynaptic β-adrenoceptors leaving an unopposed postsynaptic α-adrenoceptor-mediated vasoconstriction (Fig. 14.4).

### 4.3.2   Effect of β-adrenoceptor antagonists

Non-selective and $\beta_1$-adrenoceptor-selective antagonists are effective antihypertensive drugs. While their blood pressure-lowering activity is considered to be attributable primarily to a reduction in cardiac output, it can be surmised that blockade of facilitatory presynaptic β-adrenoceptors may also contribute to the antihypertensive effect of these agents. Indeed, acute β-adrenoceptor blockade with propranolol decreases both plasma noradrenaline levels, which might be expected following the blockade of facilitatory presynaptic β-adrenoceptors, and adrenaline levels. However, it is by no means certain that the reduction in plasma noradrenaline is caused only by an inhibition of the presynaptic facilitation of its release by propranolol: the membrane-stabilising effects, neuronal blocking and central actions of propranolol could contribute since all of these are likely to decrease sympathetic neuronal activity. The sole trial of the antihypertensive potential of a selective $\beta_2$-adrenoceptor antagonist (ICI 118,551) proved to be disappointing[20]. This may have been because the blood pressure-lowering effects of attenuated sympathetic neurotransmitter release caused by blockade of facilitatory presynaptic $\beta_2$-adrenoceptors was counteracted by the blood pressure-elevating effects of the blockade of postsynaptic vasodilator $\beta_2$-adrenoceptors. Attempts to reduce blood pressure using

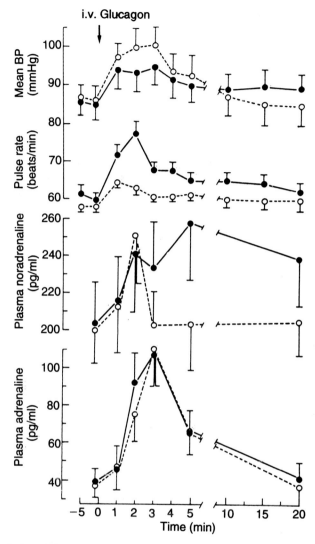

Fig. 14.4. The effect of a bolus of glucagon on mean arterial blood pressure (mean BP), pulse rate, plasma noradrenaline and plasma adrenaline concentrations under control conditions (solid line) and following β-adrenoceptor blockade with propranolol (interrupted line). Pretreatment with propranolol prevents activation of presynaptic β-adrenoceptors, and whereas this does not affect glucagon's effect on plasma adrenaline levels, it attenuates the effect of adrenaline on neuronal noradrenaline release. This is revealed by the reduced increment both in plasma noradrenaline levels and pulse rate. The enhancement by propranolol of the initial increase in mean BP is probably the result of blockade of postsynaptic vasodilator β-adrenoceptors. (Redrawn from ref. 18 and reproduced with permission.)

ICI 118,551 in adult SHR rats with established hypertension have also been disappointing, but chronic treatment with ICI 118,551 did attenuate hypertension develop-

ment in young SHRs. It may be that facilitatory presynaptic β₂-adrenoceptors play a role only in the development of hypertension and not in its maintenance.

## 4.4    The 'adrenaline hypothesis'

Brown and Macquin[7] proposed that an increased release of adrenaline from the adrenal medulla may be the underlying cause of primary hypertension. Their hypothesis was that repeated increases in circulating adrenaline cause hypertension by activating presynaptic $\beta_2$-adrenoceptors, which facilitate sympathetic neurotransmitter release and end-organ responses. Therefore, it was suggested that it is the repeated facilitation of sympathetic activity by adrenaline, rather than adrenaline's direct effects on the vasculature, that leads to a chronic elevation in blood pressure. However, adrenaline is a full agonist at both $\alpha$- and $\beta$-adrenoceptors and it might be expected that the facilitatory effects of presynaptic $\beta$-adrenoceptor stimulation would be negated by the inhibitory effects of presynaptic $\alpha$-adrenoceptor stimulation by adrenaline. To counter this argument, there is evidence that both pre- and postsynaptic $\beta$-adrenoceptors are more sensitive than their $\alpha$-adrenoceptor counterparts and, therefore, would be stimulated preferentially at lower concentrations of adrenaline. Brown and Macquin's 'adrenaline hypothesis' was a crystallisation of the long-held belief in an association between stress, adrenaline and high blood pressure. Certainly, an increased blood pressure had been described in soldiers in the desert war in North Africa, in Zulu tribesmen living in an urban compared with a rural environment and in individuals subjected to emotional stress. Also the plasma concentrations of adrenaline achieved during mental stress reach thresholds for adrenaline's cardiovascular and metabolic actions, and elevated plasma adrenaline levels have been reported in patients with essential hypertension. Furthermore, adrenaline has been shown to have presynaptic effects in humans, enhancing pressor responses to cold exposure and isometric exercise, facilitating forearm vasoconstriction in response to lower body negative pressure (Fig. 14.5) and causing a sustained elevation in plasma noradrenaline following its infusion[8]. Therefore, the concept

that adrenaline may be the physiological link between stress and hypertension and, moreover, acting via presynaptic $\beta$-adrenoceptors is attractive.

Majewski, Rand and Tung[14] were the first to demonstrate that adrenaline-induced facilitation of sympathetic activity might be important in hypertension. They showed that subcutaneous slow-release depot implants of acutely subpressor doses of adrenaline induced a chronic elevation in blood pressure in normotensive rats. Adrenaline's prohypertensive effect was attenuated by concomitant treatment with metoprolol, which indicated an involvement of $\beta$-adrenoceptors.

Whereas adrenaline supplementation induced an elevation in blood pressure, the depletion of circulating adrenaline by surgical adrenal enucleation was found to attenuate the development of raised blood pressure in young SHR rats between 4 and 16 weeks of age (Fig. 14.6). These effects appeared to involve presynaptic $\beta_2$-adrenoceptors, since treating adrenal-enucleated SHRs with slow-release depots of adrenaline, or either of the $\beta_2$-agonists salbutamol or procaterol, restored development of hypertension[6]. Moreover, adrenaline's prohypertensive effects in enucleated SHRs were abolished by concomitant treatment with the $\beta_2$-antagonist ICI 118,551 (Fig. 14.6), and ICI 118,551 itself attenuated hypertension development in young SHRs with intact adrenal medullae[6].

These observations lead to the conclusion that activation of facilitatory presynaptic $\beta_2$-adrenoceptors, by adrenaline, plays a role in the development of genetic hypertension. However, a role for adrenaline in the maintenance of hypertension is unlikely since adrenal enucleation does not significantly affect blood pressure in adult SHRs with established hypertension (Fig. 14.7), nor do $\beta_2$-adrenoceptor antagonists lower blood pressure in these rats. It is possible that there are multiple mechanisms serving to maintain hypertension and this may mask any reduction in blood pressure expected as a result of attenuation of the presynaptic $\beta_2$-adrenoceptor-mediated facilitation of sympathetic

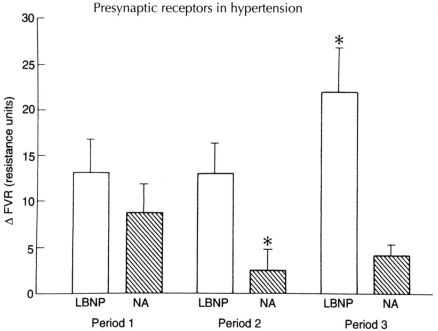

Fig. 14.5. Effects of adrenaline infusion on forearm vascular resistance (FVR) increased either by application of lower body negative pressure (LBNP), i.e. reflexly induced neurogenic vasoconstriction, or by a noradrenaline bolus (NA), i.e. direct vasoconstriction. Control stimuli prior to adrenaline infusion (period 1) indicate similar responses to each stimulus. During adrenaline infusion (period 2), the reduction in the response to noradrenaline indicates that its direct vasoconstrictor effects mediated by postsynaptic α-adrenoceptors are opposed by the direct vasodilator effects of adrenaline mediated by postsynaptic β-adrenoceptors. However, the neurogenic response is not reduced, indicating that there must be a pronounced augmentation by adrenaline (mediated by presynaptic β-adrenoceptors) of neuronal noradrenaline release that causes vasoconstriction sufficient to counteract the direct vasodilatation. Following cessation of adrenaline infusion (period 3), the noradrenaline response begins to return towards normal, indicating a waning of direct (adrenaline-mediated) vasodilatation. However, an augmentation of neurogenic vasoconstriction caused by the continued release of neuronally sequestered adrenaline, which stimulates presynaptic β-adrenoceptors, is apparent. * Indicates a significant change ($p < 0.05$). (Redrawn from ref. 9 and reproduced with permission.)

activity. An alternative possibility is that there is a period of critical sensitivity, perhaps dependent upon changes in facilitatory presynaptic $\beta_2$-adrenoceptor responsiveness, to adrenaline's prohypertensive effects during the time course of hypertension development. Therefore, attempts to modify presynaptic $\beta_2$-adrenoceptor activity at a time when these receptors are no longer involved in the hypertensive disease process would not be expected to affect blood pressure. It is worthy of note that adrenal enucleation does lead to significant reductions in blood pres-

sure and heart rate in adult normotensive rats (Fig. 14.7), suggesting a possible role for adrenaline in the maintenance of cardiovascular homeostasis in normotension.

Attempts to demonstrate differences in prejunctional $\beta_2$-adrenoceptor responsiveness between hypertensive and normotensive rats and between young and adult SHRs have, so far, been rather inconclusive. However, it appears that adrenal enucleation attenuates hypertension development only if performed in SHRs younger than 6 weeks of age[4], suggesting that the period of critical

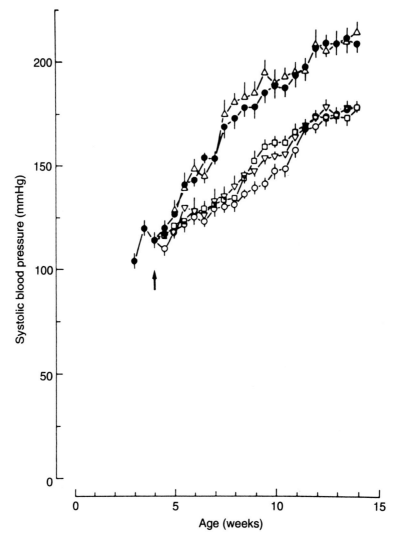

Fig. 14.6. Arterial systolic blood pressure in young SHR (3 to 14 weeks of age). Rats were sham-operated (●) or underwent bilateral adrenal enucleation (open symbols) at 4 weeks of age. Groups of enucleated rats were then left untreated (○), implanted with slow-release depots of adrenaline (△), treated with the $\beta_2$-antagonist ICI 118, 551 (▽) or implanted with depots of adrenaline and treated with ICI 118, 551 (□). Adrenal enucleation reduced plasma adrenaline levels and attenuated hypertension development. Adrenaline depots restored hypertension development in enucleated rats, but this effect was abolished by concomitant treatment with ICI 118, 551, a compound which had no direct hypotensive effect. (Redrawn from ref. 6 and reproduced with permission.)

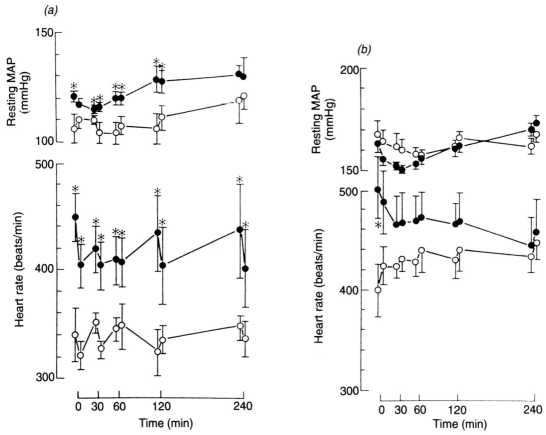

Fig. 14.7. The effect of plasma adrenaline depletion, by adrenal enucleation, on mean arterial blood pressure (MAP) and heart rate in conscious unrestrained adult normotensive (a) and spontaneously hypertensive (b) rats. At each of the time points, the values of MAP and heart rate in sham-operated (●) and adrenal enucleated (○) rats are shown immediately before and 5 min after an alerting stimulus. Adrenaline depletion reduced blood pressure and heart rate in normotensive rats but not in those with established hypertension. $p < 0.05$. (Redrawn from ref. 5 and reproduced with permission.)

sensitivity to adrenaline's prohypertensive effects occurs very early in hypertension development. Few, if any, studies of $\beta_2$-adrenoceptor responsiveness in rats younger than 6 weeks of age have, however, been performed.

### 4.5   Conclusions

Animal experiments tend to support a role for adrenaline activating facilitatory presynaptic $\beta_2$-adrenoceptors in the develop-

ment, if not maintenance, of genetic (spontaneous) hypertension. A similar role for adrenaline in the pathophysiology of human essential hypertension is an intriguing and attractive, though unproved, possibility and has been the subject of a comprehensive review by Floras[8]. Attempts to reduce blood pressure in humans by using $\beta_2$-antagonists have been disappointing. This may be because the effects of attenuated sympathetic facilitation are counteracted by the blockade of postsynaptic vasodilator $\beta_2$-adrenoceptors.

However, if facilitatory presynaptic $\beta_2$-adrenoceptors in humans exhibit a period of critical sensitivity early in hypertension development, as appears to occur in SHRs, and then lose their responsiveness as hypertension progresses, it may be unreasonable to expect blockade of these receptors to affect blood pressure in established hypertension. At this time, it is possible to state only that presynaptic $\beta_2$-adrenoceptor-mediated facilitation of sympathetic activity plays little, if any, role in blood pressure elevation. Further, blockade of presynaptic $\beta_2$-adrenoceptors may be effective only in attenuating hypertension development. However, this is, arguably, a true 'antihypertensive' effect, as distinct from the 'hypotensive' actions of present antihypertensive agents. Therefore, agents that prevent adrenaline's facilitation of sympathetic activity may prove useful as a novel strategy aimed at attenuating hypertension development rather than reducing an already elevated blood pressure.

## 5  Summary

A variety of different presynaptic receptor populations, which have been shown to modulate the release of sympathetic neurotransmitter, have been identified. The majority of these presynaptic receptors inhibit sympathetic neurotransmitter release and, thus, attenuate neurogenic end-organ responses. Of these, $\alpha$-adrenoceptors appear to be the most notable. Agonists at these receptors reduce the effects of sympathetic activity and can be expected to have antihypertensive (hypotensive) efficacy. At present, only 'centrally acting' $\alpha$-adrenoceptor agonists such as $\alpha$-methyldopa and clonidine have proved useful in the treatment of hypertension. As yet, it is by no means certain what proportion, if any, of their antihypertensive action results from stimulation of inhibitory presynaptic $\alpha$-adrenoceptors that attenuate noradrenaline release either centrally or in the periphery, and what proportion, the result of stimulation of postsynaptic $\alpha$-adrenoceptors

within the CNS that inhibit sympathetic drive.

A smaller number of presynaptic receptors, notably $\beta_2$-adrenoceptors and angiotensin II receptors, facilitate sympathetic neurogenic transmitter release and end-organ responses. Blockade of these receptors would be expected to decrease sympathetic neurotransmitter release and thereby reduce blood pressure. Certainly both ACE inhibitors, which reduce angiotensin II formation, and $\beta$-adrenoceptor antagonists are effective antihypertensive drugs. However, the contribution of presynaptic $\beta_2$-adrenoceptor blockade to the overall blood pressure-lowering effect of $\beta$-adrenoceptor antagonists, which appears to result largely from a reduction in cardiac output, is unknown. It is likely to be minimal in established hypertension. Some $\beta_2$-adrenoceptor antagonists are effective in attenuating hypertension development, indicating that developing rather than established hypertension may be relatively more amenable to pharmacological intervention at the level of presynaptic receptors.

The proportion of the antihypertensive effect caused by withdrawal of presynaptic angiotensin II receptor stimulation following depletion of angiotensin II with ACE inhibition is also unknown.

Agonists at non-adrenergic inhibitory presynaptic receptors might also be expected to possess antihypertensive efficacy. However, as with adrenoceptor agonists, the cardiovascular impact of presynaptic actions of non-adrenergic receptor agonists is likely to be complicated by postsynaptic effects of these agents. Continued studies and development of new pharmacological tools (drugs) may uncover therapeutically exploitable differences between pre- and postsynaptic receptors. The identification of such differences will, no doubt, stimulate the search for useful antihypertensive drugs with a presynaptic mechanism of action.

A reduced responsiveness of inhibitory presynaptic receptors, or an increased responsiveness of facilitatory presynaptic receptors, would be envisaged to result in augmented noradrenaline release and elevated blood pressure. Attempts to identify changes in presynaptic receptor responsiveness during hypertension development and maintenance have, so far, yielded equivocal results. Nevertheless, there appear to be changes in the responsiveness of presynaptic receptors, in particular the facilitatory $\beta_2$-adrenoceptors, early in hypertension. These receptors may, therefore, play a role in the development rather than maintenance of hypertension. Whereas present antihypertensive drugs act to reduce an already elevated blood pressure, the pharmacological manipulation of presynaptic receptors may represent an opportunity to attenuate progression of the hypertensive disease process.

## References

1. Anon (1990) Presynaptic Receptors and the Question of Autoregulation of Neurotransmitter Release. *Annals of the New York Academy of Sciences* **604**
2. Borkowski KR (1988) Pre- and postjunctional β-adrenoreceptors and hypertension. *Journal of Autonomic Pharmacology* **8:** 153–171
3. Borkowski KR (1990) Presynaptic receptors in hypertension. *Annals of the New York Academy of Science* **604:** 389–397
4. Borkowski KR (1991) The effect of adrenal demedullation and adrenaline on hypertension development and vascular reactivity in young spontaneously hypertensive rats. *Journal of Autonomic Pharmacology* **11:** 1–14
5. Borkowski KR and Kelly E (1986) The effect of adrenal demedullation on cardiovascular responses to environmental stimulation in conscious rats. *British Journal of Pharmacology* **88:** 943–945
6. Borkowski KR and Quinn P (1985) Adrenaline and the development of spontaneous hypertension in rats. *Journal of Autonomic Pharmacology* **5:** 89–100
7. Brown MJ and Macquin I (1981) Is adrenaline the cause of essential hypertension? *Lancet* **2:** 1079–1082
8. Floras JS (1992) Epinephrine and the genesis of hypertension. *Hypertension* **19:** 1–18
9. Floras JS, Aylward PE, Victor RG, Mark AL and Abboud FM (1988) Epinephrine facilitates neurogenic vasoconstriction in humans. *Journal of Clinical Investigation* **81:** 1265–1274
10. Folkow B (1982) Physiological aspects of primary hypertension. *Physiological Reviews* **62:** 347–504
11. Gillespie JS (1980) Presynaptic receptors in the autonomic nervous system. In: Sezekeres L (ed), *Handbook of Experimental Pharmacology:* vol 54: *Adrenergic Activators and Inhibitors*, pp 353–425, Springer-Verlag, Berlin
12. Langer SZ (1981) Presynaptic regulation of the release of catecholamines. *Pharmacological Reviews* **32:** 337–362
13. Majewski H (1983) Modulation of noradrenaline release through activation of presynaptic β-adrenoreceptors. *Journal of Autonomic Pharmacology* **3:** 47–60
14. Majewski H, Tung L-H and Rand MJ (1981) Adrenaline-induced hypertension in rats. *Journal of Cardiovascular Pharmacology* **3:** 179–185
15. Misu Y and Kubo T (1986) Presynaptic β-adrenoceptors. *Medical Research Reviews* **6:** 197–225
16. Nakamaru M, Jackson EK and Inagami T (1986) β-Adrenoceptor-mediated release of angiotensin II from mesenteric arteries. *American Journal of Physiology* **250:** H144–H148
17. Nakamaru M, Jackson EK and Inagami T (1986) Role of vascular angiotensin II released by β-adrenergic stimulation in rats. *Journal of Cardiovascular Pharmacology* **8** (Suppl 10): 1–5
18. Nezu M, Miura Y, Adachi M *et al.* (1985) The effects of epinephrine on norepinephrine release in essential hypertension. *Hypertension* **7:** 187–195
19. Pickering GW (1968) *High Blood Pressure*, 2nd edn. Churchill, London
20. Robb OJ, Webster J, Petrie JC, Harry JD and Young J (1988) Effects of the β2-adrenoceptor antagonist ICI 188,551 on blood pressure in hypertensive patients known to respond to β1-adrenoceptor antagonists. *British Journal of Clinical Pharmacology* **25:** 433–438
21. Rokkedal Nielsen J, Gram LF and Pedersen PK (1988) Plasma noradrenaline levels in young subjects at increased risk of developing essential hypertension. Response to a multistage exercise test. *Pharmacological Toxicology* **63** (Suppl 1): 32–34

22. Society of Actuaries and Association of Life Insurance Medical Directors of America. (1980) *Blood Pressure Study 1979*. Recording and Statistical Corp., Washington, DC

23. Starke K (1977) Regulation of noradrenaline release by presynaptic receptor systems. *Reviews of Physiology, Biochemistry and Pharmacology* **77:** 1–124

24. Stjärne L, Msghina M and Stjärne E (1991) 'Upstream' regulation of the release probability in sympathetic nerve varicosities. *Neuroscience* **36:** 571–587

25. Westfall TC (1977) Local regulation of adrenergic neurotransmission. *Physiological Reviews* **57:** 659–728

26. Westfall TC and Meldrum MJ (1985) Alterations in the release of norepinephrine at the vascular neuroeffector junction in hypertension. *Annual Reviews of Pharmacology and Toxicology* **25:** 621–641

# 15 Monoamine neurones and antidepressant treatments

Pierre Blier and Claude de Montigny

The neurochemistry of psychiatric disorder and neurological disease, considered from a perspective focused on neurotransmitter release-modulating mechanisms, is the basis of this chapter by Pierre Blier and Claude de Montigny. Besides considering the possible role of neurotransmitter release-modulating receptors at the nerve terminal in the treatment of some psychiatric conditions, the writers draw attention to the additional modulatory pathway, mediated by receptors located on the dendrites and cell body of neurones, that might be involved. Their commentary is based in large part on observations made in laboratory animals treated with a variety of neuroactive therapeutic drugs.

## 1 Dysfunction of monoamine neurones as a possible cause of neuropsychiatric disorders

For any given psychiatric disorder, there are reports suggesting the deficiency or excess of virtually every monoamine neurotransmitter as a possible aetiological factor. Rather than speculating on putative links between presynaptic receptors and biochemical anomalies reported to occur with various psychiatric disorders, this chapter covers one small area. It focuses on the effects of acute and long-term administration of psychotropic drugs on presynaptic (soma-dendritic and terminal) receptors modulating the efficacy of 5-HT, noradrenergic and, to a lesser extent, dopaminergic neurotransmission in laboratory animals. The emphasis is on the effects of antidepressant drugs. It is important to mention that most of these drugs are also effective in the treatment of anxiety disorders, such as generalised anxiety and panic disorders. Furthermore, in the obsessive–compulsive disorder, selective 5-HT-reuptake inhibitors (including the preferential 5-HT-reuptake inhibitor chlorimipramine) are the only agents among the various classes of antidepressant drug that exert a clear therapeutic effect. The neurochemical alterations produced by long-term administration of these drugs may, therefore, be germane to their delayed onset of action in anxiety and depressive disorders.

### 1.1 Dopamine and Parkinson's disease

Several CNS disorders have been linked to specific dysfunctions of chemical neurotransmission. The best documented case is certainly Parkinson's disease. The characteristic tremors of this disorder generally appear when about 80% of the dopaminergic neurones of the substantia nigra have degenerated. Effective treatment consists either in administering a postsynaptic dopamine agonist or, more commonly, since dopamine does not penetrate the blood–brain barrier, in giving the immediate dopamine precursor L-dopa. This is converted to dopamine by a non-specific aromatic amino acid decarboxylase present in monoaminergic nerve terminals in the basal ganglia. The increased availability of dopamine is generally sufficient to alleviate the symptoms. Unfortunately, the pathophysiology and the therapeutic strategies linked to this disease are too often extrapolated inappropriately to provide a general model for psychiatric illnesses. That is, researchers who have identified a neurobiological modification produced by a class of psychotropic drugs in a given system often assume that a dysfunction of that particular system is responsible for the disease. For example, in the case of schizophrenia, it has often been assumed that psychotic symptoms must result from a hyperactive dopaminergic system because of the well-documented effectiveness of most antipsychotic drugs presently available to block dopamine receptors. Although there is considerable evidence supporting this hypothesis, the relationship between the aetiology and the therapeutics of schizophrenia is certainly not as straightforward as for Parkinson's disease. In particular, while antipsychotic drugs block dopaminergic $D_2$ receptors in the human brain within minutes to hours, as documented by positron-emission tomography, they begin to exert their therapeutic effect only after several days.

## 1.2  Depression and 5-HT

In the case of major depression, there is evidence indicating that the 5-HT system might be hypofunctioning, perhaps consistently so in subgroups of patients. For example, Åsberg et al.[4] were the first to report low levels of the main metabolite of 5-HT, 5-hydroxyindole acetic acid, in a subgroup of depressed patients who had attempted to commit suicide by violent means (gun shot or hanging as distinct from drug intoxication).

Rather than using baseline parameters, another approach to assess the function of a specific system has been to use pharmacological challenges. For the 5-HT system, four probes have been widely used in depressed subjects. The intravenous injection of a bolus of L-tryptophan, the amino acid precursor of 5-HT, and the oral administration of the 5-HT-releasing agent fenfluramine have both been used to trigger neuroendocrine responses (e.g. altered plasma levels of prolactin). In general, such studies indicate that these responses, which are mediated by $5\text{-HT}_{1A}$ receptors in the case of tryptophan and by $5\text{-HT}_2$ receptors in the case of fenfluramine, are blunted in depressed patients. However, the observations have to be interpreted from a 'postsynaptic' as well as a 'presynaptic' viewpoint, because tryptophan is converted to 5-HT within 5-HT terminals and fenfluramine releases endogenous 5-HT from these terminals, which can then cause an increased activation of postsynaptic 5-HT receptors.

Another approach consists of administering a 5-HT agonist. In the case of selective $5\text{-HT}_{1A}$ agonists, while it is generally accepted that the neuroendocrine responses (see above) result from the activation of postsynaptic $5\text{-HT}_{1A}$ receptors, it has been claimed that the hypothermic response reflects the sensitivity of (presynaptic) soma-dendritic $5\text{-HT}_{1A}$ autoreceptors. However, there is now considerable evidence against this claim, and data have been gathered recently that show that it is postsynaptic $5\text{-HT}_{1A}$ receptors which mediate the hypothermic response to the administration of $5\text{-HT}_{1A}$ agonists[7], even in humans[18].

Finally, m-chlorophenylpiperazine (a metabolite of the antidepressant trazodone) has also been used extensively in depressed subjects as a probe to assess 5-HT responsiveness. However, this drug acts as a $5\text{-HT}_{1A/1B/1D}$ agonist and as a $5\text{-HT}_{2/3}$ antagonist (see Table 15.1). The effects of m-chlorophenylpiperazine, therefore, cannot be attributed solely to its capacity to interact selectively with a single subtype of 5-HT receptor at a pre- or postsynaptic location.

Therefore, we presently lack selective tools and experimental paradigms to study specifically the actions of presynaptic 5-HT receptors in humans, whether it be the

Table 15.1. *Subtypes of central serotonin (5-HT) receptors with their effector mechanisms and cellular localisation*

|  | Subtype | Effector mechanism | Cellular location |
|---|---|---|---|
| 5-HT$_1$ | 5-HT$_{1A}$ | Phosphatidylinositol metabolism, K$^+$ channels, adenylyl cyclase (+/−) | Soma-dendritic autoreceptor and postsynaptic receptor |
|  | 5-HT$_{1B}$ | Adenylyl cyclase (−), phosphatidylinositol metabolism, Ca$^{2+}$ channels | Terminal autoreceptor in rats and mice, heteroreceptor and postsynaptic receptor |
|  | 5-HT$_{1C}$ | Phosphatidylinositol metabolism | Postsynaptic receptor and choroid plexus |
|  | 5-HT$_{1D}$ | Adenylyl cyclase (−) | Terminal autoreceptor in guinea pigs and humans, and postsynaptic receptor |
|  | 5-HT$_{1E}$ | Adenylyl cyclase (−) |  |
| 5-HT$_2$ |  | Phosphatidylinositol metabolism |  |
| 5-HT$_3$ |  | Na$^+$/K$^+$ channels |  |
| 5-HT$_4$ |  | Adenylyl cyclase (+) |  |

Note that these receptors have all been cloned. Different subpopulations most probably exist for each subtype of 5-HT receptor. (+/–) indicates a stimulatory and inhibitory effect, respectively, on the activity of adenylyl cyclase to generate the second messenger cAMP.

5-HT$_{1A}$ autoreceptor on the cell body of 5-HT neurones, which regulates their firing activity, or the autoreceptor on 5-HT terminals, which regulates the release of the neurotransmitter.

## 1.3   Noradrenaline and depression

With regard to the indices available to assess the function of the noradrenergic system (e.g. measurement of the catecholamine content of peripheral or CNS fluids), there are no clear trends suggesting a modification of noradrenergic function in depressed patients. Furthermore, there is as yet no pharmacological agent or method available to assess specifically the function of brain presynaptic α$_2$-adrenoceptors *in vivo*. Currently available α$_2$-adrenoceptor agonists not only bind to presynaptic receptors to attenuate noradrenaline release but also activate postsynaptic α$_2$-adrenoceptors, the latter tending to have the opposite effect on noradrenergic transmission. Furthermore, the interpretation of challenge studies carried out with the α$_2$-adrenoceptor agonist clonidine is complicated by the recent discovery of the imidazoline receptors, which

are clearly distinct from α$_2$-adrenoceptors and to which clonidine binds with a high affinity.

A similar problem is encountered with studies of the dopaminergic system, since the drugs presently available neither discriminate between the soma-dendritic and the terminal autoreceptors, which are both of the D$_2$ subtype, nor between these and the D$_2$ receptors that are located on postsynaptic neurones.

## 1.4 Summary

At present there are no tools to assess reliably the responsiveness of presynaptic monoamine receptors in the human brain. However, it is clear that perturbations of the function of monoamine neurones and of receptors present on their cell body and/or their terminals may contribute to the pathophysiology of psychiatric disorders, such as schizophrenia, anxiety and depressive disorders, as with Parkinson's disease. What follows is a review of some of the abundant animal-derived data, obtained mainly *in vivo* using the electrophysiological paradigm depicted in Fig. 15.1, which indicate that

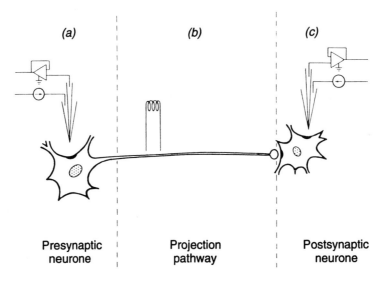

Fig. 15.1. Electrophysiological paradigm used to assess the net effect of drugs on monoaminergic neurotransmission[11]. (a) Firing activity of the presynaptic neurone and sensitivity of the soma-dendritic autoreceptor, assessed by either micro-iontophoretic or systemic administration of agonists. (b) Effect of the electrical activation of the projection pathway on the firing activity of the postsynaptic neurone and responsiveness of the terminal autoreceptor, assessed by determining the effectiveness of the antagonist methiothepin in prolonging the suppression of firing produced by the stimulation. (c) Responsiveness of the postsynaptic neurone to microiontophoretic application of agonists.

modifications of the function of presynaptic receptors may lead to therapeutic benefit. In some cases, these data are supported by clinical observations.

## 2    Soma-dendritic autoreceptors in the brain

Dopaminergic, noradrenergic and 5-HT neurones are endowed with soma-dendritic autoreceptors, i.e. autoreceptors located on their cell body and dendrites that exert a negative feedback control on firing activity and release, respectively[42]. 5-HT neurones discharge at a relatively low and regular rate. Their firing activity is highest in freely moving animals, particularly during certain feeding and grooming behaviours, lower during slow-wave sleep and silent during REM (rapid eye movement) sleep periods[32]. In general, the firing activity of noradrenergic neurones is similar to that of 5-HT neurones

across the sleep–wake–arousal cycle, but, in addition, noradrenergic neurones are highly responsive to a variety of environmental stimuli, especially nociceptive ones. Finally, dopaminergic neurones display stability in both rate and pattern across the sleep–wake–arousal cycle and may also respond to phasic sensory stimuli without habituation, unlike noradrenergic neurones[31]. For these three types of neurone, firing activity is positively correlated with neurotransmitter release, thus alterations of the degree of activation, and/or of the sensitivity of their soma-dendritic autoreceptors, following administration of psychotropic drugs may have profound physiological repercussions.

### 2.1    Soma-dendritic 5-HT autoreceptors

The amount of 5-HT in the vicinity of the cell body of 5-HT neurones can be increased by either acutely blocking its reuptake with drugs, such as fluoxetine, or by inhibiting

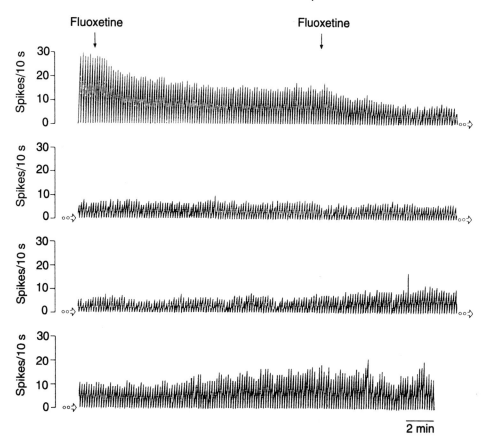

Fig. 15.2. Integrated firing rate histogram showing the suppressant effect of the 5-HT-reuptake blocker fluoxetine (0.4 mg/kg, i.v.) on the firing rate of a dorsal raphe 5-HT-neurone. This extracellular recording was obtained in a rat anaesthetised with chloral hydrate. The four traces are continuous.

monoamine oxidase (MAO) type A, which normally metabolises 5-HT. This local increase causes suppression of the firing activity of 5-HT neurones (Fig. 15.2) mediated by 5-HT stimulation of soma-dendritic autoreceptors. The resultant attenuated impulse flow reaching the nerve terminals would be expected to reduce 5-HT release, but it appears that synaptic 5-HT (in forebrain regions) is not significantly altered, probably because of compensatory mechanisms present on the 5-HT terminals. Indeed, Adell and Artigas[1] were the first to show that systemic administration of chlorimipramine, a 5-HT-reuptake-blocking drug, did not invariably enhance the extracellular concentration of 5-HT as measured by microdialysis in the rat frontal cortex. However, the extracellular concentration of 5-HT is increased in the dorsal raphe as a result of 5-HT-reuptake blockade by the same drug.

In contrast, when the soma-dendritic autoreceptor is activated with a selective 5-HT$_{1A}$ agonist, 5-HT levels decrease drastically in innervated forebrain structures. Therefore, the degree of activation of all subtypes of postsynaptic 5-HT receptor is attenuated except 5-HT$_{1A}$ because of the presence of the exogenous 5-HT$_{1A}$ agonist in the synaptic cleft (Fig. 15.3). The complementary

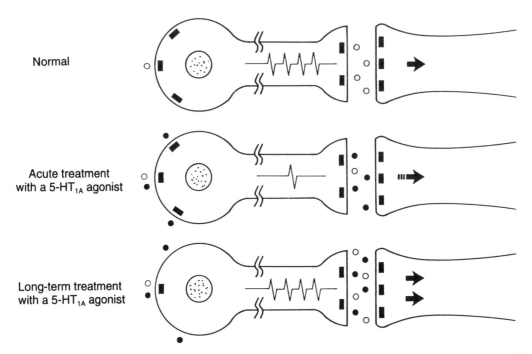

Fig. 15.3. The effect of acute administration of a 5-HT$_{1A}$ agonist on the 5-HT system and the adaptation of the firing activity of dorsal raphe 5-HT neurones as a result of soma-dendritic 5-HT autoreceptor desensitisation. The diagrams indicate the resultant modifications in the degree of the tonic activation of postsynaptic 5-HT$_{1A}$ receptors in the dorsal hippocampus. The open circles represent endogenous 5-HT molecules and the closed ones the exogenous 5-HT$_{1A}$ agonist. The broken arrow in the middle diagram indicates that the degree of the tonic activation of the postsynaptic receptors depends on the dose of agonist used[23].

experiment, that of blocking selectively the soma-dendritic 5-HT$_{1A}$ autoreceptors, has not been performed because sufficiently selective antagonists are not yet available. However, on present indications, it would appear that activation of this autoreceptor subtype by endogenous 5-HT would be physiologically significant only during high levels of activity because it is only in this condition, when a substantial amount of 5-HT is present, that a 5-HT$_{1A}$ antagonist increases the firing activity of 5-HT neurones in freely moving animals[32].

## 2.2  Soma-dendritic noradrenaline autoreceptors

The soma-dendritic autoreceptor on locus coeruleus noradrenergic neurones is of the $\alpha_2$-subtype. When activated by an increased

presence of noradrenaline, as a result of reuptake blockade or MAO-A inhibition, there is a suppression of firing. However systemic administration of a noradrenaline reuptake blocker, despite producing a suppression of noradrenergic neurone firing activity, actually increases noradrenaline in innervated forebrain structures, as measured by *in vivo* microdialysis (see Chapter 12). Interestingly, when the $\alpha_2$-adrenoceptors are blocked as well as the noradrenaline-reuptake process, then a massive increase in extracellular noradrenaline occurs[24]. This secondary increase most probably results not only from the blockade of soma-dendritic noradrenaline autoreceptors (which would restore noradrenergic impulse flow) but also from blockade of the release-inhibiting $\alpha_2$-adrenoceptors located on noradrenergic terminals. Unlike for 5-HT autoreceptors, there are several effective antagonists for $\alpha_2$-adrenoceptors, some of which have been used in humans. For example, a 20 mg dose of yohimbine can induce anxiety in healthy volunteers, increase the symptomatology in patients with anxiety disorders and may even trigger panic attacks[30]. This presumably results from an enhanced noradrenaline release in the CNS, because peripheral markers of noradrenaline turnover are increased following administration of this drug.

### 2.3 Soma-dendritic dopamine autoreceptors

Systemic administration of $D_2$ receptor agonists decreases and that of antagonists increases, respectively, the firing activity of two populations of dopaminergic neurones: that of substantia nigra neurones projecting to the basal ganglia and that of ventromedial tegmentum neurones projecting to the cerebral cortex and limbic structures. The increase in firing activity results, at least in part, from the interaction of such drugs with soma-dendritic $D_2$ autoreceptors. Antagonists of $D_2$ receptors not only enhance firing activity, but also increase the number of dopaminergic neurones displaying a bursting firing pattern. It has been elegantly demonstrated that, for a given number of impulses, this bursting mode of firing of dopaminergic neurones produces a greater amount of dopamine release in postsynaptic structures than does a regular firing pattern[29].

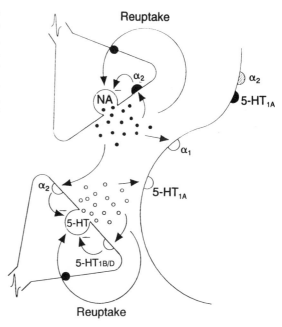

Fig. 15.4. Schematic representation of the modulation of 5-HT and noradrenergic (NA) neurotransmission in the hippocampus by presynaptic receptors located on 5-HT and noradrenergic terminals. Note that different symbols are used to depict $\alpha_2$-adrenoceptors on the 5-HT terminal on the noradrenergic terminal and on the postsynaptic pyramidal neurone because several lines of evidence indicate that they are pharmacologically different. There might also be two distinct populations of 5-HT$_{1A}$ receptors on these postsynaptic neurones: those located intrasynaptically on their dendritic tree and those located extrasynaptically on their cell body (upper right corner).

## 3 Presynaptic receptors on nerve terminals

It is important to remember that the number of presynaptic receptors is probably infinitesimal in any given brain structure relative to that of their postsynaptic congeners. It is, therefore, virtually impossible to study them using radioligand-binding techniques. The existence of nerve-terminal presynaptic receptors in CNS structures, however, is gen-erally accepted despite this technical drawback, since their function is readily observable in any neurotransmitter release paradigm (see Fig. 15.4).

### 3.1 Presynaptic receptors on serotoninergic neurones

Nerve terminal autoreceptors play a major role in controlling release from central 5-HT neurones. In the rat brain, the 5-HT-release-

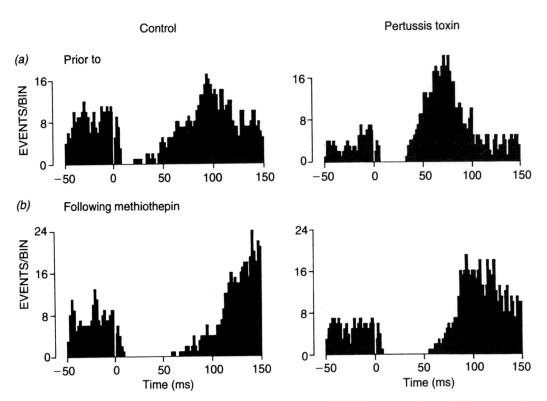

Fig. 15.5. Peristimulus time histograms illustrating the response of CA3 hippocampal pyramidal neurones to electrical stimulation of their afferent 5-HT pathway prior to (*a*), and following (*b*), injection of the 5-HT autoreceptor antagonist methiothepin (1 mg/kg, i.v.) in a control rat and in a rat pretreated with pertussis toxin (1 μg injected into the hippocampus 10 days prior to recording). Each histogram was constructed from 200 consecutive stimuli of 0.5 ms delivered at time 0. The efficacy of pertussis toxin to inactivate $G_{i/o}$-proteins was confirmed by a greater than 90% decrease in sensitivity to microiontophoretic application of 5-HT onto the cell body of the same neurones. The suppression of firing produced by the stimulation is mediated by intrasynaptic $5-HT_{1A}$ receptors on the dendritic tree of the pyramidal neurones. It was not altered by pertussis toxin, thereby indicating that these postsynaptic receptors are not coupled to $G_{i/o}$-proteins, unlike the extrasynaptic $5-HT_{1A}$ receptors located on the cell body[15].

modulating autoreceptor displays a $5-HT_{1B}$ pharmacological profile, whereas in other species, such as guinea-pigs and humans, it has a $5-HT_{1D}$ profile[28]. In the rat hippocampus, the terminal $5-HT_{1B}$ autoreceptor is not coupled to $G_{i/o}$- or $G_s$-protein, as indicated by the lack of effect of pertussis toxin (Fig. 15.5), cholera toxin or the non-selective alkylating agent *N*-ethylmaleimide[6]. These results, although surprising, have parallels elsewhere: prejunctional $\alpha_2$-adrenergic adrenoceptors in peripheral tissues, such as

the mouse atrium, have been found to be insensitive to pertussis toxin (see Chapter 9; see also refs. 2, 26, 39). The nerve-terminal 5-HT autoreceptors appear to be tonically activated by locally prevailing 5-HT levels since the 5-HT antagonist methiothepin can approximately double the stimulation-induced release of 5-HT both in the *in vitro* slice preparation (whether this is from rat[17], guinea-pig[7], or human brain[28]) and in *in vivo* electrophysiological experiments carried out in the rat dorsal hippocampus[15] (Fig. 15.5).

5-HT terminals are also endowed with heteroreceptors, including $\alpha_2$-adrenoceptors (see Fig. 15.4). In the rat hypothalamic slice preparation, the $\alpha_2$-adrenoceptor agonist UK 14,304 can produce a complete inhibition of the electrically evoked release of [$^3$H]-5-HT from prcloaded slices, and an 85% inhibition of the electrically evoked release of [$^3$H]-noradrenaline from preloaded slices of the same structures[13]. These results indicate that $\alpha_2$-adrenergic heteroreceptors located on 5-HT terminals are at least as effective in suppressing 5-HT release as are $\alpha_2$-adrenergic autoreceptors in suppressing noradrenaline release. The results also indicate that $\alpha_2$-adrenergic heteroreceptors are as effective as 5-HT autoreceptors in suppressing 5-HT release. In fact, these two types of presynaptic receptor on 5-HT terminals may share common transducing mechanism(s). This possibility is supported by the observation that, when the degree of activation of the 5-HT autoreceptor is enhanced by a 5-HT-reuptake blocker, the activation of $\alpha_2$-heteroreceptors is much less effective[13]. Consistent with this, it has been observed that, by concurrently blocking the 5-HT autoreceptor and the 5-HT-reuptake process, the responsiveness of the $\alpha_2$-adrenergic heteroreceptor was normalised. Finally, it is important to note that this $\alpha_2$-adrenergic heteroreceptor is likely to be activated *in vivo* by endogenous noradrenaline, despite the fact that several studies carried out in rat brain slices have generally yielded negative results. For example, superfusion with $\alpha_2$-adrenoceptor antagonists failed to enhance the release of 5-HT. In *in vivo* electrophysiological experiments, however, the intravenous administration of (−)mianserin, a drug acting preferentially on the $\alpha_2$-adrenergic heteroreceptor, prolonged the period of suppression of firing of rat hippocampus neurones produced by electrical stimulation of the 5-HT pathway[36]. This also appears to be the case in the human brain[25,28].

There are data from *in vivo* and *in vitro* studies indicating that the release of 5-HT can be modulated also by presynaptic 5-HT$_3$ receptors. Galzin and Langer[27] were the first to report that activation of 5-HT$_3$ receptors enhances the electrically evoked release of 5-HT from preloaded slices of the guinea-pig frontal cortex and hypothalamus. The same modulation has been found in the hippocampus, and a functional characterisation of the receptor involved has been performed[9]. In brief, activation of the 5-HT$_3$ receptor is more effective when the synaptic availability of 5-HT is low, the receptor desensitises rapidly (as is to be expected for a positive feedback system) and it can be activated by endogenous 5-HT. However, the 5-HT$_3$ receptor may not be located on 5-HT terminals[16]. The neurotransmitter release-enhancing effect of the activation of this receptor has also been documented in *in vivo* microdialysis experiments carried out in the rat hippocampus[35].

## 3.2 Presynaptic receptors on noradrenergic neurones

Terminals from central noradrenergic neurones are endowed with $\alpha_2$-adrenergic autoreceptors. These have been shown to be tonically activated in experiments using both the *in vitro* slice preparation and *in vivo* electrophysiological and microdialysis paradigms. In one *in vivo* electrophysiological experiment, the ascending noradrenergic bundle was electrically stimulated and the effect of the resulting release of noradrenaline was assessed indirectly by measuring the suppression of the firing activity of postsynaptic hippocampal CA3 neurones[21]. An 80% decrease in the suppression of firing was obtained when the frequency of stimulation was increased from 1 Hz to 5 Hz (Fig. 15.6). Using the same experimental protocol to study the 5-HT system, a 25% to 50% decrease was obtained when the stimulating frequency was increased from 0.8 to 5 Hz (see Fig. 15.9). These results suggest that nerve terminal $\alpha_2$-adrenergic autoreceptors play a greater role in noradrenaline release than do 5-HT autoreceptors in modulating the release of 5-HT.

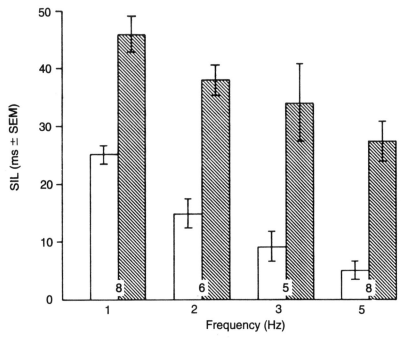

Fig. 15.6. Effects of different frequencies of electrical stimulation (200 consecutive 0.5 ms pulses at an intensity of 800 μA) of the rat locus coeruleus on the duration of the suppression (SIL) of firing of hippocampal CA3 pyramidal neurones prior to (open columns), and following (shaded columns), the injection of the $\alpha_2$-adrenoceptor antagonist idazoxan (500 μg/kg, i.v.). The number of neurones tested (before and after idazoxan) at each frequency is given at the bottom of each pair of columns[21].

## 4    Effect of long-term antidepressant treatment on soma-dendritic autoreceptors

### 4.1    Soma-dendritic 5-HT autoreceptors

Antidepressant drugs that enhance the synaptic availability of 5-HT produce a suppression of the firing activity of 5-HT neurones at the beginning of the treatment. After two days of treatment with either the potent 5-HT-reuptake blockers zimelidine, indalpine, and citalopram or the MAO inhibitors phenelzine, clorgyline and amiflamine, the activity of dorsal raphe 5-HT neurones was reduced by 50% or more (Fig. 15.7). With prolonged treatment, 5-HT neurones progressively regain their normal firing activity after two or three weeks. With all of the six drugs listed above, the respon-siveness of the soma-dendritic 5-HT auto-receptor to an exogenous agonist was attenuated even after 5-HT neurones had regained their normal firing activity. In terms of cause and effect, these results suggest that soma-dendritic 5-HT autoreceptors desensitise following long-term exposure to an increased concentration of 5-HT, allowing the 5-HT neurones to recover their normal firing rate despite sustained blockade of reuptake or MAO-A inhibition[11].

Since these autoreceptors are of the 5-HT$_{1A}$ type (see Section 2.1), it was thought crucial to study particularly the effects of long-term administration of 5-HT$_{1A}$ agonists, some of which are known to have both anxiolytic and antidepressant properties (see Table 15.2). Sustained administration of the selective 5-HT$_{1A}$ agonists gepirone, tandospirone and flesinoxan was found to

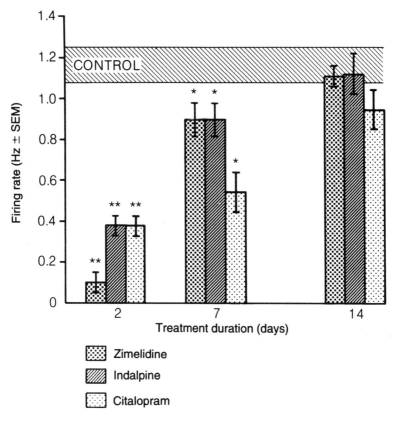

Fig. 15.7. Effects of treatment for 2, 7 and 14 days with the selective 5-HT-reuptake inhibitors zimelidine and indalpine (5 mg/kg per day, i.p.) and citalopram (20 mg/kg per day, i.p.) on the firing rate of dorsal raphe 5-HT neurones recorded by systematic electrode descents through the dorsal raphe in anaesthetised rats. The shaded area represents the range (SEM × 2) of the firing activity of these neurones in control rats. Significant differences from control are shown as *$p < 0.05$; **$p < 0.001$, using the two-tailed Student's $t$-test[11].

produce an initial decrease in the firing activity of dorsal raphe 5-HT neurones. As with 5-HT-reuptake blockers and MAO-A inhibitors, this decrease was followed by a gradual and complete recovery after 14 days of treatment and, at the same time, a decreased responsiveness of 5-HT neurones to direct microiontophoretic application of 5-HT agonists (Fig. 15.8)[23]. Electroconvulsive shocks and tricyclic antidepressants, which are weak inhibitors of 5-HT reuptake or which are rapidly metabolised into preferential noradrenaline-reuptake inhibitors, did not alter the sensitivity of soma-dendritic 5-HT autoreceptors[10,11]. The mechanism of the autoreceptor desensitisation is not clear. Down-regulation of the number of autoreceptors may be involved[43], but in one study, the electrophysiological responsiveness of the autoreceptors to the 5-HT$_{1A}$ agonist ipsapirone was attenuated despite an unchanged density of binding sites for [$^3$H]-8-OH-DPAT (a selective 5-HT$_{1A}$ ligand)[40].

### 4.2   Soma-dendritic noradrenaline autoreceptors

The effects of antidepressant treatments on central noradrenergic neurones are different from those on 5-HT neurones. Sustained

Table 15.2. *Site of action of some drugs acting on monoamine neurones and on selected postsynaptic receptors*

| Type of neurone | Soma-dendritic autoreceptor | Terminal receptor | Postsynaptic receptor | Uptake blocker |
|---|---|---|---|---|
| Serotonergic | 5-HT$_{1A}$ agonists: 8-OH-DPAT, LSD, buspirone, gepirone, flesinoxan | 5-HT antagonist: methiothepin | 5-HT$_{1A}$-agonists: 8-OH-DPAT, buspirone, gepirone, flesinoxan | Chlorimipramine, citalopram, fluoxetine, fluvoxamine, paroxetine, sertraline |
| Noradrenergic | $\alpha_2$-Agonist: clonidine | $\alpha_2$-Agonist: clonidine | $\alpha_2$-Agonist: clonidine | Desipramine, nomifensine |
| | $\alpha_2$-Antagonists: yohimbine, mianserin | $\alpha_2$-Antagonists: yohimbine, mianserin | $\alpha_2$-Antagonists: yohimbine, mianserin | Mazindol |
| Dopaminergic | D$_2$ agonist: apomorphine D$_2$ antagonist: haloperidol | D$_2$ agonist: apomorphine D$_2$ antagonist: haloperidol | D$_2$ agonist: apomorphine D$_2$ antagonist: haloperidol | Bupropion, nomifensine |

inhibition of MAO-A by clorgyline and phenelzine produces a decrease in firing activity of noradrenergic neurones after 2 days of treatment but this is not followed by any recovery after 3 weeks of treatment. At this time, the suppressing effect of the $\alpha_2$-adrenoceptor agonist clonidine on noradrenergic neurones is unaltered. Therefore, the reduced firing activity of noradrenergic neurones persists during long-term MAO-A inhibition, probably because their soma-dendritic autoreceptors do not desensitise[11]. Following long-term treatment with the selective noradrenaline-reuptake blocker desipramine, several groups of investigators have reported a decreased effectiveness of intravenous injection or microiontophoretic application of clonidine in suppressing the firing activity of noradrenergic neurones in the locus coeruleus. However, the responsiveness to microiontophoretic application of noradrenaline itself onto the same noradrenergic neurones that presented an attenuated responsiveness to clonidine was unchanged[34]. This discrepancy may be attributable to the capacity of clonidine to activate two populations of receptors, namely the recently identi-

fied imidazoline receptors in addition to the $\alpha_2$-adrenoceptors. It is, therefore, possible that long-term blockade of noradrenaline reuptake desensitises clonidine-sensitive imidazoline receptors but not the noradrenaline-sensitive $\alpha_2$-adrenoceptors. Identical results were obtained following long-term treatment with the antidepressant drug milnacipran. It is intriguing that sustained administration of a MAO inhibitor, or of a noradrenaline-reuptake blocker, both produced a continuous attenuation of the firing activity of locus coeruleus neurones, presumably by enhancing synaptic availability of noradrenaline, but that their responsiveness to clonidine was altered only by the noradrenaline-reuptake blocker.

### 4.3 Soma-dendritic dopamine autoreceptors

Several studies carried out in animals have shown that long-term antidepressant drug administration can alter neurochemical and behavioural parameters involving brain dopaminergic functions. The antidepressant efficacy of the dopamine-reuptake blockers

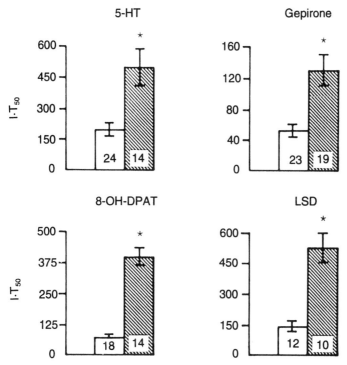

Fig. 15.8. Sensitivity of dorsal raphe 5-HT neurones to microiontophoretic application of 5-HT, gepirone, 8-OH-DPAT and lysergic acid diethylamide (LSD) in control rats (open columns) and in rats treated with gepirone for 14 days (shaded columns). Gepirone was administered at 15 mg/kg daily using an osmotic minipump implanted subcutaneously. The baseline firing rate was the same in controls and in gepirone-treated rats. Sensitivity is expressed as $I \bullet T_{50}$ values (mean $\pm$ SEM, I, current in nA, T, time in s). $I \bullet T_{50}$ corresponds to the charge necessary to eject from the micropipette a quantity of drug sufficient to inhibit by 50% the firing activity of the neurones. Therefore, the higher the column, the less sensitive are the neurones. The number of neurones tested is given at the bottom of each column. Significant differences from control are shown as $*p < 0.05$ using the two-tailed Student's $t$-test[23].

nomifensine and buproprion suggests that the dopaminergic system may be mediating their therapeutic efficacy. These two drugs, however, are also noradrenaline-reuptake blockers. It has been reported that treatments with tricyclic antidepressants, MAO inhibitors or electroconvulsive shocks produce a desensitisation of the soma-dendritic dopamine autoreceptor of substantia nigra dopaminergic neurones. This, surprisingly, appears to depend more on the passage of time than on repeated administration of these treatments[3]. Other groups[33], have been unable to replicate the finding. In addition,

the clinical relevance of this neurobiological effect remains doubtful because, in humans, it is recognised that repeated administration of antidepressant treatments is essential to induce a remission. Furthermore, there is no evidence of increased dopamine turnover in the cerebrospinal fluid of depressed patients treated with antidepressant drugs, an increase that would be expected to result from inactivation of presynaptic negative feedback systems. It is well known clinically that antipsychotic drugs (dopamine receptor antagonists) do not prevent or reverse the therapeutic effect of antidepressant drugs.

## 5    Effect of long-term antidepressant treatment on presynaptic receptors

### 5.1    Presynaptic receptors on serotoninergic neurones

Long-term administration of 5-HT-reuptake blockers produces a desensitisation of the terminal 5-HT$_{1B}$ autoreceptor in the rat brain, thus allowing more 5-HT to be released per impulse reaching the synaptic boutons[11]. This phenomenon was observed in an *in vivo* electrophysiological paradigm using two approaches. First, the effect of the terminal 5-HT autoreceptor antagonist methiothepin in suppressing the firing activity of postsynaptic neurones caused by electrical stimulation of the 5-HT pathway was abolished following long-term administration of the 5-HT-reuptake blockers citalopram and paroxetine. These results imply that the 5-HT$_{1B}$ autoreceptor is no longer functional under these experimental conditions, because its blockade no longer produces a prolongation of the period of suppression of firing of hippocampal neurones. The second approach consisted of comparing the efficacy of electrical stimulation of the 5-HT pathway at a low (1 Hz) and a high (5 Hz) frequency. The period of suppression of firing of postsynaptic neurones was shorter at 5 Hz than at 1 Hz. The attenuated release of 5-HT per impulse at 5 Hz probably occurs because the autoreceptor is still being activated by 5-HT at the time of arrival of the next stimulation-triggered action potential. In rats treated with paroxetine or fluoxetine, the degree of attenuation of the suppression of firing obtained by increasing the frequency of stimulation from 1 to 5 Hz was significantly smaller than in non-treated animals. This desensitisation of the terminal 5-HT$_{1B}$ autoreceptor was subsequently documented using *in vitro* superfusion of rat hypothalamic slices[38]. The slices were prepared from rats treated with citalopram and were preloaded with [$^3$H]-5-HT. The inhibition of electrically evoked release of [$^3$H]-5-HT produced

by a 5-HT autoreceptor agonist was attenuated. It is noteworthy that in the guinea-pig hypothalamus, where the terminal 5-HT autoreceptor is of the 5-HT$_{1D}$ subtype as in humans, a desensitisation is also produced by long-term treatment with the potent 5-HT-reuptake blocker paroxetine[9].

Since 5-HT neurones regain their normal firing activity and the effectiveness of the stimulation of the ascending 5-HT pathway is increased following treatment for two weeks with a 5-HT-reuptake blocker (see also Section 15.4.1), it is clear that 5-HT neurotransmission is enhanced at this point in time. Such a desensitisation of the presynaptic 5-HT receptors is not produced by long-term administration of tricyclic antidepressant drugs, possibly because they do not produce a sufficient degree of 5-HT-reuptake blockade and, hence, a sufficiently increased intrasynaptic concentration of 5-HT. MAO inhibitors increase the synaptic availability of 5-HT but, surprisingly, are ineffective. The possibility that 5-HT-reuptake blockers increase 5-HT in the biophase much more than MAO inhibitors is unlikely since treatment for 21 days, with the potent and selective MAO-A inhibitor clorgyline does desensitise the postsynaptic 5-HT$_{1A}$ receptors in the rat hippocampus. This attenuated postsynaptic responsiveness almost certainly results from the sustained increase, by more than two-fold, in the brain concentration of 5-HT caused by the long-term MAO inhibition. Therefore, there remains the possibility of an interaction between the 5-HT-reuptake carrier and the terminal 5-HT autoreceptor during a long-term treatment with a 5-HT-reuptake blocker[8,11].

It is important to emphasise that the net effect of repeated administration of 5-HT-reuptake blockers and of MAO inhibitors on 5-HT neurotransmission is similar, but achieved through different mechanisms. In the case of the former drugs, both soma-dendritic and terminal 5-HT autoreceptors would desensitise as a result of increased extracellular availability of 5-HT, thus allowing 5-HT neurones to release more neurotransmitter because of the inactivation of the negative feedback elements. In the case of the MAO inhibitors, it is the size of the releasable pool of 5-HT that is increased and it is this presumably that leads to increased release of 5-HT. However, another mechanism may also be involved in enhancing 5-HT neurotransmission. It has been noted that the sensitivity of the $\alpha_2$-adrenergic heteroreceptor of 5-HT terminals is attenuated (but not the soma-dendritic $\alpha_2$-autoreceptor, see Section 4.2) following long-term treatment with a MAO inhibitor and with noradrenaline-reuptake blockers[9,37]. From the evidence that this heteroreceptor is tonically activated *in vivo* and the knowledge that it exerts a potent regulatory role on 5-HT release[9,25,28,36], it may well contribute to the enhanced 5-HT neurotransmission following long-term treatment with MAO inhibitors.

Activation of 5-HT$_3$ receptors can produce an enhancement of 5-HT release, but only acutely since they appear to desensitise rapidly[8,27]. However, it is important to note that these receptors are not located presynaptically since the modulation is tetrodotoxin sensitive in brain slices and is absent in synaptosomes[16]. The responsiveness of these receptors following long-term antidepressant treatments has been assessed in guinea-pigs. Their sensitivity remains unaltered following repeated electroconvulsive shocks and long-term treatment with an MAO inhibitor[7,9]. Unexpectedly, treatment for 21 days, but not for 2 days, with a 5-HT-reuptake blocker desensitised these 5-HT$_3$ receptors in the hypothalamus, hippocampus and frontal cortex. The enhancement of 5-HT release observed following a long-term treatment with a 5-HT-reuptake blocker, therefore, cannot be linked to an altered capacity of 5-HT$_3$ receptors to modulate 5-HT release. However, of clinical relevance, it is likely that the nausea often reported during the initiation of a treatment of patients with a 5-HT-reuptake blocker, and its subsequent disappearance upon prolonged treatment, may be attributable to the desensitisation of 5-HT$_3$ receptors. This possibility is reinforced by the observation that a 5-HT$_3$ antagonist can eliminate the nausea caused by 5-HT-reuptake blockers[5].

## 5.2 Presynaptic noradrenergic autoreceptors

The responsiveness of the $\alpha_2$-adrenergic autoreceptor on noradrenergic nerve terminals appears not to be altered following long-term treatment with an MAO inhibitor. Initial reports described an attenuated capacity of the $\alpha_2$-adrenoceptor agonist clonidine to inhibit the evoked release of noradrenaline following long-term treatment with the selective MAO-A inhibitor clorgyline. However, it was later demonstrated that the attenuated effect of the exogenous agonist was merely caused by competition of this partial agonist with the increased levels of endogenous noradrenaline resulting from MAO inhibition[19]. Consistent with this interpretation, it has been observed recently that following long-term treatment with the reversible type A MAO inhibitor befloxatone, the efficacy of an exogenous noradrenaline agonist to inhibit the electrically evoked release of [$^3$H]-noradrenaline from preloaded slices of guinea-pig hippocampus and hypothalamus was unaltered[9]. However, the terminal $\alpha_2$-adrenergic autoreceptor can desensitise: in an *in vivo* electrophysiological paradigm, the ability of the $\alpha_2$-adrenoceptor agonist clonidine to attenuate the effect of stimulation of the dorsal noradrenergic bundle is decreased following long-term administration of the noradrenaline-reuptake blocker desipramine[34]. This desensitisation could produce an enhancement of noradrenergic neurotransmission, at least under certain physiological conditions when noradrenergic neurones have a high frequency of firing.

## 6   Clinical observations supporting monoamine neurone involvement in the therapeutic action of antidepressant drugs

### 6.1   Serotoninergic neurones

There are four lines of evidence that are consistent with the possibility that the therapeutic effect obtained with certain types of antidepressant drug are mediated by presynaptic 5-HT mechanisms[11]. First, it was reported that administration of a 5-HT-synthesis inhibitor produced a rapid relapse of depressed patients successfully treated with the MAO inhibitor tranylcypromine. The capacity of 5-HT depletion to produce a relapse in MAO inhibitor-treated patients was later confirmed using a tryptophan-free diet. Second, the combination of tryptophan supplementation with a MAO inhibitor is more effective in the treatment of depression than is a MAO inhibitor used alone. Third, the addition of lithium to the therapeutic regimen of depressed patients treated with, but not responding to, a 5-HT-reuptake blocker or a MAO inhibitor produces a marked improvement within a week in many cases. Since lithium has been shown to enhance 5-HT release following short-term administration (Fig. 15.9), but by a mechanism different from that of 5-HT-reuptake blockers and MAO inhibitors[12], it is possible that this therapeutic improvement results from potentiation of these actions on 5-HT terminals. Finally, it was shown that the enhancement in prolactin release induced by an intravenous injection of L-tryptophan was increased following a long-term treatment of depressed patients with the 5-HT-reuptake blocker fluvoxamine and the MAO inhibitor tranylcypromine. Obviously, these four series of results provide only indirect indications. Nevertheless, they clearly show that when the function of 5-HT neurones is decreased, a relapse occurs, whereas an increased function is associated with a therapeutic benefit. It is not until selective 5-HT-autoreceptor agonists and/or antagonists are

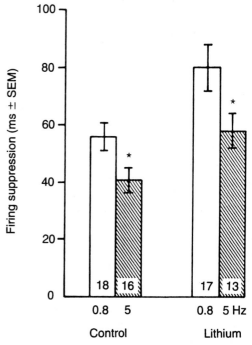

Fig. 15.9.  Duration of suppression of firing of hippocampal pyramidal neurones caused by 200 consecutive stimulations at 320 µA of the ascending 5-HT pathway at frequencies of 0.8 and 5 Hz in control rats and in rats treated with lithium (added to their diet for three days). The plasma levels of lithium were in the same range as those obtained in humans (0.4–1.1 mEq/l) during lithium teatment. Note that the period of suppression of firing was longer in the treated rats, and that the degree of attenuation produced by increasing the frequency of stimulation from 0.8 to 5 Hz was identical in control and in lithium-treated rats, thus indicating an unaltered responsiveness of the terminal 5-HT autoreceptor. The number of neurones tested is given at the bottom of each column. Significant differences from control are shown as *$p < 0.05$ using the two-tailed Student's $t$-test[12].

developed that it will be possible to establish whether there is a direct relationship between the antidepressant response to certain drugs in humans and alterations of presynaptic receptor function.

## 6.2   Noradrenergic neurones

Preliminary evidence suggests that an enhancement of noradrenergic transmission may play a crucial role in mediating the antidepressant response obtained with noradrenaline-reuptake blockers. Using the catecholamine synthesis inhibitor $\alpha$-methyl-$p$-tyrosine, in a double-blind procedure, a rapid relapse was observed in depressed patients successfully treated with desipramine or mazindol[22]. These results, however, stand in contrast with the negative results of two studies reporting the lack of efficacy of the $\alpha_2$-adrenoceptor antagonist yohimbine in depressed patients treated with, but not responding to, desipramine treatment[20,41]. It would be expected that yohimbine, by blocking inhibitory $\alpha_2$-adrenergic autoreceptors, should further enhance noradrenergic transmission and, thus, should have provided a therapeutic effect. The expectation is not unwarranted as it has been observed in animals that the combination of these two types of drug induce a massive release of noradrenaline[24]. These negative results could, of course, be explained by the capacity of yohimbine to block the postsynaptic population of $\alpha_2$-adrenoceptors present in various regions of the limbic forebrain, which may contribute in some way to the antidepressant response.

## 7   Summary

In recent years, there has been intensive investigation of the idea that the clinical efficacy of certain psychotropic drugs may result from the alteration of the ability of presynaptic receptors to modulate neurotransmitter release. In the case of antidepressant drugs, it appears that 5-HT-reuptake-blocking drugs, by increasing the synaptic concentration of 5-HT, desensitise both the soma-dendritic and the terminal 5-HT autoreceptors. MAO inhibitors, however, by increasing the concentration of unmetabolised monoamine transmitter extrasynaptically, could also act by desensitising the 5-HT autoreceptors and possibly the $\alpha_2$-adrenergic heteroreceptors on 5-HT terminals. These effects could be relevant also to the therapeutic efficacy of these drugs in certain anxiety disorders. It is striking that, among the antidepressant drugs, only the 5-HT-reuptake blockers are effective in the treatment of obsessive compulsive disorders and they are the only drugs which result in desensitisation of the terminal 5-HT autoreceptors. Given the crucial role these autoreceptors play in controlling 5-HT release, it could be hypothesised that this therapeutic effect of 5-HT-reuptake blockers results from their capacity to enhance 5-HT release by this mechanism in regions of the brain responsible for the symptoms of obsessive compulsive symptoms, such as the orbital frontal cortex or the anterior part of the caudate nucleus.

In the case of noradrenaline-reuptake blockers, the enhancement of noradrenergic neurotransmission produced by the desensitisation of terminal $\alpha_2$-autoreceptors resulting from increased synaptic concentration of noradrenaline could be important clinically.

With antipsychotic drugs, the prolonged blockade of the soma-dendritic $D_2$ autoreceptors they produce leads to a depolarisation block of the firing activity of mesolimbic dopaminergic neurones, which could explain their delayed onset of action in alleviating psychosis.

Obviously, these are only hypotheses at present and they cannot be verified in the absence of selective agents for the various presynaptic receptors (which present pharmacological properties different from their postsynaptic congeners[14,15]). Nevertheless, they are valuable working hypotheses that have already formed the basis for the development of augmentation strategies, such as lithium addition, in treatment-resistant patients. The availability of a full spectrum of such selective pharmacological agents should further improve the efficacy of the treatments for psychiatric disorders.

# References

1. Adell A and Artigas F (1991) Differential effects of clomipramine given locally or systemically on extracellular 5-HT in raphe nuclei and frontal cortex. An in vivo brain dialysis study. *Naunyn-Schmiedeberg's Archives of Pharmacology* **343:** 237–244

2. Allgaier C, Feuerstein TJ, Jackish R and Hertting G (1985) Islet-activating protein (pertussis toxin) diminishes $\alpha_2$-adrenoceptor mediated effects on noradrenaline release. *Naunyn-Schmiedeberg's Archives of Pharmacology* **331:** 235–239

3. Antelman SM, Chiodo LA and de Giovanni LA (1982) Antidepressants and dopamine autoreceptors: implications for both a novel means of treating depression and understanding bipolar illness. In: Costa E and Racagni G (eds), *Typical and Atypical Antidepressants*, pp 121–132, Raven Press, New York

4. Åsberg M, Traskman L and Thoren P (1976) 5-HIAA in the cerebrospinal fluid: a biochemical suicide predictor? *Archives of General Psychiatry* **33:** 1193–1197

5. Bergeron R and Blier P (1994) Cisapride for the treatment of nausea produced by selective serotonin reuptake inhibitors. *American Journal of Psychiatry* **151:** 1084–1086

6. Blier P (1991) Terminal serotonin autoreceptor function in the rat hippocampus is not modified by pertussis and cholera toxins. *Naunyn-Schmiedeberg's Archives of Pharmacology* **344:** 160–166

7. Blier P and Bouchard C (1992) Effects of repeated electroconvulsive shocks on serotonin neurons. *European Journal of Pharmacology* **211:** 365–373

8. Blier P and Bouchard C (1993) Functional characterization of a 5-HT$_3$ receptor which modulates the release of 5-HT in the guinea pig brain. *British Journal of Pharmacology* **108:** 13–22

9. Blier P and Bouchard C (1993) Presynaptic modulation of 5-HT release in the guinea pig brain following long-term administration of antidepressant drugs. *British Journal of Pharmacology* **113:** 485–495

10. Blier P and de Montigny C (1980) Effect of chronic tricyclic antidepressant treatment on the serotonergic autoreceptor. *Naunyn-Schmiedeburg's Archives of Pharmacology* **314:** 123–128

11. Blier P and de Montigny C (1994) Current advances and trends in the treatment of depression. *Trends in Pharmacological Sciences* **15:** 220–226

12. Blier P, de Montigny C and Tardif D (1987) Short-term lithium treatment enhances responsiveness of postsynaptic 5-HT$_{1A}$ receptors without altering 5-HT autoreceptor sensitivity: an electrophysiological study in the rat brain. *Synapse* **1:** 225–232

13. Blier P, Galzin A-M and Langer SZ (1990) Interaction between serotonin uptake inhibitors and alpha-2 adrenergic heteroreceptors in the rat hypothalamus. *Journal of Pharmacology and Experimental Therapeutics* **254:** 236–244

14. Blier P, Lista A and de Montigny C (1993) Differential properties of pre- and postsynaptic 5-hydroxytryptamine$_{1A}$ receptors in the dorsal raphe and hippocampus: I. Effect of spiperone. *Journal of Pharmacology and Experimental Therapeutics* **265:** 7–15

15. Blier P, Lista A and de Montigny C (1993) Differential properties of pre- and postsynaptic 5-hydroxytryptamine$_{1A}$ receptors in the dorsal raphe and hippocampus: II. Effect of pertussis and cholera toxins. *Journal of Pharmacology and Experimental Therapeutics* **265:** 16–23

16. Blier P, Monroe PJ, Bouchard C, Smith DC and Smith DJ (1993) 5-HT$_3$ receptors which modulate [$^3$H]5-HT release in the guinea pig hypothalamus are not autoreceptors. *Synapse* **15:** 143–148

17. Blier P, Ramdine R, Galzin A-M and Langer SZ (1989) Frequency-dependence of serotonin autoreceptor but not $\alpha_2$-adrenoceptor inhibition of [$^3$H]-serotonin release in rat hypothalamic slices. *Naunyn-Schmiedeberg's Archives of Pharmacology* **339:** 60–64

18. Blier P, Seletti B, Benkelfat C, Young S and de Montigny C (1994) Serotonin$_{1A}$ receptor activation and hypothermia: evidence for a postsynaptic mechanism in humans. *Neuropsychopharmacology* **10:** 92

19. Campbell IC and McKernan RM (1986) Clorgyline and desipramine alter the sensitivity of [$^3$H] noradrenaline release to calcium but not to clonidine. *Brain Research* **372:** 253–259

20. Charney DS, Price LH and Heninger GR (1986) Desipramine–yohimbine combination treatment of refractory depression. *Archives of General Psychiatry* **43:** 1155–1161

21. Curet O and de Montigny C (1989) Electrophysiological characterization of adrenoceptors in the rat dorsal hippocampus. III. Evidence for the physiological role of terminal $\alpha_2$-adrenergic autoreceptors. *Brain Research* **499**: 18–26

22. Delgado PL, Miller HL, Salomon RM *et al.* (1992) The mechanism of antidepressant action in depression. *Society for Neuroscience, Abstracts* **18**: 727

23. de Montigny C and Blier P (1992) Electrophysiological properties of 5-HT$_{1A}$ receptors and of 5-HT$_{1A}$ agonists. In: Stahl SM, Gastpar M, Keppel Hesselink JM and Traber J (eds) *Serotonin 1A Receptors in Depression and Anxiety*, pp 83–98, Raven Press, New York

24. Dennis T, L'Heureux R, Carter C and Scatton B (1987) Presynaptic alpha-2 adrenoceptors play a major role in the effects of idazoxan on cortical noradrenaline release (as measured by *in vivo* dialysis) in the rat. *Journal of Pharmacology and Experimental Therapeutics* **241**: 642–649

25. Feuerstein TJ, Mutschler A, Lupp A, van Veltoven V, Schlicker E and Göthert M (1993) Endogenous noradrenaline activates $\alpha_2$-adrenoceptors on serotoninergic nerve endings in human and rat neocortex. *Journal of Neurochemistry* **61**: 474–480

26. Fredholm BB and Lindgren E (1987) Effects of *N*-ethylmaleimide and forskolin on noradrenaline release from rat hippocampal slices. Evidence that prejunctional adenosine and $\alpha$-receptors are linked to N-proteins but not to adenylate cyclase. *Acta Physiologica Scandinavica* **130**: 95–105

27. Galzin AM and Langer SZ (1991) Modulation of 5-HT release by presynaptic inhibitory and facilitatory 5-HT receptors in brain slices. *Advances in Bioscience* **82**: 59–62

28. Galzin AM, Poirier MF, Lista A *et al.* (1992) Characterization of the 5-hydroxytryptamine autoreceptor modulating the release of [$^3$H]-5-hydroxytryptamine in slices of the human neocortex. *Journal of Neurochemistry* **59**: 1293–1301

29. Gonon FG (1988) Nonlinear relationship between impulse flow and dopamine release by rat midbrain dopaminergic neurons as studied by in vivo electrochemistry. *Neuroscience* **24**: 19–28

30. Gorman JM, Fyer MR, Liebowitz MR and Klein DF (1987) Pharmacologic provocation of panic attacks. In: Meltzer HY (ed) *Psychopharmacology: The Third Generation of Progress*, pp 985–994, Raven Press, New York

31. Jacobs BL (1986) Single unit activity of brain monoamine-containing neurons in freely moving animals. *Annals of the New York Academy of Sciences* **473**: 70–77

32. Jacobs BL and Fornal CA (1991) Activity of brain serotonergic neurons in the behaving animal. *Pharmacological Reviews* **43**: 563–578

33. Jimerson DC (1987) Role of dopamine mechanisms in the affective disorders. In: Meltzer HY (ed) *Psychopharmacology: The Third Generation of Progress*, pp 505–511, Raven Press, New York

34. Lacroix D, Blier P, Curet O and de Montigny C (1991) Effects of long-term desipramine administration on noradrenergic neurotransmission: electrophysiological studies in the rat brain. *Journal of Pharmacology and Experimental Therapeutics* **257**: 1081–1090

35. Martin KF, Hannon S, Phillips I and Heal DJ (1992) Opposing roles for 5-HT$_{1B}$ and 5-HT$_3$ receptors in the control of 5-HT release in rat hippocampus *in vivo*. *British Journal of Pharmacology* **106**: 139–142

36. Mongeau R, Blier P and de Montigny C (1993) *In vivo* electrophysiological evidence for a tonic inhibitory action of endogenous norepinephrine on $\alpha_2$-adrenergic heteroreceptors on 5-hydroxytryptamine terminals in the rat hippocampus. *Naunyn-Schmiedeberg's Archives of Pharmacology* **347**: 266–272

37. Mongeau R, de Montigny C and Blier P (1993) Electrophysiological evidence for desensitization of $\alpha_2$-adrenergic heteroreceptors on 5-HT terminals following long-term treatment with drugs increasing noradrenaline synaptic availability. *Neuropsychopharmacology* **10**: 41–52

38. Moret C and Briley M (1990) Serotonin autoreceptor subsensitivity and antidepressant activity. *European Journal of Pharmacology* **180**: 351–356

39. Murphy TV and Majewski H (1990) Pertussis toxin differentiates between $\alpha_1$- and $\alpha_2$-adrenoceptor-mediated inhibition of noradrenaline release from rat kidney cortex. *European Journal of Pharmacology* **179**: 435–439

40. Schechter LE, Bolaños FJ, Gozlan H *et al.* (1990) Alterations of central serotoninergic

and dopaminergic neurotransmission in rats chronically treated with ipsapirone: biochemical and electrophysiological studies. *Journal of Pharmacology and Experimental Therapeutics* **255:** 1335–1347

41. Schmauss M, Laakmann G and Dieterle D (1988) Effects of $\alpha_2$-receptor blockade in addition to tricyclic antidepressants in therapy-resistant depression. *Journal of Clinical Psychopharmacology* **8:** 108–111

42. Starke K, Göthert M and Kilbinger H (1989) Modulation of neurotransmitter release by presynaptic autoreceptors. *Physiological Reviews* **69:** 864–969

43. Welner SA, de Montigny C, Desroches J, Desjardins P and Suranyi-Cadotte BE (1989) Autoradiographic quantification of serotonin$_{1A}$ receptors in rat brain following antidepressant drug treatment. *Synapse* **4:** 347–352

# 16 Modulation of neurotransmitter release by some therapeutic and socially used drugs

Nicotine  Susan Wonnacott
Ethanol (alcohol)  Manfred Göthert
Exogenous opiates  Loris A. Chahl
Amphetamines  Max Willow and Graham M. Nicholson
Barbiturates  Graham M. Nicholson and Max Willow

Human beings deliberately choose to expose themselves to a wide range of substances that can produce desirable changes in mood or behaviour. The substances inevitably bring about these effects by causing neurochemical changes. Although multiple mechanisms are often involved, it is clear that some of the effects come about as a result of changes in the availability of neurotransmitter in the synaptic cleft caused by drug actions at receptors that modulate release. In this chapter, the contributors consider the mode of action of some of the more commonly used substances: their consideration is focused primarily on the possible neurotransmitter release-modulating activity of these drugs, though it is clear that in most cases this activity may only be one of a spectrum of pharmacological activities. Susan Wonnacott considers the actions of nicotine, Manfred Göthert those of ethanol (alcohol), Loris Chahl describes the possible release-modulating actions of opioids and Max Willow and Graham Nicholson consider amphetamines and barbiturates. There are, of course, many others that could have been included: these are but a few examples to illustrate the underlying concepts.

## 1  Nicotine

Nicotine, the principal psychoactive agent in the tobacco plant, *Nicotiana tabacum,* can elicit the release of many neurotransmitters in various brain regions. It is probable that this action underlies the drug's perceived effects and contributes to its addictiveness. Similar actions of nicotine occur in peripheral tissues: nicotine releases catecholamines from adrenal chromaffin cells and acts on sympathetic neurones, for example, but these effects are minimal in smokers, reflecting heterogeneity in the receptor targets for nicotine at different loci. This review focuses on the CNS as the locus of nicotine's psychoactive effects.

The ability of nicotine to release neurotransmitters has been recognised for a long time: for example in 1969 Armitage[1] showed that nicotine caused acetylcholine release in the cat cerebral cortex. More recently, the techniques of *in vivo* microdialysis and *in vivo* voltammetry (see Chapter 12) have confirmed that nicotine, given either systemically (by subcutaneous injection) or locally (via a stereotaxically positioned canula or the dialysis probe), results in transmitter release in the brain[22]. These studies, as well as *in vitro* investigations, have tended to focus on

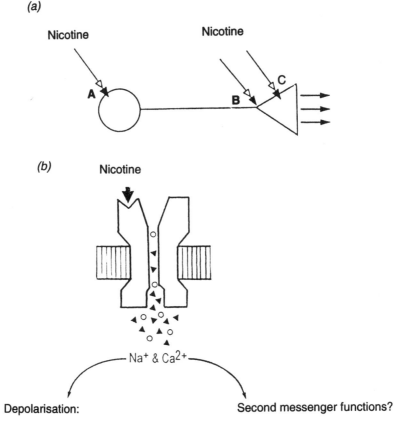

Fig. 16.1. (*a*) Schematic representation of a neurone showing sites at which nicotine may act: (A) soma and dendrites; (B) preterminal areas; (C) terminal (i.e. presynaptic area). (*b*) Section through a nicotinic acetylcholine receptor (nAChR) illustrating cation influx in response to agonist binding (the concomitant efflux of K+ is omitted for clarity; K+ is not considered to significantly contribute to nAChR function).

ascending dopaminergic pathways, inspired by the role of dopamine in locomotor and reward systems that are activated by psychomotor stimulants like nicotine. Using electrophysiological techniques, nicotine has been shown to act at the perikarya of dopaminergic neurones in the substantia nigra[14]. Biochemical studies, first using slices and subsequently synaptosomes, have established that nicotine also has direct actions on dopaminergic nerve terminals in the striatum, resulting in dopamine release (reviewed by Wonnacott *et al.*[93]). A similar picture is seen with the mesolimbic pathway, with nicotine acting on cell bodies in the ventral tegmentum and on terminals in the nucleus accumbens, again with enhanced dopamine release as the result. The mesolimbic pathway is particularly implicated in reward responses[22], and it may be significant that dopamine release from the nucleus accumbens is apparently more sensitive to modulation by nicotine than that from the nigrostriatal pathway[40,93].

Pre- and postsynaptic actions of nicotine have also been discerned in the habenulo-interpeduncular system, by electrophysiological recording (see ref. 48 and references therein). This is a well-defined pathway, projecting from the medial habenula to the interpeduncular nucleus via the fasciculus retroflexus (which is partly cholinergic). Several sites of action of nicotine have been documented in this system.

1. Somata of medial habenular neurones. Stimulation by nicotine here results in the generation of tetrodotoxin-sensitive action potentials and subsequent synaptic transmission.
2. Terminals of the medial habenular neurones in the interpeduncular nucleus. Nicotine acts presynaptically, leading to transmitter release and a tetrodotoxin-insensitive enhancement of synaptic transmission.
3. Somata of interpeduncular nucleus neurones. Nicotine acts postsynaptically, as in (1). The term 'postsynaptic' here relates to the anatomical arrangement of neurones in the pathway under study.
4. Axons of intrinsic GABAergic neurones in the interpeduncular nucleus. This is a 'preterminal' locus, at which nicotine produces the same effects as at presynaptic sites, except that its actions are blocked by tetrodotoxin, implicating the generation of action potentials.

The demonstration of 'preterminal' sites of action on projecting axons[48] introduces a novel locus for effecting transmitter release, although analogous preterminal modulation of acetylcholine release has been postulated to occur at the neuromuscular junction[7]. The cellular loci of nicotine's actions are illustrated schematically in Fig. 16.1.

## 1.1 Nicotinic acetylcholine receptors: molecular targets for nicotine

The actions of nicotine outlined above are mediated by nicotinic acetylcholine receptors (nAChR). The evidence for this comes from the pharmacology of nicotine's effects: responses recorded electrophysiologically and *in vivo* and *in vitro* measures of transmitter release are blocked by nicotinic antagonists, such as mecamylamine and dihydro-β-erythroidine. Furthermore, other nicotinic agonists can elicit similar responses. It is assumed that, physiologically, nAChR are activated by acetylcholine released at conventional cholinergic synapses on somata and dendrites, at axo-axonic synapses and by that released from cholinergic terminals (see below). It is possible that some nAChR are extrasynaptic, at these acetylcholine would act in a paracrine manner.

Nictotinic acetylcholine receptors are ligand-gated cation channels: five membrane-spanning subunits create a notional 'cylinder' with a central pore permeable to $Na^+$, $K^+$ and $Ca^{2+}$ when opened by agonist binding (Fig. 16.1). Nicotine binds to a presently ill-defined site in the large extracellular N-terminal domain of α (agonist-binding) subunits. However, the nicotine-binding site may overlap adjacent subunits, and neighbouring subunits may influence agonist binding.

The prototype nAChR that has been extensively characterised is that found in *Torpedo* electroplax and its counterpart in skeletal muscle. Four different subunits (α, β, γ and δ, with two copies of the agonist-binding α subunit) constitute the *Torpedo* and embryonic or denervated muscle nAChR. In nervous tissues, a plethora of distinct nAChR subunits are expressed (for a comprehensive review, see ref. 78). This was unexpected, especially in view of the low abundance of nAChR in the brain. Currently six distinct α subunits (α2–α7, the muscle α subunit being α1, defined by the presence of a pair of adjacent cysteine residues) and three β subunits (β2–β4, which lack the pair of cysteines) have been found in mammalian brain. In *Xenopus* oocytes, expression of α2, α3 or α4 with either β2 or β4 results in the formation of functional nicotinic channels that resemble the muscle nAChR in having a pentameric structure with two copies of the α subunit. The α7

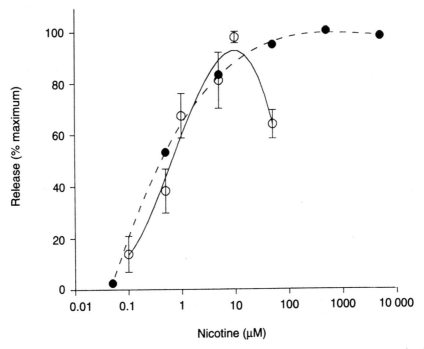

Fig. 16.2. Dose–response curves for nicotine-evoked transmitter release from synaptosomes *in vitro*. ○—○ [³H]-acetylcholine release from rat hippocampal synaptosomes (see ref. 78); ●- - -● [³H]-dopamine release from mouse striatal synaptosomes (see ref. 34).

subunit is exceptional in that it can form channels when expressed in oocytes in the absence of any additional subunit.

The combinations of subunits that make up the native nAChRs that occur in the brain have generally not been identified but may be more complex. Certainly, numerous different subtypes of nAChR exist and a consequence of this heterogeneity is the different pharmacological profiles of various nAChR-mediated responses. For example, in the interpeduncular nucleus, presynaptic nAChR are some 10 times more sensitive to nicotine than postsynaptic nAChR (see ref. 48). Therefore, nicotine concentrations in smokers may preferentially activate certain subtypes of nAChR: nicotine in the brains of smokers has been estimated to reach 0.1–0.5 µM (see ref. 93), so only the more sensitive nAChR may be activated.

Some nAChR can be discriminated by radioligand binding and with this technique two major classes of nicotinic ligand-binding site have been characterised in mammalian brain. High-affinity agonist-binding sites have been found using either [³H]-nicotine, [³H]-cytosine or [³H]-acetylcholine. The neuronal nAChR identified by high-affinity radiolabelled agonist binding is thought to comprise α4 and β2 subunits[29], although recent evidence suggests the association of additional subunits, at least in the chick brain[17]. The second class of site is specifically labelled by [¹²⁵I]-α-bungarotoxin[15], a snake toxin that also acts at the muscle nAChR, thus enabling the snake to paralyse its prey. In terms of subunit composition, nAChR labelled by [¹²⁵I]-α-bungarotoxin in the brain contain α7 subunits, so these receptors are different from those in muscle. However, it must be emphasised that other nAChR in central and autonomic neurones are not labelled by any of these radioligands. Another snake toxin, neuronal- or κ-bungarotoxin, shows a preference for nAChR containing α3 and β4 subunits. The pattern of labelling of brain sections by [$^{125}$I]-labelled neuronal bungarotoxin is quite distinct from the distributions of [$^3$H]-nicotine or [$^{125}$I]-α-bungarotoxin-binding sites, consistent with the notion that each of these radioligands identifies a different subtype of nAChR that has a unique anatomical localisation and that may serve different functions[12]. Evidence for the presynaptic localisation of [$^3$H]-nicotine-binding sites includes the loss of binding after lesions that destroy axons and terminals, the enrichment of [$^3$H]-nicotine-binding sites in synaptosome fractions on subcellular fractionation of brain tissue, and the loss of binding sites together with presynaptic markers in neurodegenerative diseases (for review see ref. 93).

The present limitations in correlating cloned nAChR subunits, nicotinic ligand-binding sites and functional nAChR make it difficult to assign molecular subtypes to physiological roles.

With respect to nicotine's influence on transmitter release, it would be of interest to know if nAChR on cell somata are of a different subtype from those present on nerve terminals. However, it would be naive to assume a simple pre- versus postsynaptic allocation of nAChR subtypes. For example, in rat hippocampus, presynaptic nicotinic autoreceptors elicit the release of acetylcholine. This response exhibits sharply bell-shaped agonist dose–response curves (Fig. 16.2), signifying marked receptor desensitisation at higher agonist concentrations[89]. In contrast, presynaptic nicotinic heteroreceptors that modulate dopamine release in the striatum give hyperbolic agonist dose–response curves (Fig. 16.2)[34]. One interpretation of these data is that the two responses are mediated by different subtypes of nAChR. The inhibition of nicotine-evoked dopamine release by neuronal bungarotoxin[34] favours the presence of α3-containing nAChR on striatal terminals. Another possibility is that more than one subtype of nAChR is associated with striatal nerve terminals, producing a compound dose–response curve.

## 1.2 Mechanisms of nicotine-evoked transmitter release

The fact that nAChR are ligand-gated cation channels explains why nicotine increases (rather than decreases) neurotransmitter release. Activation of nAChR on cell somata can cause neurones to fire action potentials[14] that invade the nerve terminals and activate VSCC to promote $Ca^{2+}$ influx. This in turn triggers neurotransmitter release (see Chapter 1). Therefore, nicotine-evoked transmitter release via somatic nAChR is both tetrodotoxin sensitive and $Ca^{2+}$ dependent. The tetrodotoxin sensitivity of 'pre-terminal' nAChR[48] indicates that their localisation is not at synaptic boutons but probably on terminal portions of the axon where they can trigger action potentials.

In contrast, activation of presynaptic nAChR elicits tetrodotoxin-insensitive transmitter release (see ref. 93). Dependence on $Ca^{2+}$ is observed, suggesting that release proceeds directly, via exocytosis. The $Ca^{2+}$ dependence raises an interesting, and as yet unresolved, question. Neuronal nAChR are more permeable to $Ca^{2+}$ than their counterparts in skeletal muscle[78]. If presynaptic nAChR were strategically localised near active zones, the sites of vesicle exocytosis, their activation might provide sufficient $Ca^{2+}$ to trigger transmitter release. Alternatively, if the $Ca^{2+}$ influx via the nicotinic channels is insufficient, or they are not optimally located, the $Na^+$ current passing through the nAChR might result in sufficient local depolarisation to open VSCC, which provides the $Ca^{2+}$ for transmitter release (Fig. 16.1). Attempts to distinguish between these two mechanisms have not provided clearcut answers so far (see also Section 3.1).

Calcium-independent and mecamylamine-insensitive dopamine release from striatal preparations has been observed at high nicotine concentrations (above 0.1 mM, see refs. 34 and 93). This is most probably because of a tyramine-like effect[34] exerted by nicotine, where high concentrations of the lipophilic drug can displace catecholamines from vesicle stores. This phenomenon is not observed at the submicromolar nicotine concentrations relevant to human smoking.

### 1.3    Effects of *in vivo* chronic nicotine treatment on nicotine-evoked transmitter release

A feature of tobacco smoking is the intermittent but frequent intake of nicotine with each puff of cigarette smoke. Consequently, rather constant plasma nicotine levels (typically 10–50 ng/ml) are sustained throughout the smoking day. The continuous presence of nicotine may have quite different effects from discrete (acute) doses. In experimental animals, it is difficult to reproduce the complex pattern of nicotine intake exhibited by humans (who are the only animals that will voluntarily inhale!). However, chronic treatment of rats and mice by daily injection or continuous infusion of nicotine results in an up-regulation of [³H]-nicotine-binding sites in the brain[92], and similar up-regulation has been reported for human brain samples taken postmortem from smokers versus non-smokers[5]. However, very few studies have been undertaken to ascertain the functional significance of receptor up-regulation. It has been proposed that up-regulation is a consequence of receptor desensitisation by nicotine, such that the agonist inactivates the receptor and elicits a response more commonly associated with antagonist treatment. The functional consequences could be that up-regulation maintains the *status quo*, with no net change in responsiveness, there could be a loss of function, or a propensity for increased responsiveness if the increased number of receptors can be activated. Furthermore, while up-regulation of high-affinity [³H]-nicotine-binding sites has been extensively documented, other nAChR subtypes occur in the CNS (as discussed above) and their response to chronic nicotine is gen-

erally not known. Behaviourally, some nicotine-mediated responses measured in animals show tolerance to repeated doses of nicotine whereas others are apparently unchanged or may be increased.

With respect to transmitter release, a recent *in vitro* study has found *increased* release of [³H]-dopamine and [³H]-5-HT from rat striatal slices stimulated with nicotine, following twice-daily injections of nicotine for 10 days prior to sacrifice[95]. This result corroborates an earlier observation of enhanced nicotine-evoked [³H]-dopamine release from striatal synaptosomes (which paralleled an increase in [³H]-nicotine-binding sites) following continuous infusion for 7 days of a very low dose of the potent nicotinic agonist (+)anatoxin-A (ref. 75). However, chronic infusion of nicotine in the mouse resulted in dose-related *decreases* in nicotine-evoked [³H]-dopamine release from striatal synaptosomes[53]. Nicotine-evoked release of [³H]-acetylcholine from striatal and hippocampal slices is also decreased following chronic nicotine administration[47,95]. Therefore, there is no consistent picture of whether transmitter release is more or less sensitive to nicotine after chronic exposure to the drug. Factors complicating these experiments include drug doses (both chronically, which may determine the extent of nAChR desensitisation, and acutely, which will determine which nAChR subtypes are stimulated), tissue preparation and delay after death (which will determine the extent of recovery from desensitisation).

*In vivo*, a lack of tolerance to chronic nicotine treatment of nicotine-evoked dopamine release has been seen, using microdialysis to sample dopamine release in the nucleus accumbens[29] (i.e. dopamine release elicited by an acute dose of nicotine was the same in animals that had received nicotine chronically as in chronically saline-treated controls). A subsequent microdialysis study[4] found *increased* dopamine release in response to a nicotine challenge following 5 days of nicotine injections, compared with the response to nicotine of chronically saline-treated controls. The lack of tolerance to sustained exposure to nicotine displayed by the ascending dopaminergic pathways may be pertinent to the propensity of this drug to produce dependence: the mesolimbic dopaminergic pathway (the 'reward' pathway) is considered to be a primary substrate for the reinforcing properties of drugs of abuse[22].

### 1.4  Summary

The heterogeneity of nAChR subtypes in the brain, and their differential expression and regulation, results in complex responses to both acute and chronic nicotine. A primary consequence of nAChR activation is neurotransmitter release at the cellular level, but the dose dependency, desensitisation and modulation of this response will be influenced not only by the transmitter system in question but also by the subtype(s) of nAChR involved. The scale of this issue is only now being appreciated: much more effort will be necessary before we can rationally explain why nicotine is such an addictive drug.

### 2  Ethanol

Many investigations support the hypothesis that the effects of ethanol in the nervous system result from changes in synaptic transmission[21,64]. Ethanol has been reported to act at both pre- and postsynaptic sites in the CNS and periphery, but many effects only occur at lethal concentrations. This holds particularly true for presynaptic effects, i.e. alterations of transmitter release observed in synaptosomes, brain slices or peripheral tissues. Such isolated preparations are very suitable for examining the effects of ethanol on the release mechanism itself, on presynaptic receptors as well as on ion fluxes and/or biochemical events underlying depolarisation of the axon terminals and stimulus–release coupling.

In addition to such *in vitro* investigations, an increasing number of *in vivo* studies have been carried out. Animals, in most cases rats, have been injected with ethanol and its effects on neurotransmitter release in various brain areas were checked by the microdialysis technique or, in very few cases, by voltammetry (see Chapter 12). The advantages of such investigations are that they were carried out with non-lethal doses leading to physiologically relevant blood concentrations and that both acute responses and effects of chronic exposure were examined. A disadvantage is that the response measured is the result of a complex interplay of many processes, which comprise not only effects on transmitter release from the respective axon terminals but also effects on their cell bodies and the variety of neurones innervating them. However, such integrated responses are not the subject of this book; therefore, only a few examples of such effects are included in this section. In many, if not all, cases, the integrated responses are mainly consequences of influences on receptors and ion channels of the soma-dendritic area of the neurone or even other neurones, rather than changes that occur at the level of the respective nerve terminals themselves. Even when the latter are experimentally depolarised by locally applied high $K^+$, the possibility of the activation of neuronal circuits, feeding back to the neurones under investigation, cannot be entirely excluded. Accordingly, the results obtained in such *in vivo* studies in many cases are contradictory[64].

This section focuses mainly on acute influences of ethanol on axon terminals themselves, which are reflected by changes in neurotransmitter release in isolated preparations (see Göthert[31] for investigations before 1978). As already mentioned above and will be outlined in more detail below, these experiments have revealed that changes in the nerve terminals themselves mainly occur at ethanol concentrations above 100 mM; hence, these changes probably contribute to its lethal effect, since the average ethanol concentration in the blood of fatal cases has been found to be in this range, or even slightly lower[70]. Changes relevant for 'social drinking', acute non-lethal intoxication or chronic alcoholism would come into play at concentrations below 100 mM. However, it is obvious that no clear-cut borderline can be drawn between ethanol concentrations caused by 'social drinking' and those characteristic of intoxication, since the ethanol dose that is tolerated without producing CNS symptoms varies from individual to individual. It depends, among other factors, on the degree of habituation. It has been observed that more than 50% of persons are grossly intoxicated when their blood ethanol concentration is 150 mg/dl (33 mM)[70], but that, on the other hand, some alcoholics can perform well in difficult tasks when their blood ethanol concentrations are above 200 mg/dl (43 mM)[41]. Interestingly, it has been observed that ethanol in the concentration range below 100 mM is capable of selectively inhibiting neurotransmitter release evoked by stimulation of excitatory presynaptic receptors such as nicotinic or ionotropic glutamate receptors. These investigations have significantly contributed to the elucidation of the sites and mechanisms underlying the neuronal effects of ethanol and, therefore, these findings are included in this chapter.

The simplistic view that ethanol is a non-specific drug that exclusively acts by perturbing lipids of the neuronal cell membrane is no longer tenable[33]. A number of studies have provided evidence to support the hypothesis that ligand-gated ion channels, to which nicotinic, 5-HT$_3$ and ionotropic glutamate receptors belong, are the selective targets for ethanol. Among the channel proteins, quantitative differences appear to exist with respect to their sensitivity to ethanol. It is also clear that ethanol, although it has much in common with general anaesthetics, does not act exactly as do the latter agents. This can be deduced, for example, from influences on 5-HT$_3$ receptor-mediated cation influx in neuroblastoma cell lines, in which anaesthetics and ethanol exert opposite effects, the former

acting in an inhibitory fashion and the latter facilitatory (see below).

## 2.1  Effects of ethanol in peripheral tissues

In view of potential cardiovascular implications, the influence of ethanol on noradrenaline release from postganglionic sympathetic nerve terminals has been investigated in detail[31]. Very high concentrations of ethanol (in the range of 1 M) were found to be necessary to increase the spontaneous release of endogenous noradrenaline. This effect is probably caused by an impairment of the cell membrane of the varicosities and/or of the storage vesicle membrane, leading to leakage of the neurotransmitter molecules. Similarly, high concentrations were required for the inhibition of noradrenaline release in response to electrical nerve stimulation or depolarisation by high K$^+$ levels. This inhibitory effect may have resulted from blockade of either Na$^+$ or Ca$^{2+}$ influx, thus reducing membrane depolarisation and/or inhibiting stimulus–release coupling. Such impairment in the function of voltage-sensitive ion channels may be brought about by an interaction of ethanol with hydrophobic regions of the channel proteins or they may be secondary to the action of the drug on membrane lipids.

At much lower concentrations, which are comparable with those achieved during non-lethal intoxication, ethanol inhibits noradrenaline release evoked by activation of presynaptic nicotinic receptors on the sympathetic nerve terminals. The physiological role of these receptors is unknown, but they have been assumed to be activated during tobacco smoking (see Section 1). The threshold concentration for ethanol-induced inhibition determined in perfused rabbit hearts has been reported to be 36 mM and the IC$_{50}$ 129 mM. In order to obtain clues for the mechanism underlying the inhibitory effect of ethanol on the noradrenaline release evoked by stimulation of presynaptic nicotinic receptors, 1-propanol, 1-butanol and

1-pentanol were also investigated. These substances shared the inhibitory effect of ethanol on the noradrenaline release induced by nicotinic receptor stimulation, and the potency of the alcohols in inhibiting release was correlated with their lipophilicity, suggesting that the effect may result from an interaction with hydrophobic regions of the receptor protein.

An inhibitory effect at much lower concentrations than those necessary for the inhibition of electrically evoked noradrenaline release was also observed when noradrenaline release was stimulated in isolated rabbit hearts by activation of presynaptic 5-HT$_3$ receptors, which like nicotinic receptors are ligand-gated ion channels (IC$_{50}$ for ethanol inhibition of 5-HT evoked release: 195 mM). The 5-HT$_3$ receptor on sympathetic axon terminals has, until now, not been identified in species other than the rabbit and even in this species it is found exclusively in the heart. The ability of ethanol at relatively low concentrations to decrease selectively the noradrenaline release evoked by nicotinic and 5-HT$_3$ receptor stimulation implies that the ligand-gated ion channels are particularly sensitive to the inhibitory effect of ethanol, suggesting that it is these channels that are sites of action of ethanol.

The inhibitory effect of ethanol on noradrenaline release evoked by 5-HT$_3$ receptor stimulation is to a certain extent surprising when considering recent data with 5-HT and ethanol in the neuroblastoma cell line N1E-115, which is also endowed with 5-HT$_3$ receptors. As mentioned above, ethanol increased cation influx through the 5-HT$_3$ receptor channel of these cells. However, this discrepancy may perhaps be explained by the pronounced species differences in the pharmacological properties of 5-HT$_3$ receptors. Furthermore, it has been reported that, under certain experimental conditions, ethanol indeed inhibits rather than facilitates cation influx through the 5-HT$_3$ receptor channel of neuroblastoma cells.

Acute ethanol intoxication has been shown to increase adrenaline and noradrena-line concentrations in blood. This effect has been ascribed to an increase in catecholamine release from the adrenal medulla. The increased release probably results from increased central stimulation by ethanol of the sympatho-adrenal system, leading to increased impulse traffic in splanchnic nerves. This view is supported by two findings. First, it has been shown that in animals the ethanol-induced increase in plasma catecholamines was abolished by treatment with a ganglion-blocking drug. Second, exposure of isolated adrenal glands or chromaffin cells to ethanol at concentrations up to 100 mM did not increase (but rather tended to decrease) catecholamine release evoked by nicotine or depolarising stimuli.

## 2.2 Effects of ethanol in the CNS

### 2.2.1 Effects of ethanol on depolarisation-evoked release

An important investigation of the influence of ethanol on neurotransmitter release in cerebral cortical slices was carried out by Carmichael and Israel[10]. They found that concentrations above 100 mM had to be applied in order to obtain an inhibition of the electrically evoked release of neurotransmitters, acetylcholine being the most sensitive. The order of sensitivity to ethanol (in parentheses, IC$_{50}$ values in mM) was acetylcholine (170) > 5-HT (320) > dopamine (410) > noradrenaline (420) > glutamate (500) > GABA (660). The authors speculated that the inhibitory effect might be caused by blockade of Na$^+$ conductance or of stimulus–release coupling and that the differences in sensitivity of the various types of neurone might be related to differences in nerve fibre size or in 'sensitivity of excitation–coupling blockade' in the various nerve endings releasing the different transmitters. The alcohols 1-butanol and 1-hexanol mimicked ethanol in inhibiting acetylcholine and noradrenaline release. The inhibitory potency of the alcohols was correlated with their octanol/water partition coefficient, again pointing to an interaction with

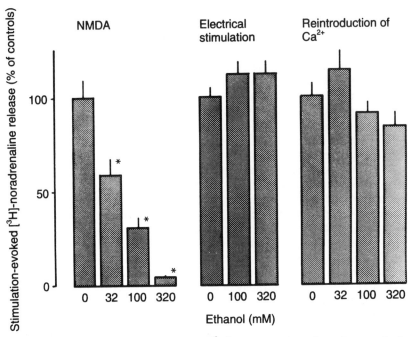

Fig. 16.3. Influence of ethanol on stimulation-evoked [³H]-noradrenaline release from rat brain cortical slices superfused with Krebs' solution. Stimulation was achieved with either NMDA (300 μM, slices superfused with Mg²⁺-free Krebs' solution), electrical impulses (3 Hz) or reintroduction of Ca²⁺ (1.3 mM) to K⁺-depolarised slices (slices superfused with Ca²⁺-free Krebs' solution containing K⁺ 25 mM throughout). Note that ethanol selectively inhibited (* $p < 0.01$) the NMDA-evoked release. (From ref. 32, with permission.)

hydrophobic compounds of the cell membrane as the mechanism underlying their inhibitory effect.

**Dopamine release.** Subsequent to the investigation of Carmichael and Israel[10], the effect of ethanol on dopamine release has attracted particular interest. Accordingly, a large number of both *in vitro* and *in vivo* studies have been carried out. In rat striatal slices, administration of ethanol was found to *increase* basal dopamine release. Interestingly, this response was diminished by compounds that block δ-opioid receptors. In agreement with these findings, microdialysis and voltammetric studies revealed that acute ethanol stimulates dopamine release in the corpus striatum and nucleus accumbens of the rat. This effect is probably the result of stimulation of the firing activity of the dopaminergic neurones. Blockade of δ-opioid and 5-HT receptors

diminished the effect of ethanol, indicating that such receptors and their endogenous agonists are probably involved in modulating the stimulatory effect on dopaminergic neurones. After withdrawal of ethanol, dopamine release was decreased.

In studies of K⁺-evoked dopamine release in rat striatal slices, the results obtained resembled those in the cerebral cortical slices[10] (see above) in that high concentrations of ethanol acted in an inhibitory manner. This effect was lost, or even reversed to a facilitation, after long-term (5–7 days) exposure of rats to ethanol. In striatal synaptosomes from rats chronically treated with ethanol, a reduced depolarisation-induced dopamine release was observed, whereas Ca²⁺ entry into the same synaptosomes was found to be unaltered. These results suggest that chronic ethanol may change coupling between $Ca^{2+}$ entry and dopamine release (see Chapter 11).

**Noradrenaline release.** The low potency of ethanol in inhibiting noradrenaline release from cerebral cortical slices in response to electrical impulses[10] (see above) has been confirmed repeatedly (see, for example, Fig. 16.3: ethanol up to 320 mM was ineffective in inhibiting the electrically evoked [$^3$H]-noradrenaline release[32]). In a microdialysis study in the rat frontal cortex, an ethanol dose of 2 g/kg was necessary to inhibit noradrenaline release. An inhibition of $K^+$-evoked noradrenaline release by very high ethanol concentrations was also observed in cerebellar slices, but not in hypothalamic slices where an increase in $K^+$-evoked release of noradrenaline occurred. Accordingly, differences appear to exist between brain areas with respect to the acute effect of ethanol on noradrenaline release. In cerebral slices from rats treated chronically with ethanol, its effect on the noradrenaline release evoked by high $K^+$ or electrical impulses was reversed to a facilitation.

**Release of 5-HT.** Whereas the low-potency inhibition of 5-HT release by ethanol, which was earlier observed in rat cortical slices[10] (see above), could be confirmed in rat hippocampal synaptosomes, an increasing effect of ethanol was found in microdialysis studies in the rat nucleus accumbens and corpus striatum. This increase, which resembles the influence of ethanol on dopamine release observed in analogous experiments (see above), may be assumed to be caused by an increase in impulse flow in the serotoninergic neurones. Accordingly this increase in release probably does not reflect changes that occur in the respective axon terminals.

**Acetylcholine release.** The finding that ethanol inhibited the electrically evoked acetylcholine release from cortical slices at higher potency than the release of the other neurotransmitters[10] (see above) stimulated other authors to re-examine this effect and to extend the finding. The inhibition of electrically evoked acetylcholine release was consistently found, but, interestingly, ethanol did not affect the $K^+$-evoked release. This finding suggests that ethanol may primarily act to inhibit $Na^+$ influx during action potentials.

**GABA release.** As already observed by Carmichael and Israel[10], the electrically evoked GABA release from cortical slices was even less sensitive to the inhibitory effect of ethanol than the release of the other neurotransmitters investigated (see above). This low sensitivity has been confirmed by more recent investigations with cortical slices. However, ethanol at concentrations that did not affect the impulse-evoked GABA release did inhibit the $K^+$-evoked release. This pattern is the opposite to that observed for acetylcholine release, suggesting here that ethanol at the high concentrations applied does not primarily influence $Na^+$ conductance but may exert a direct action on stimulus–release coupling or on the transmitter-release process for GABAergic neurones. An inhibitory effect of ethanol on GABA release was also observed in rat hippocampal CA1 slices.

**Glutamate release.** The inhibitory effect of ethanol on the electrically evoked glutamate release from rat cortical slices[10] (see above) was confirmed for $K^+$-evoked release, not only from neocortical but also from hippocampal CA1 slices. In contrast, in striatal slices, the $K^+$-evoked release of glutamate was found to be increased. The reason for this regional difference in the effect of ethanol on $K^+$-evoked glutamate release is unknown.

### 2.2.2 Modulation of neurotransmitter release evoked by stimulation of (presynaptic) excitatory receptors

Whereas in most investigations mentioned so far ethanol concentrations above 100 mM had to be applied in order to modify (in most cases to inhibit) the electrically or $K^+$-evoked

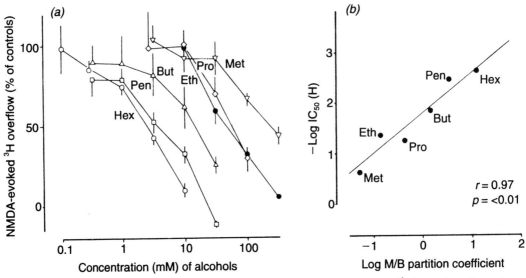

Fig. 16.4. (*a*) Inhibitory effect of aliphatic alcohols on NMDA (300 μM)-evoked [³H]-noradrenaline release from rat brain cortical slices superfused with Krebs' solution. (*b*) Correlation ($r = 0.97$; $p < 0.001$) of their inhibitory potency ($-\log IC_{50}$) with their membrane/buffer (M/B) partition coefficient. Methanol (▽, Met), ethanol (●, Eth), 1-propanol (◇, Pro), 1-butanol (△, But), 1-pentanol (□, Pen) and 1-hexanol (○, Hex). (From ref. 26, with permission.)

neurotransmitter release from brain preparations, the release in response to stimulation of presynaptic excitatory receptors was inhibited at much lower concentrations. In this respect, the central neurones resembled those in the periphery (see Section 16.2.1). As in the periphery, the physiological importance of the presynaptic excitatory receptors in the CNS (in particular glutamate receptors) that are relevant in this context is unknown, but again the investigation of the receptor-mediated transmitter release has provided important insight into the subcellular site of action of ethanol.

The most comprehensive investigations of the effect of ethanol on neurotransmitter release evoked by activation of excitatory receptors were carried out for noradrenergic neurones. Thus, when noradrenaline release was evoked by stimulation of the NMDA receptor (an important subtype of ionotropic glutamate receptors), ethanol at concentrations compatible with mild intoxication

($< 50$ mM) acted in an inhibitory manner[32]. This inhibition was observed in rat brain cortical slices irrespective of whether NMDA (Figs. 16.3 and 16.4) or glutamate was used to stimulate ($IC_{50}$ 45 and 37 mM, respectively)[32]. Similarly, an inhibition of the [³H]-noradrenaline release evoked by NMDA (but not by high K⁺, veratridine and/or reintroduction of $Ca^{2+}$ after superfusion with $Ca^{2+}$-free solution containing high K⁺ throughout) was observed in human cortical slices[27] and in rat brain synaptosomes. This suggests that the NMDA receptor itself is a site of action of ethanol. The process of secretion and stimulus–release coupling in the noradrenergic axon terminals are not affected by ethanol at such (relatively) low concentrations. Other aliphatic alcohols share the inhibitory property of ethanol on NMDA-evoked [³H]-noradrenaline release. The inhibitory potency of the alcohols was correlated with their membrane/buffer partition coefficients[26] (Fig. 16.4).

As a rule, the experiments with NMDA were carried out in the absence of $Mg^{2+}$ in the superfusion fluid, since $Mg^{2+}$ is well known to block the NMDA receptor channel when the cell membrane is in a non-depolarised state. The $Mg^{2+}$ block can be removed by depolarisation and, accordingly, NMDA evokes noradrenaline release even in the presence of physiological $Mg^{2+}$ concentrations when the cell membrane is continuously kept partially depolarised by, for example, veratridine. In rat brain cortical slices, the NMDA-evoked noradrenaline release in the presence of veratridine and a physiological $Mg^{2+}$ concentration was found to be inhibited by ethanol with similar potency to that seen in the experiments on slices superfused with $Mg^{2+}$- and veratridine-free solution; whereas the noradrenaline release evoked by veratridine alone was again not affected[32].

Ethanol at concentrations lower than 100 mM also inhibited the NMDA-evoked acetylcholine release from rat striatal slices. In agreement with the *in vitro* findings reported so far, a microdialysis study in the corpus striatum of awake rats treated with 2 g/kg ethanol revealed a decrease of neurotransmitter release, in this particular case, of glutamate release.

Since the NMDA receptor is known to be a ligand-gated $Ca^{2+}$ channel, it is interesting to note that ethanol, in the concentration range in which it inhibited NMDA-evoked neurotransmitter release, caused an inhibition of NMDA-evoked $Ca^{2+}$ influx into cultured rat cortical neurones.

coupling, respectively. This conclusion can be drawn from the failure of ethanol concentrations lower than 100 mM to modify the release evoked by electrical impulses, high $K^+$, veratridine or reintroduction of $Ca^{2+}$. The ethanol-induced changes observed in microdialysis or voltammetric studies *in vivo* in most cases reflect changes in impulse flow resulting from effects exerted in the soma-dendritic area of the neurone.

However, ethanol at concentrations below 100 mM does affect neurotransmitter release in response to activation of excitatory receptors on the axon terminals themselves. Clearly the ligand-gated ion channels are important sites of action of ethanol and may come into play at concentrations compatible with those achieved during 'social drinking'. Accordingly, the central and peripheral nerve terminals have become valuable models for the elucidation of the site and mechanism of action of ethanol. The selective inhibition of the neurotransmitter release in response to nicotinic or NMDA receptor stimulation by ethanol and the correlation of the inhibitory potency of various alcohols with their lipophilicity are compatible with the suggestion that ethanol at low concentrations (those which produce behavioural alterations without other symptoms of acute intoxication) interacts with hydrophobic regions of important classes of excitatory receptor in the brain and periphery, namely the NMDA and nicotinic receptor channels, or with their surrounding lipids.

## 2.3  Summary

Inhibition of neurotransmitter release is the most consistent effect of ethanol on various nerve endings in the central and peripheral nervous systems. However, as a rule, lethal concentrations, or at least concentrations characteristic for severe acute intoxication, are necessary to inhibit both the process of transmitter release and the voltage-sensitive $Na^+$ and $Ca^{2+}$ channels involved in propagation of action potentials and stimulus–release

## 3  Exogenous opiates

The opiate or narcotic drugs are the most potent analgesic agents known and are indispensable in clinical medicine for the treatment of severe pain. Opiates used clinically comprise a number of naturally occurring alkaloids from the opium poppy, the most notable of which are morphine and codeine, and a number of synthetic and semi-synthetic drugs. The synthetic opiate drugs have structures unrelated to morphine and include the phenylpiperidines (pethidine and fentanyl), the methadone series (methadone and dextropropoxyphene), the benzomorphans (pentazocine and cyclazocine) and the semi-synthetic thebaine derivatives (etorphine and buprenorphine). Semi-synthetic analogues of morphine include heroin and the narcotic antagonist naloxone[42,71]. As well as producing analgesia, the opiate agonist drugs share with the prototype drug morphine the ability to produce mood changes, physical dependence, tolerance and a phenomenon known as 'reward', which may lead to compulsive drug use and 'addiction'[87]. Cessation of administration of an opiate, or administration of an opiate antagonist, leads to a withdrawal or abstinence response which is a reflection of physical dependence[94]. The interrelationships between these various actions of opiate drugs and the brain pathways involved in mediating the actions is an area of intensive investigation[24,38,45].

## 3.1　Endogenous opioid peptides

Prior to 1975, the existence of high-affinity receptors for opiates was known, but it was not until endogenous peptides with opiate-like activity were discovered in the brain[39], that an understanding of the mechanism of action of opiate drugs began to emerge. It is now known that there are three families of these endogenous peptides, the enkephalins, the endorphins and the dynorphins, which derive from the three large protein precursor molecules, pro-enkephalin, pro-opiomelanocortin, and pro-dynorphin, respectively[42]. They are known collectively as opioid peptides. Although there are several members of each family, the opioid peptides that have been most studied are [Met-5]- and [Leu-5]-enkephalin, β-endorphin and dynorphin A (1–17).

## 3.2　Opioid receptors

Three major types of opioid receptor, namely, μ, δ and κ, were defined pharmacologically several years ago. Recently three opioid receptors have been cloned and their molecular structures described[72]. These receptors belong to the superfamily of receptors possessing seven transmembrane-spanning domains of amino acids. The pharmacology of the cloned receptors has confirmed the results from the older pharmacological studies. All three types of cloned receptor have been shown to associate with G-proteins and to couple to adenylyl cyclase to inhibit its activity, thereby reducing cAMP formation (see Section 3.4.2.2). In addition, the cloned κ-opioid receptor has been found to mediate agonist inhibition of $Ca^{2+}$ channel activity.

Pharmacological studies have shown that the naturally occurring opioid peptide β-endorphin interacts preferentially with μ-opioid receptors, the enkephalins with δ-opioid receptors and dynorphin with κ-opioid receptors. The prototype opiate drug, morphine, has considerably higher affinity for μ-opioid receptors than for other opioid receptors. The opiate antagonist naloxone inhibits all opioid receptors but with different affinities. Selective agonists and antagonists are now known for each of the three opioid receptor types and these have been used extensively in investigating opioid mechanisms (Table 16.1).

## 3.3　Sites of action of opiates

Two major sites of pharmacological action of opiate drugs are the central and enteric nervous systems. Within the CNS opiates have been found to have effects in many areas, including the cortex, hippocampus, thalamus, hypothalamus, nigrostriatal and mesolimbic systems, periaqueductal grey, locus coeruleus, medulla oblongata and the spinal cord[25]. However, the sites and pathways involved in analgesia and the other central actions of opiates have not yet been fully elucidated. Within the enteric nervous system, opiates act in both the myenteric plexus and submucous plexus, these actions being responsible for the powerful constipating effect of opiates. In recent years, considerable

**Table 16.1.** *Commonly used selective agonists and antagonists for opioid receptors*

| Receptor | Agonists | Antagonists |
| --- | --- | --- |
| Mu (μ) | [D-Ala$^2$,*N*-Me-Phe$^4$, Gly-ol$^5$]-enkephalin (DAMGO; DAGO) Morphine Fentanyl | [Cys$^2$,Tyr$^3$,Orn$^5$,Pen$^7$ amide] (CTOP-somatostatin analogue) |
| Delta (δ) | [D-Pen$^{25}$]-enkephalin (DPDPE) [D-Ala$^2$,D-Leu$^5$]-enkephalin (DADLE) | Naltrindole |
| Kappa (κ) | U50488 U62066 U69593 | Nor-binaltorphimine |

evidence has also been obtained for an action of opiates on primary afferent neurones in the periphery[82].

At the neuronal level, opiates have actions at one or both of two sites; the presynaptic nerve terminal and the postsynaptic neurone. The postsynaptic actions of opiates have usually been found to be inhibitory, although excitatory actions, as shown by increased action-potential duration, have been observed with low concentrations of opioids in dorsal root ganglion neurones in culture[80]. The major presynaptic action of opiates is to inhibit neurotransmitter release and the mechanisms involved in this action are the subject of this review. However, it must be remembered that the final effect of an opiate drug in the brain is the result not only of its action at multiple interacting presynaptic sites on both inhibitory and excitatory neurones but also of its postsynaptic effects.

### 3.4   Presynaptic modulation of neurotransmitter release by opiates

Many of the pharmacological effects of opiates are considered to result from modulation of neurotransmitter release in the nervous system. The most marked modulatory effect of opiates is inhibition of neurotransmitter release, although facilitation has also been observed. Neurotransmitters that have been extensively studied with respect to presynaptic modulatory effects of opiates include noradrenaline, acetylcholine, dopamine and substance P, and these are discussed below. It must be stressed that the majority of studies have been conducted on rat tissues. Results from the few experiments that have been carried out in other animals have demonstrated marked species differences. Therefore, the relevance of the experimental findings described below to the effects of opiates in humans has yet to be established. For a comprehensive literature survey on the modulatory effects of opiates on neurotransmitter release, the reader is referred to the review by Mulder and Schoffelmeer[56].

### 3.4.1   Inhibitory effects of opiates on release of neurotransmitters

**Noradrenaline release.** During the 1970s, it was observed that morphine inhibited depolarisation-induced release of [$^3$H]-noradrenaline from rat brain cortex slices, an effect that was later found to be caused by activation of μ-opioid receptors located on noradrenergic varicosities. It has subsequently been found that this effect of morphine and other opiates is not restricted to the cortex but occurs in several other regions of the rat brain, including the hippocampus, amygdala, cerebellum, periaqueductal grey and nucleus tractus solitarius, all of which receive projections from the locus coeruleus. Noradrenaline release from the mediobasal hypothalamus, which regulates pituitary function and which receives its noradrenergic innervation from a different brain region (the A1 and A2 nuclei in the brain stem), was not affected by opiates. Therefore, not all noradrenergic varicosities, even in the same species, are similar in their response to opiates. Furthermore, striking species differences exist. For example, inhibition of depolarisation-induced [$^3$H]-noradrenaline release from rabbit hippocampus and from guinea-pig cortex, hippocampus and cerebellum is mediated predominantly by κ-opioid receptors. It is possible that the effect of opiates in some regions of the guinea-pig brain might reflect more closely the effects in human brain since the guinea-pig, like the human, has a high proportion of κ-opioid receptors[52].

**Acetylcholine release.** Major regional differences in the effects of opiates and opioids on depolarisation-induced release of acetylcholine from rat brain slices have been found. Acetylcholine release from the frontal cortex is not affected by opioids, whereas inhibition of release occurs in the striatum and is mediated by δ-opioid receptors. In the nucleus accumbens and olfactory tubercle, inhibition is mediated by μ- and δ-opioid receptors, and in the hippocampus and amygdala by μ-opioid receptors. Therefore, the distribution of opioid receptors on particular cholinergic neurones apparently depends on neuronal type and origin. However, as with the effect of opioids on noradrenaline release, there are marked species differences in the effects of opioids on acetylcholine release: κ-opioid receptors, for example, are the predominant receptor involved in rabbit hippocampus and in several regions of guinea-pig brain.

**Dopamine release.** There is general agreement from recent *in vitro* and *in vivo* studies

with rat and guinea-pig brain that dopamine release is inhibited by κ-opioid receptor agonists acting presynaptically. In *in vitro* experiments, variable effects of δ-opioid receptor agonists and no effect of μ-opioid receptor agonists have been found. However, *in vivo* brain microdialysis studies (see Chapter 12) have found an enhanced release of dopamine in the rat striatum and nucleus accumbens during administration of μ- and δ-opioid receptor agonists, an effect that has been suggested to result from the inhibitory action of opioids on other neurones that normally tonically inhibit dopamine neurones.

**Substance P release.** In a classic study, Jessell and Iversen[43] showed that morphine and [Met-5]-enkephalinamide (an analogue of [Met-5]-enkephalin) inhibited K$^+$ depolarisation-evoked release of substance P from primary afferent terminals in the spinal trigeminal ganglion. They suggested that opioid-containing nerve terminals made axo-axonic synapses with primary afferent terminals. This proposal was of considerable importance, since it provided an explanation for the well-known spinal analgesic actions of opioids[23]. Several *in vivo* and *in vitro* studies in trigeminal ganglion and spinal cord have confirmed that opiates inhibit substance P release, although the site and mechanism of this action is still not clear. More recent studies have shown that morphine produces complex bidirectional effects on substance P release, depending on the concentration used and the receptor subtype activated[83]. Thus, very low nanomolar and low micromolar concentrations of morphine, acting preferentially on μ$_1$- and δ-opioid receptors, respectively, suppressed release, whereas higher nanomolar and high micromolar concentrations enhanced release by acting on a postulated μδ-complex receptor and on κ-opioid receptors, respectively. It is not known, however, whether the observed effects were the result of pre- or postsynaptic actions of morphine.

### 3.4.2 Neuronal mechanisms involved in the inhibitory effects of opioids

**G-proteins.** It has been widely accepted for several years that μ- and δ-opioid receptors are coupled to G-proteins. The recent cloning of these opioid receptors has confirmed this and, furthermore, has demonstrated that κ-opioid receptors are also coupled to G-proteins[72]. The G-proteins are heterotrimers comprising α-, β- and γ-subunits (see Chapters 9 and 10). Receptor-mediated activation of G-proteins results in the α-subunit exchanging a GDP molecule for GTP. Having bound GTP, the α-subunit is able to interact with components of the effector system. The interaction is terminated by the hydrolysis of GTP to GDP (by the intrinsic GTPase activity of the G-protein), which leads to the dissociation of the α-subunit from the effector system and its reassociation with the β- and γ-subunits, thus returning the G-protein to its original state[6,18]. Two major properties of G-protein-coupled receptor mechanisms are first, that activation of a G-protein GTPase activity is associated with receptor-mediated activation of the G-protein, and, second, that guanine nucleotides in the presence of Na$^+$ regulate the binding of agonists, whereas antagonist binding is not so regulated.

Pertussis toxin, which inhibits $G_i$ and $G_0$ subtypes by ADP-ribosylation of their α-subunits, has been used extensively in studies of opioid mechanisms. The toxin has been found to inhibit μ- and δ-opioid receptor-mediated effects and, more recently, a cloned κ-opioid receptor has been shown to associate with pertussis toxin-sensitive G-proteins.

**Inhibition of adenylyl cyclase.** Several effector systems coupled through G-proteins have been implicated in the actions of opioids (Fig. 16.5). The most widely studied is adenylyl cyclase, which mediates cAMP formation (see also Chapters 9 and 11). Collier and Roy[16] first reported that morphine inhibited prostaglandin E$_1$-stimulated adenylyl cyclase activity of rat striatal membranes in a naloxone-sensitive manner. Since then,

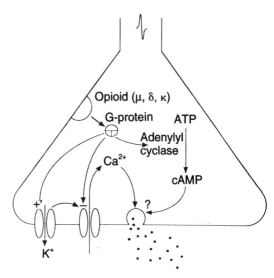

Fig. 16.5. Proposed mechanisms of inhibition of neurotransmitter release by opiates. It has been suggested that opiates administered acutely inhibit neurotransmitter release by inhibiting adenylyl cyclase activity, by inhibiting Ca$^{2+}$ influx, either directly or indirectly by increasing K$^+$ outward currents.

studies on the effects of opioids on adenylyl cyclase have been made on many tissues, most notably on NG108-15 cells (which have δ-opioid receptors only), pituitary tumour cells 7315C (μ-opioid receptors only) and guinea-pig cerebellum (predominantly κ-opioid receptors). It is now known that all three types of cloned opioid receptor couple to adenylyl cyclase[72]. However, despite extensive investigation, the role of adenylyl cyclase in the presynaptic inhibitory effect of opioids on neurotransmitter release is unclear. Since some studies have shown no role of adenylyl cyclase in modulating neurotransmitter release whereas others have, it is possible that the contribution of adenylyl cyclase to the presynaptic effects of opioids differs between neuronal types (see also Chapter 9).

**Mechanism by which inhibition of adenylyl cyclase might inhibit neurotransmitter release.** Recently, Fleming and Childers[13] identified two phosphoproteins, corresponding to synapsin I and synapsin II, the phosphorylation of which are inhibited by opioids that inhibit adenylyl cyclase in rat striatal membranes. Since stimulation of the phosphorylation of these proteins has been shown to increase neurotransmitter release in the squid giant axon, it has been suggested that acute inhibition of synapsin phosphorylation by opioid agonists, mediated by inhibition of adenylyl cyclase, might be involved in inhibition of neurotransmitter release by opioids. It is perhaps of importance that, in rats chronically treated with morphine, stimulation of synapsin phosphorylation, which should increase neurotransmitter release, was found in the thalamus, an area rich in μ-opioid receptors. Stimulation of synapsin phosphorylation following chronic opioid treatment has been suggested to reflect changes that occur in tolerance and/or dependence.

**Effect of opioids on other second messenger systems.** Opioids have been reported to affect other second messenger systems in addition to adenylyl cyclase, although the significance of these effects is not known[13]. An increase in cGMP, as well as a decrease in cAMP mediated by δ-opioid receptors, has been reported to occur in N4TG1 cells.

Several G-protein-coupled receptors are linked to inositol phospholipid turnover. In this second messenger system, the G-protein–receptor complex is linked via phospholipase C to formation of inositol trisphosphate and diacylglycerol (see Chapters 1 and 9). However, at present it appears that this second messenger system does not play a major role in the actions of opioids. The significance of the reported effects of κ-opioid receptor agonists to stimulate inositol phospholipid turnover in rat hippocampal slices and to inhibit GTP-stimulated, but not basal, phospholipase C remains to be evaluated.

**Action on ion channels.** Neurotransmitter release from nerve terminals or varicosities is normally preceded by depolarisation of the terminal and $Ca^{2+}$ entry through VSCC (see Chapters 1 and 10). Drugs may inhibit neurotransmitter release by reducing $Ca^{2+}$ entry directly, by an effect on VSCC, or indirectly by increasing outward $K^+$ current thus shortening repolarisation time and reducing action-potential duration. Both $K^+$ channels and VSCC have been shown to be involved in the actions of opioids (see also Chapter 10).

**Decreased $Ca^{2+}$ conductance.** Direct inhibition of voltage-sensitive $Ca^{2+}$ currents at nerve terminals is one mechanism that has been proposed to underlie the presynaptic inhibition of neurotransmitter release induced by opioids. However, as opioids are much more effective at inhibiting neurotransmitter release than at inhibiting $Ca^{2+}$ currents, the proposal has not received full acceptance.

Electrophysiological evidence has shown that activation of μ- and δ-opioid receptors on SH-SY5Y cells (derived from human neuroblastoma), μ- and κ-opioid receptors on dorsal root ganglion neurones and δ-opioid receptors on submucous plexus neurones decrease voltage-sensitive $Ca^{2+}$ currents[61]. Studies in submucous plexus neurones at the single channel level have shown definitively that in these neurones the type of VSCC affected by opioids is the N-type channel, which may be distinguished from other VSCCs by its intermediate conductance. This contrasts with the T (small conductance)-type channel, and with the L (large conductance)-type channel sensitive to dihydropyridines ('$Ca^{2+}$-channel blockers'). Although the precise mechanism of action of opioids on $Ca^{2+}$ currents is not yet known, it is clear that in some neurones it is mediated via pertussis toxin-sensitive G-proteins (possibly $G_o$ and $G_i$) and is independent of the action of opioids on adenylyl cyclase.

**Increased $K^+$ conductance.** There is now considerable evidence that μ-opioid receptor agonists increase membrane $K^+$ conductance in neurones from several CNS regions commonly associated with opioid actions, including the locus coeruleus, hypothalamic nuclei, inhibitory interneurones of the hippocampus, substantia nigra, ventral tegmental area, raphe magnus and substantia gelatinosa of the spinal cord, as well as in the guinea-pig myenteric plexus[61]. Activation of δ-opioid receptors in submucous plexus neurones also produces an increase in $K^+$ conductance. Activation of κ-opioid receptors has recently been shown to increase membrane $K^+$ conductance in guinea-pig substantia gelatinosa neurones[36].

The properties of single $K^+$ channels opened by opioids in rat locus coeruleus neurones (μ-opioid receptors) and guinea-pig submucous plexus neurones (δ-opioid receptors) have been studied in patch-clamp studies, which allow the characteristics of single conductances to be studied[61]. There are many types of $K^+$ channels, some of which are voltage sensitive while others are gated by intracellular ligands such as G-proteins, ATP and $Ca^{2+}$. Opioids modulate voltage-sensitive $K^+$ channels but not ligand-gated channels. Functionally, two main types of voltage-sensitive $K^+$ channel are known, those that remain open during a maintained depolarisation (delayed rectifier type) and those that close during a maintained depolarisation (transient or A currents). It has been observed that the hyperpolarisation resulting from opioid-mediated opening of $K^+$ channels increases the effectiveness of opioids to open remaining $K^+$ channels. This property, which is known as inward rectification, leads to amplification of opioid action.

The properties of the $K^+$ conductances activated by opioids appear to vary considerably between neurones in different regions of the nervous system. In locus coeruleus neurones, a single small conductance $K^+$ current was activated in the presence of a μ-opioid receptor agonist, whereas in submucous plexus neurones, [Met[5]]-enkephalin, acting on δ-opioid receptors, increased the conductances of several different $K^+$ channels. Hippocampal neurones have been reported to show two different responses to opioids. Some neurones exhibited an inwardly rectify-

ing current as described above, while the majority exhibited no effect of opioids at resting membrane potential but showed an increase in the outward current produced on membrane depolarisation, that is in the delayed rectifier. Increase in the delayed rectifier would explain the finding that opioids reduce action-potential duration. Thus opioids do not appear to have a selective effect on any one type of $K^+$ channel. Note that agonists acting at several other G-protein-coupled receptors, including α₂-adrenoceptors and $M_2$ muscarinic receptors, are also capable of increasing the same $K^+$ conductances as opioid agonists. There is considerable evidence that opioids couple to the several types of $K^+$ channel via the pertussis toxin-sensitive G-proteins, $G_i$ and $G_o$, without the intervention of the adenylyl cyclase system or any other freely diffusible second messenger.

Although increase in $K^+$ conductance is the likely mechanism of the hyperpolarisation and inhibition of neurones throughout the nervous system[62] induced by opioids, particularly by those acting on μ- and δ-opioid receptors, it remains to be definitively established that this is the mechanism involved in the presynaptic action of opioids to inhibit neurotransmitter release.

## 3.5   Opioid tolerance and dependence

No discussion of the actions of opiates is complete without some mention of tolerance and dependence, since these phenomena are induced by chronic exposure to morphine and other opioids to a greater extent than by any other group of drugs[45]. Tolerance is reflected in a shift to the right of the dose–response curve to the opioid such that higher concentrations are required to produce a given effect. The maximum response attainable is also reduced following pretreatment with high concentrations of opioids, indicating that there is inactivation of the receptor response that becomes apparent only when the receptor reserve (spare receptor population) is abolished. Such an effect could be produced either by a reduction in the number of functional receptors (receptor down-regulation) or by receptor desensitisation, where agonist action results in the formation of non-functional receptors. It is now established that modest μ- and δ-opioid receptor down-regulation is induced in cells in culture and in rat brain slices *in vitro* on chronic treatment with high doses of opioids over a prolonged period of time. However, the extent of μ-opioid receptor down-regulation is inadequate to explain the degree of functional tolerance that is observed following chronic opioid treatment. Furthermore, tolerance is observed before a significant reduction in receptor number is observed. It is now considered that tolerance is the result of receptor desensitisation, induced by functional uncoupling of opioid receptors from G-proteins. This would result in uncoupling of the receptors from their effector systems[18]. Although the subject of many studies, the mechanism of this desensitisation is still not fully understood. An agonist-induced change in receptor conformation has been suggested, and there is some evidence that inactivation of μ-opioid receptors by phosphorylation may be induced by a kinase that phosphorylates agonist-occupied receptors. Desensitisation of cloned κ-opioid receptors involves β-adrenoceptor-like kinase, an enzyme that is also responsible for desensitisation of several other receptors. However, it is not clear how these mechanisms are related to the functional uncoupling of receptors from G-proteins that occurs with tolerance. Chronic opioid exposure has also been found to produce tissue-specific changes in G-protein subunits, the α-subunits in general being more susceptible than the β- or γ-subunits. These changes may contribute to tolerance in some tissues and to changes in sensitivity of effector systems to agonists acting on other receptors sharing the same G-proteins as opioids.

Although dependence usually accompanies tolerance, it is a distinct phenomenon. Dependence is covert until the opiate drug is removed from its receptors, either by cessation of administration or by administration of an opioid receptor antagonist such as naloxone. Dependence is then revealed by the occurrence of a withdrawal response, which is opposite in nature to the acute effect of the opiate. Dependence occurs much more rapidly than tolerance, and naloxone-precipitated withdrawal can be seen in the guinea-pig ileum 2 min after addition of a single dose of morphine[11]. It has been known for many years that chronic exposure of NG108-15 cells to morphine and other opioids produces an initial inhibition of adenylyl cyclase activity followed by a gradual return to normal levels. On addition of naloxone to induce withdrawal, an increase in adenylyl cyclase activity occurs. These effects are considered to be a model of opioid tolerance and dependence. Although the mechanisms involved in these changes in adenylyl cyclase activity are not known, they appear to be a general response of NG108-15 cells to inhibition of $G_i$, since a similar effect is observed following addition of an α-adrenoceptor antagonist following chronic α-adrenoceptor agonist treatment of these cells.

Increased adenylyl cyclase activity following chronic morphine treatment has been observed in the locus coeruleus, a central noradrenergic cell group that is considered to play a major role in opioid withdrawal. Furthermore, increased activity in cAMP-dependent kinase, increased levels of tyrosine hydroxylase and increased levels of $G_i$ and $G_o$ have been found in the locus coeruleus following chronic morphine treatment. These biochemical changes, which are specific for the locus coeruleus, are not considered to be the only factors involved in withdrawal, as they return to normal many hours before the withdrawal signs disappear.

The withdrawal response is very complex and, presumably, many brain regions, each exhibiting specific changes in tissue sensitivity and release of multiple neurotransmitters, participate in the response. However, the mechanisms involved in the integrated functioning brain *in vivo* remain to be elucidated.

### 3.6 Summary

Inhibition of neurotransmitter release is considered to be the major mechanism of action of opiates that is responsible for their clinical effects. Nevertheless, despite extensive investigations over many years, understanding of the cellular actions of morphine and other opioids is incomplete. This is surprising for a group of drugs with such powerful effects and is a reflection both of the multiple actions of opiates and of the complexity of the mechanisms involved in neurotransmitter release. In the CNS, where opiates might inhibit release of inhibitory as well as excitatory neurotransmitters onto the same postsynaptic neurone, determination of the mechanisms involved in altering neurotransmitter release is particularly difficult. A major limitation to studies on the effects of opioids on neurotransmitter release is that changes in conductances measured at the cell soma do not necessarily reflect those occurring on axons and dendrites. Only recently have techniques been developed to measure currents in single varicosities (see Chapter 3), and confirmation of current hypotheses regarding mechanisms of modulating neurotransmitter release must await the application of these new techniques.

## 4 Amphetamines

Unlike the other substances considered in this chapter, the effects of amphetamine probably are not mediated by presynaptic receptors. The amphetamine-like drugs are classified as indirect amine agonists, since they exert little if any direct agonist activity on monoamine receptors (pre- or postsynaptic) *per se*. It is now clear that the major factors which determine the acute central pharmacological effects of amphetamine and related substances are an enhancement of monoamine release and/or an inhibition of transmitter reuptake[55]. Hence amphetamine is included here for interest, and as an example of a neuroactive drug that has a mechanism of action independent of membrane-associated receptors.

### 4.1 Pharmacology of amphetamine

Amphetamine and related stimulants, in small to moderate doses (in humans, ingestion of 5–15 mg), exert a number of well-characterised effects in the CNS including an increase in alertness, locomotor activity, elevation in mood, euphoria, hyperthermia and reduced appetite. In humans, the plasma level range of amphetamine following these therapeutic/recreational doses is 5–10 μg/100 ml (cf. ref. 63). At higher single doses (ingestion of $\geq$ 20–30 mg in humans), or with continuous intake of smaller doses over several days, amphetamine can induce a toxic psychosis characterised by delusional thinking and auditory hallucinations that resemble closely the positive symptoms seen in acute paranoid schizophrenia. In laboratory animals, amphetamine administration produces increased locomotor activity at low doses (1.0–2.5 mg/kg), while higher doses ($\geq$ 2.5 mg/kg) are associated with well-characterised patterns of stereotyped behaviour[19]. In both animals and humans, tolerance develops to some, but not all, of the pharmacological effects of amphetamine. The requirement for dose escalation in order to maintain the euphoric effects of amphetamine is an important factor which contributes to the substance-abuse potential of this agent.

### 4.2 Effects of amphetamine on the release and/or reuptake of central monoamines

A variety of experimental studies, both in animals and humans, has established the critical role of monoamine neurotransmitters (dopamine, noradrenaline and 5-HT) in the expression of psychopharmacological and behavioural effects following amphetamine administration. Furthermore, the results of these experiments have identified a number of neuro-anatomical substrates associated with specific neurotransmitter projections that are critical for the expression of altered locomotor activity and stereotyped behaviour, for example. The projection of dopamine-containing neurones from the substantia nigra/ventral tegmental area (A9 and A10 regions) of the midbrain to the corpus striatum (nigrostriatal tract) has been identified as the operational component responsible for mediating the stereotyped behavioural responses following amphetamine administration[19]. In contrast, the increased locomotor activity seen following low doses of amphetamine has been shown to result from the effects of inceased dopamine released from terminals of nigrostriatal neurones located in the nucleus accumbens. In humans, it is likely that a number of specific nuclei, which are functionally classified as belonging to the so called 'limbic system' (including the amygdala, medial prefrontal/anterior cingulate cortex and nucleus accumbens) and which receive afferent input from midbrain dopaminergic cells, are responsible for mediating the psychotomimetic effects of amphetamine. These projections, which traditionally have been referred to as the 'mesolimbic' and 'mesocortical' dopaminergic projections, are now grouped together as the 'mesolimbocortical' pathway. While it is now apparent that specific behavioural responses to amphetamine are probably the result of complex interactions involving the participation of several types of transmitter/neuromodulator at various CNS locations, these seminal experiments were important in identifying the role of monoamine release as a primary permissive requirement.

Early neurochemical studies established the characteristic potency of amphetamine to enhance the release of radiolabelled monoamines and/or inhibit monoamine reuptake in brain slice or synaptosomal preparations. It appears that noradrenaline and dopamine release are affected by low concentrations of amphetamine while higher concentrations are required to increase 5-HT release[55]. Methamphetamine appears to be slightly more potent than amphetamine in its ability to enhance the release of dopamine from central nerve terminals. In addition, the effects on dopamine release show stereoselectivity, in as much as the (+) isomer of amphetamine (commonly referred to as dexamphetamine) is somewhat more potent in comparison to the (−) isomer (commonly referred to as laevoamphetamine). Substituted amphetamines, such as 3,4,-methylenedioxyamphetamine (MDA) and 3,4,-methylenedioxymethamphetamine (MDMA, 'Ecstasy'), which exert mild hallucinogenic actions in addition to their stimulant effects, act with greater potency on 5-HT release/uptake in comparison to their effects on dopamine systems[76].

## 4.3  Role of transmitter reuptake in regulating synaptic activity

It is now well established that reuptake of released neurotransmitter into the presynaptic terminal is an important process in the termination of transmitter action at certain central synapses. The pioneering work from the laboratories of Burn[8] and Axelrod (see ref. 2) established the existence of an effective and rapid uptake process for noradrenaline in sympathetic nerve endings. The uptake of noradrenaline against its concentration gradient was shown to be by a high-affinity, saturable process. This demonstration led to the postulate of a carrier-mediated transporter, analogous to the membrane transport mechanism that had already been described for amino acids and sugars. Confirmation of the existence of specific macromolecular monoamine transporters has been made possible with the recent advent of molecular cloning techniques[30]. Further investigations demonstrated that the uptake mechanism could, under certain conditions, transport monoamines in the reverse direction (see Section 4.3.1), giving rise to an apparent increase in release of transmitter into the extracellular space. A close relationship between the uptake mechanism and release was re-inforced by the experimental findings in which it was shown that amphetamine could exert the dual actions of inhibiting dopamine/noradrenaline uptake as well as enhancing release of these catecholamines.

### 4.3.1  Dopamine release and reuptake in brain neurones

In order to understand the functional role of the uptake carrier for dopamine and related monoamines and its relationship to the pharmacological actions of amphetamine, it is useful to provide a brief overview of the processes by which these neurotransmitters are released from central nerve terminals. The release of monoamines from central nerve terminals occurs by two main mechanisms. In part, release occurs by the classical $Ca^{2+}$-dependent exocytotic process described for other transmitters such as acetylcholine (see Chapter 1 and ref. 91). However, monoamines can also be released from central nerve terminals by a second process which is both $Ca^{2+}$-independent and independent of impulse conduction[3]. This second process can be produced experimentally when either (i) the normal inwardly directed $Na^+$ current pathway across the neuronal membrane (which mediates the initial phase of impulse conduction) is blocked by a specific $Na^+$-channel blocker, such as tetrodotoxin or (ii) extracellular $Na^+$ is isotonically replaced with sucrose or an impermeant cation such as choline. In general, the increase in $Ca^{2+}$-dependent release of transmitter in brain slices, or from synaptosomes induced by depolarisation, is unaffected by drugs that block the uptake transporter. However, the release of monoamines through the $Ca^{2+}$-independent process is sensitive to uptake-transport inhibitors (Fig. 16.6).

### 4.3.2  Intraneuronal storage of monoamines: vesicular and cytoplasmic pools

There is now considerable evidence to support the existence of at least two intraneuronal pools of dopamine (and other monoamines) in central nerve terminals. An in-depth coverage of this area is beyond the scope of this review, but sufficient details are provided here to assist the reader to assess the relative importance of the two pools as determinants of the pharmacological actions of amphetamine and related CNS stimulants.

It is now clear that the release of dopamine in response to low to moderate doses of amphetamine is dependent on an adequate cytoplasmic pool of the transmitter. Pretreatment of experimental animals with α-methyl-*p*-tyrosine, (a drug that inhibits the activity of tyrosine hydroxylase, the rate-limiting enzyme involved in catecholamine biosynthesis), produces a dose-dependent depletion of cytoplasmic stores of neuronal dopamine and a concomitant attenuation of most of the behavioural responses to amphetamine. In contrast, most of the behavioural effects of amphetamine are relatively resistant to the effects of reserpine (see ref. 73), a drug which depletes vesicular stores of catecholamines.

### 4.3.3  Differential drug effects on transmitter uptake and release

Many drugs that have been shown to block the reuptake of monoamines have also been described as being effective inducers of release[55]. However, the ability to discriminate whether increased extracellular neurotransmitter concentration has resulted either from uptake blockade or from enhanced release remains a difficult problem. Early studies used brain tissue slices or synaptosomes suspended in an incubation medium containing radiolabelled dopamine in the presence or absence of the drug of interest. After a fixed time interval (10–30 min), portions of the incubation medium were sampled and counted for the amount of radioactivity present. An increase in the amount of radiolabelled dopamine in comparison with controls could be attributed equally well to either inhibition of uptake or enhancement of release. A number of experimental paradigms have, therefore, been employed in an attempt to discriminate 'pure' uptake blockers from drugs

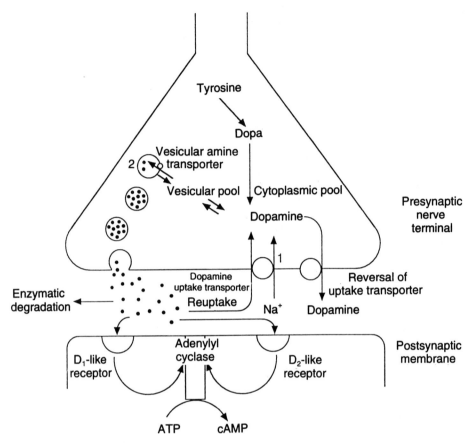

Fig. 16.6. Primary site of amphetamine action at monoamine synapses. Schematic representation of a typical dopaminergic synapse, which demonstrates the indirect agonist effects of amphetamine. At low concentrations, amphetamine (**1**) interacts with the dopamine-reuptake transporter and by an exchange–diffusion mechanism causes a $Ca^{2+}$-independent increase of dopamine release (similar effects would be seen at noradrenergic terminals). The dopamine released by this process can interact in the normal way with pre- and postsynaptic $D_1$-like ($D_1$ and $D_5$) or $D_2$-like ($D_2$, $D_3$, and $D_4$) dopamine receptors. At higher concentrations, amphetamine (**2**), having accumulated in the nerve terminal via exchange–diffusion or passive diffusion, may block vesicular amine storage via an interaction with the vesicular membrane transporter and/or by dissipation of the vesicular transmembrane proton gradient.

that act primarily by enhancing release. In particular, the development of superfusion techniques, in which the rate of perfusion of a synaptosomal or brain slice preparation is too rapid to allow significant reuptake, has further assisted in discriminating uptake blockers from release inducers[68]. For example, Heikkila, Orlansky and Cohen[37] demonstrated that cocaine, which acts primarily as an uptake blocker, blocks the accumulation of [³H]-dopamine into rat brain slices without inducing release of previously accumulated [³H]-dopamine. The use of this technique has also assisted in the determination that nomifensine (an atypical antidepressant) is a drug that acts primarily as an inhibitor of dopamine-uptake while drugs like amphetamine block uptake, and additionally enhance release of dopamine[69]. Recent experiments employing *in vivo* dialysis techniques (see Chapter 12) have provided further information concerning the basis of apparent increases in transmitter release following drug treatment.

In the intact nervous system, *exocytotic* ($Ca^{2+}$-dependent) release of transmitter occurs in response to neuronal action potentials. The reuptake process that follows returns dopamine to the interior of the nerve terminal; this process is the one mainly responsible for the rapid reduction in transmitter concentration in the synaptic cleft. 'Apparent' increases in transmitter release that are secondary to inhibition of reuptake would be expected to diminish in association with reduced neuronal action-potential frequency, since the rate of reuptake would slow in proportion to demand. In contrast, *transport-mediated* release of dopamine from the terminal cytoplasm should be largely unaffected by variation in the frequency of action potentials. However, the increase in concentration of extracellular dopamine seen in response to administration of cocaine, nomifensine and bupropion can be virtually abolished by tetrodotoxin, which, by blocking voltage-sensitive $Na^+$ channels, prevents invasion of the nerve terminal by action potentials[60]. This suggests that these drugs interfere with mechanisms associated with maintaining the availability of dopamine in the vesicular pool, in addition to their action on cytoplasmic stores. In contrast, the amphetamine-induced increase in extracellular dopamine levels is essentially unaffected by tetrodotoxin[60] or γ-butyrolactone, a drug that is a relatively specific inhibitor of dopamine cell firing[9]. Taken together, these findings suggest that amphetamine acts primarily to increase carrier-mediated release of dopamine derived from the cytoplasmic pool.

## 4.4  Exchange-diffusion models of amphetamine-induced dopamine release

An exchange-diffusion process has been proposed to account for the ability of amphetamine to induce dopamine release[28,50]. In this model, it is postulated that amphetamine binds to the dopamine uptake transporter on the extracellular side of the neuronal plasma membrane to block inwardly directed dopamine-transport. Subsequently, the transporter moves amphetamine into the neuronal cytoplasm where it dissociates in exchange for the binding of a dopamine molecule. The transporter, now binding dopamine, reorients in an outwardly facing direction causing release of the transmitter into the extracellular space. The model proposes that there is a net accumulation of intracellular amphetamine in exchange for a net increase in extracellular dopamine. Inherent in the interpretation of this model is the notion that, while amphetamine may enter the nerve terminal via the uptake transporter or by diffusion, it is only the fraction of amphetamine that enters the cytoplasm via the transporter that can participate in the dopamine-exchange process. In contrast, Liang and Rutledge[50] suggest that dopamine release can occur in response to amphetamine that accumulates both via the uptake mechanism and by passive diffusion into the nerve terminal. They argued that, as amphetamine concentrations in the terminal are increasing, a fraction of dopamine stored in vesicles is displaced into the cytoplasm, making more dopamine available for release.

In this latter context, there is a reasonable body of experimental evidence to suggest that amphetamine and related compounds can, under certain conditions, release dopamine from reserpine-sensitive vesicular stores[66]. This action could occur by a direct interaction of the drugs with the vesicular dopamine transporter and/or via amphetamine-induced dissipation of the proton gradient across the vesicular membrane. It has been proposed that the latter effect results from the ability of amphetamine to act as a weak base, resulting in alkalinisation of the storage vesicle, which in turn causes vesicle disruption[44,84]. Experiments with MDMA suggest that relatively low concentrations of this drug block vesicular 5-HT transport in a stereoselective manner, the (+) isomer being considerably more potent than the (−) isomer[76]. At higher concentrations, MDMA can release vesicular 5-HT in a non-stereoselective manner. The relationship between the $pK_a$ of a drug and its ability to alkalinise transmitter storage vesicles remains unclear. Like amphetamine and its congeners, 5-HT is a weak base, but it lacks potency to disrupt the pH gradient across the vesicular membrane. While further experimentation is required to substantiate this hypothesis of vesicular alkalinisation, it is clear, nonetheless, that disruption of amine stores can occur in response to amphetamine. However, these effects, which have been seen in brain slices, chromaffin granules, and synaptosomes, require very high concentrations of the drug to have entered the vesicle by diffusion[77]. At somewhat lower concentrations, amphetamine analogues may disrupt vesicular monoamine stores via a direct interaction with the vesicular membrane transporter[79]. Taken together, these results are consistent with the reserpine-insensitive behavioural effects of amphetamine seen following low to moderate doses (1–5 mg/kg) but also account for reserpine-sensitive responses (e.g. 5-HT 'wet dog shake' syndrome) seen following very large doses (> 10–15 mg/kg) of the drug (cf. ref. 73).

### 4.5   Summary

Amphetamines appear to exert their acute pharmacological effects via a relatively selective effect on monoamine uptake/exchange mechanisms, with little, if any, direct agonist–receptor interaction. This relative degree of specificity is somewhat surprising considering the relatively simple structure of amphetamine and the resemblance of its ethylamine side chain to that of dopamine. The phenylethylamine skeleton is clearly an important feature for effective carrier exchange of both dopamine and amphetamine across the nerve terminal. In contrast, the *absence* of the two hydroxyl substituents at positions 3 and 4 on the phenyl ring of the

amphetamine molecule (compared with their presence in catecholamine compounds) clearly helps in restricting the specificity of its molecular sites of action. Further detailed molecular studies, taking advantage of the existence of these simple differences in chemical structure, may reveal important details which advance our understanding of the physiological function of dopamine transporter proteins and receptors, and their modulation by pharmacologically active agents.

## 5   Barbiturates

Barbiturate drugs have a wide spectrum of action in the nervous system. They were developed as clinical agents to promote sleep, produce anaesthesia, treat seizure disorders and to reduce anxiety. They still continue to play an important role as anaesthetics (methohexitone and thiopentone) and anticonvulsants (phenobarbitone and methylphenobarbitone), although they are no longer the drugs of choice as sedative–hypnotics, having been replaced by the less toxic benzodiazepines. In spite of the therapeutic use of barbiturates for over 80 years, it is only more recently that pharmacological studies have revealed the cellular and molecular mechanisms of action of these drugs.

### 5.1   Differential effects of barbiturates on synaptic transmission

It is now generally accepted that the activity of the CNS is dependent on a balance between excitatory and inhibitory synaptic activity. Therefore, in considering the mechanism of action of drugs affecting CNS function, it is the relative effect on these two processes that is critical. Numerous electrophysiological studies investigating the effects of barbiturates in a variety of *in vivo* and *in vitro* neuronal preparations have provided evidence suggesting that depressant barbiturates can suppress excitatory synaptic

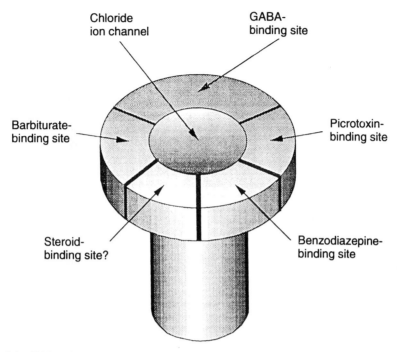

Fig. 16.7. Model of the GABA$_A$ receptor–Cl$^-$ channel complex. Schematic representation of the binding sites of various drug and toxin molecules and the central Cl$^-$ channel. The model is not meant to convey any underlying protein subunit structure of the receptor complex (modified from ref. 965).

transmission[59,85,86] and/or enhance inhibitory transmission, especially at synapses that use GABA as a neurotransmitter[57,59,81].

## 5.2 Postsynaptic actions of barbiturates

The most potent and consistent effect of barbiturates is a potentiation of postsynaptic inhibition mediated by GABA in a number of regions of the CNS[59]. This potentiation is likely to be therapeutically relevant; it occurs at plasma concentrations known to produce anaesthesia (the plasma concentration following a single dose of phenytoin sufficient to produce unconciousness ranges between 30 and 120 $\mu$M). Potentiation of the GABA-mediated postsynaptic inhibition is not caused by an inhibition of GABA uptake (which nevertheless can occur at higher barbiturate concentrations), but appears to result from enhancement by barbiturates of GABA binding, specifically at the high-affinity GABA-binding site on the postsynaptic membrane[90]. Electrophysiological studies have shown that barbiturates, at low concentrations (10–50 $\mu$M), prolong GABA$_A$-induced Cl$^-$ currents by binding to a site which allosterically regulates the postsynaptic receptor–Cl$^-$ channel complex (see Fig. 16.7) and results in an increase in mean channel-open time[51]. In addition, at slightly higher but still clinically relevant concentrations, barbiturates directly activate Cl$^-$ channels associated with the GABA receptor complex through a bicuculline-sensitive GABA-mimetic mechanism[54]. These actions result in profound hyperpolarisation of the membrane and, as a consequence, inhibit the activity of the postsynaptic neurone.

## 5.3    Presynaptic actions of barbiturates

In addition to the well-established postsynaptic actions, Nicoll[59] has suggested that there may be two presynaptic mechanisms by which barbiturates cause a change in neurotransmitter release and thereby modulate postsynaptic neuronal activity. First, they could alter the amplitude or duration of the presynaptic action potential and/or prevent invasion into the nerve terminal by the action potential. Second, the barbiturates could directly affect the neurotransmitter release mechanism, possibly by actions at presynaptic receptors and/or by blocking $Ca^{2+}$ influx or action[35].

### 5.3.1    Effects of barbiturates on nerve-terminal excitability

One of the critical factors determining the magnitude of neurotransmitter release is the amplitude of the presynaptic spike, since it is now acknowledged that there is a linear relationship between this and EPSP amplitude, at least at the squid giant synapse. Using voltage-clamp techniques, barbiturates have been shown to reduce conductance through neuronal voltage-sensitive $Na^+$ channels in a variety of axonal preparations, in a fashion similar to local anaesthetics[74]. In addition, barbiturates increase $K^+$ conductance probably via $Ca^{2+}$-activated or inward rectifying $K^+$ channels[46]. This action would be expected to reduce nerve terminal excitability, and thereby reduce transmitter release, but probably does not contribute to the sedative/hypnotic properties of barbiturates since the effects are only seen at supra-therapeutic concentrations. Indeed it is now well accepted that barbiturates at anaesthetic concentrations (100–200 μM for pentobarbitone) do not affect impulse conduction in axons.

### 5.3.2    General effects on transmitter release

The effect of barbiturates on the release of neurotransmitter has been studied electrophysiologically at only two sites; in the spinal cord at the synapse between primary afferent neurones and α-motoneurones and at the neuromuscular junction. The most compelling evidence for a presynaptic action of barbiturates was demonstrated at the first of these synapses[88]. It was shown that subanaesthetic doses (10 mg/kg) of thiopentone or pentobarbitone decreased the quantal content of the EPSP in cat triceps surae motoneurones without altering the amplitude of the miniature EPSP. This occurred in the absence of any change in the input resistance of the motoneurone or the strength–duration relationship, strongly implying that the reduction in monosynaptic reflex transmission was caused by a decrease in transmitter release from the terminals of the Group 1a primary afferent fibres[88].

At the vertebrate neuromuscular junction, the actions of barbiturates are somewhat more complicated. Barbiturates have been shown to both enhance and depress evoked transmitter release, depending on the $Ca^{2+}$ level in the bathing solution[67]. At low $Ca^{2+}$ concentrations, barbiturates increase the quantal content and EPP amplitude. At normal $Ca^{2+}$ concentrations, barbiturates depress the EPP without altering quantal content. However, the reduction in the EPP amplitude seen at normal $Ca^{2+}$ concentrations probably reflects a reduction in the amplitude of the response to acetylcholine, since the amplitude of spontaneous miniature EPPs is reduced. This inability to alter transmitter release at the neuromuscular junction at normal $Ca^{2+}$ concentrations is, therefore, in conflict with that observed at the primary afferent synapse of the cat[88].

Other neurochemical studies, in which the release of radiolabelled transmitter from brain slices or synaptosomes has been measured, have found a variety of actions of barbiturates, largely dependent on the techniques used to elicit release and the tissue used. In general, the presynaptic effects of barbiturates differ both quantitatively and qualitatively at different synapses (see ref. 90) and it seems that, although a reduction in transmitter release has been reported at the primary afferent synapse in the spinal cord, there is little support for the notion that barbiturates at anaesthetic concentrations produce a reduction of transmitter release at all synapses. It appears that the action of barbiturates to reduce release is dependent on the presence of presynaptic GABA receptors (see Section 5.3.4). Presynaptic GABA receptors are found in the spinal afferent pathway but there are many synapses that do not have a presynaptic GABA receptor representation, such as the neuromuscular junction.

### 5.3.3   Inhibition of transmitter release by blockade of presynaptic VSCC

Since it is well established that $Ca^{2+}$ entry through VSCC is required for excitation–secretion coupling during most types of evoked transmitter release, blockade of $Ca^{2+}$ channels is a possible mechanism by which barbiturates could exert their anaesthetic actions. Indeed anaesthetic concentrations (100–200 μM range) of pentobarbitone have been shown to block both L- and N- (but not T-) type $Ca^{2+}$ currents in cultured mouse dorsal root ganglion neurones[35,59] and relatively high concentrations of barbiturates (200–400 μM) have also been shown to decrease the entry of $^{45}Ca^{2+}$ into synaptosomes (pinched-off nerve terminals) induced by depolarising agents[49]. Willow and colleagues[90] were able to demonstrate a number of additional modulatory effects of barbiturates on intraneuronal $Ca^{2+}$ sequestration processes and suggested that these effects, acting in concert, may play a role in accelerating the reduction in intra-terminal $Ca^{2+}$ following $Ca^{2+}$ influx and, consequently, cause a decrease in transmitter release. These modulatory effects include an enhancement of synaptosomal plasma membrane $Ca^{2+}/Mg^{2+}$-ATPase activity (associated with the membrane $Ca^{2+}$ pump) in the presence of amylobarbitone or pentobarbitone, and also a barbiturate-induced stimulation in the initial rate of $Ca^{2+}$ uptake by metabolically active intra-terminal mitochondria in neurones from the CNS[90].

Therefore, barbiturates, at concentrations achieved during general anaesthesia (100–400 μM range), exert profound effects on $Ca^{2+}$ fluxes across synaptic plasma membranes. The influx process is inhibited, but a barbiturate-induced enhancement of efflux may also be an important mechanistic factor in reducing transmitter release.

### 5.3.4   Barbiturate-induced enhancement of GABA-mediated presynaptic inhibition

Presynaptic inhibition in the spinal cord is a phenomenon quite distinct from presynaptic modulation of neurotransmitter release as the concept has been applied elsewhere in this book. However, it still involves a reduction in neurotransmitter release arising from the depolarisation of nerve terminals. For example, sensory information from muscle spindles in the periphery is conveyed by primary afferent fibres (Group 1a) via the dorsal root of the spinal cord. Neurotransmitter release from the terminals of these fibres, evoked by sensory afferent activity can be modulated because of the presence of axo-axonic synapses at the afferent terminals (see Fig. 16.8). These axo-axonic synapses are formed from the terminals of inhibitory interneurones that release GABA. The GABA then combines with presynaptic GABA receptors and causes a resultant depolarisation of the primary afferent terminals (depolarisation rather than hyperpolarisation since the reversal potential for $Cl^-$ at the GABA receptor–$Cl^-$ channel complex is less negative than the resting membrane potential of the terminal membrane). The depolarisation results in reduction of transmitter release from the primary afferent terminal, probably by reducing the amplitude of the presynaptic action potential. This inhibition without any change in the membrane properties of the postsynaptic neurone is termed presynaptic inhibition.

Such presynaptic inhibition can be demonstrated experimentally by stimulation of spinal ventral roots, which activates a pathway that synaptically depolarises the primary

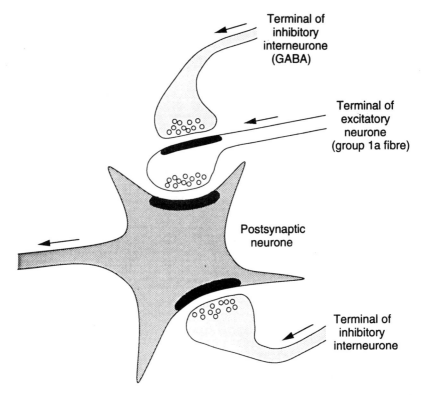

Fig. 16.8. Schematic representation of presynaptic and postsynaptic inhibition of neurones. In the upper portion of the diagram, a terminal from an inhibitory interneurone forms an axo-axonic synapse with the terminal of an excitatory fibre. Release of the neurotransmitter GABA from the inhibitory fibre onto GABA receptors on the terminal of the excitatory fibre causes depolarisation and thus, possibly, a reduction in excitatory transmitter release onto the postsynaptic neurone. The reduction of the resultant EPSP without any change in the membrane properties of the postsynaptic neurone is termed presynaptic inhibition. In the lower portion of the diagram, an inhibitory interneurone forms an axo-somatic synapse directly with the postsynaptic cell. Release of an inhibitory neurotransmitter here (either glycine or GABA) produces a direct hyperpolaristation of the postsynaptic neurone. The resultant reduction in excitability of the soma or dendrites is termed postsynaptic inhibition. Barbiturates have been shown to increase pre- and postsynaptic inhibition by enhancing GABAergic neurone activity (see text for further information).

afferent nerve terminals. This depolarisation, a direct correlate of presynaptic inhibition, is manifested as the dorsal root potential and can be recorded from dorsal roots.

In their pioneering work in 1946, Eccles and Malcolm (see ref. 90) showed that pentobarbitone markedly prolonged the dorsal root potential in the isolated frog spinal cord. Since that time, similar findings have been observed in numerous preparations, including the spinal cord and the cuneate nucleus

(see ref. 90). It has also been demonstrated that, in the presence of barbiturates, presynaptic inhibition of the spinal monosynaptic reflex (which results in reduced transmitter release and consequently a reduction in the amplitude of the EPSP) is prolonged to the same extent as the dorsal root potential. This action to reduce transmitter release by prolonging the dorsal root potential can occur at concentrations of pentobarbitone as low as 5 $\mu$M[58]. Furthermore, a direct barbiturate-induced depolarisation of primary afferent fibres (independent of GABA), which occurs at 40 μM, also directly depolarises the presynaptic terminal to reduce release. This barbiturate-induced depolarisation appears to be mediated through an interaction with $GABA_A$ receptors, on the basis of the attenuated effects seen in the presence of the $GABA_A$ antagonists bicuculline and picrotoxin[58].

## 5.4 Summary

Barbiturates exert their effects via diverse cellular and molecular mechanisms. The available evidence suggests that GABA-mediated pre- and postsynaptic inhibition is much more sensitive to the actions of barbiturates than are voltage-gated $Na^+$ and $K^+$ channels, which are blocked only at supratherapeutic concentrations. It appears that barbiturates, at low to moderate concentrations (10–50 μM) produce, first, a profound enhancement of the postsynaptic actions of GABA, an effect which is mediated at the level of the $GABA_A$ receptor–$Cl^-$ channel complex to decrease postsynaptic excitability (i.e. mediate postsynaptic inhibition); and, second, an enhancement of GABA binding at $GABA_A$ receptors on presynaptic terminals to increase the degree of presynaptic inhibition and reduce excitatory transmitter release. These actions alone are sufficient to account for the sedative–hypnotic actions of barbiturates. A more profound degree of GABA-mediated pre- and postsynaptic inhibition following direct activation of the GABA receptor-linked $Cl^-$ channel probably underlies the main mechanism for barbiturate anaesthesia at higher concentrations. Reduction in $Ca^{2+}$-dependent transmitter release may contribute to the anaesthetic actions of barbiturates. This comes about by barbiturate blockade of presynaptic VSCC or by enhancement of $Ca^{2+}$ uptake by intraterminal mitochondria. Other effects of barbiturates on receptor-mediated processes can be seen at synapses that use transmitter substances other than GABA. It remains to be established, however, if barbiturates exert differential potencies for blocking the release of different types of central transmitter.

## References

1. Armitage AG, Hall GH and Sellars CM (1969) Effects of nicotine on electrocortical activity and acetylcholine release from cat cerebral cortex. *British Journal of Pharmacology* **35**: 152–160
2. Axelrod J, Weil-Malherbe H and Tomchick R (1959) The physiological disposition of $^3$H-epinephrine and its metabolite metanephrine. *Journal of Pharmacology and Experimental Therapeutics* **127**: 251–256
3. Axelrod J, Whitby LJ and Hertting G (1961) Effects of psychotropic drugs on the uptake of $^3$H-norepinephrine by tissues. *Science* **133**: 383–384
4. Benwell ME and Balfour DJK (1992) The effects of acute and repeated nicotine treatment on nucleus accumbens dopamine and locomotor activity. *British Journal of Pharmacology* **105**: 849–856
5. Benwell MEM, Balfour DJK and Anderson JM (1988) Evidence that tobacco smoking increases the density of $(-)[^3H]$-nicotine binding sites in human brain. *Journal of Neurochemistry* **50**: 1243–1247
6. Birnbaumer L (1990) Transduction of receptor signal into modulation of effector activity by G protcins: the first 20 years or so. *Federation of American Societies for Experimental Biology Journal* **4**: 3068–3078
7. Bowman WC, Prior C and Marshall IG (1990) Presynaptic receptors in the neuromuscular junction. *Annals of the New York Academy of Sciences* **604**: 69–81
8. Burn JH (1932) The action of tyramine and ephedrine. *Journal of Pharmacology and Experimental Therapeutics* **46**: 75–95
9. Carboni E, Imperato A, Perezzani L and Di Chiara G (1989) Amphetamine, cocaine, phencyclidine and nomifensine increase extracellular dopamine concentrations preferentially in the nucleus accumbens of freely moving rats. *Neuroscience* **28**: 653–661
10. Carmichael FJ and Israel Y (1975) Effects of ethanol on neurotransmitter release by rat brain cortical slices. *Journal of Pharmacology and Experimental Therapeutics* **193**: 824–834

11. Chahl LA (1986) Withdrawal responses of guinea-pig isolated ileum following brief exposure to opiates and opioid peptides. *Naunyn-Schmiedeberg's Archives of Pharmacology* **333**: 387–392

12. Chiappinelli VA (1993) Neurotoxins acting on acetylcholine receptors. In: Harvey AL (ed), *Natural and Synthetic Neurotoxins*, pp 65–128, London, Academic Press

13. Childers SR (1993) Opioid receptor-coupled second messenger systems. In: Akil H and Simon EJ (eds), *Handbook of Experimental Pharmacology*, vol 104, *Opioids I* , pp 189–216, Springer-Verlag, Berlin

14. Clarke PBS, Hommer DW, Pert A and Skirboll LR (1985) Electrophysiological actions of nicotine on substantia nigra single units. *British Journal of Pharmacology* **85**: 827–835

15. Clarke PBS, Schwartz RD, Paul SM, Pert CB and Pert A (1985) Nicotinic binding in rat brain: autoradiographic comparison of [$^3$H]acetylcholine, [$^3$H]nicotine and [$^{125}$I] bungarotoxin. *Journal of Neuroscience* **5**: 1307–1315

16. Collier HOJ and Roy AC (1974) Morphine-like drugs inhibit the stimulation by E prostaglandins of cyclic AMP formation by rat brain homogenates. *Nature* **248**: 24–27

17. Conroy WG, Vernallis AB and Berg DK (1992) The α5 gene product assembles with multiple acetylcholine receptor subunits to form distinctive receptor subtypes in brain. *Neuron* **9**: 679–691

18. Cox BM (1993) Opioid receptor-G protein interactions: acute and chronic effects of opioids. In: Akil H and Simon EJ (eds), *Handbook of Experimental Pharmacology*, vol 104, *Opioids I*, pp 145–188, Springer-Verlag, Berlin

19. Creese I and Iversen SD (1974) The role of dopamine forebrain systems in amphetamine-induced stereotyped behaviour in the rat. *Psychopharmacologia* **39**: 345–357

20. Damsma G, Day J and Fibiger HC (1989) Lack of tolerance to nicotine-induced dopamine release in the nucleus accumbens. *European Journal of Pharmacology* **168**: 363–368

21. Deitrich RA, Dunwiddie TV, Harris RA and Erwin VG (1989) Mechanism of action of ethanol–initial central nervous system actions. *Pharmacological Reviews* **41**: 489–537

22. Di Chiara G, Acquas E, Tanda G and Cadoni C (1994) Drugs of abuse: biochemical surrogates of specific aspects of natural reward? In: Wonnacott S and Lunt GG (eds), *Neurochemistry of Drug Dependence*, pp 65–82, Portland Press, Colchester, UK

23. Duggan AW and Fleetwood-Walker SM (1993) Opioids and sensory processing in the central nervous system. In: Akil H and Simon EJ (eds), *Handbook of Experimental Pharmacology*, vol 104, *Opioids I*, pp 731–771, Springer-Verlag, Berlin

24. Dworkin SI, Porrino LJ and Smith JE (1993) Neurobiological substrates of opioid abuse. In: Hammer RP (ed), *The Neurobiology of Opiates*, pp 333–360, CRC Press Boca Raton, FL

25. Fields HL (1993) Brainstem mechanisms of pain modulation: anatomy and physiology. In: Akil H and Simon EJ (eds), *Handbook of Experimental Pharmacology*, vol 104, *Opioids II*, pp 3–20, Springer-Verlag, Berlin

26. Fink K and Göthert M (1990) Inhibition of N-methyl-D-aspartate-induced noradrenaline release by alcohols in proportion to their hydrophobicity. *European Journal of Pharmacology* **191**: 225–229

27. Fink K, Schultheiß R and Göthert M (1992) Inhibition of N-methyl-D-aspartate- and kainate-evoked noradrenaline release in human cerebral cortex slices by ethanol. *Naunyn-Schmiedeberg's Archives of Pharmacology* **345**: 700–703

28. Fischer JF and Cho AK (1979) Chemical release of dopamine from striatal homogenates: evidence for an exchange diffusion model. *Journal of Pharmacology and Experimental Therapeutics* **208**: 203–209

29. Flores CM, Rogers SW, Pabreza LA, Wolfe BB and Kellar KJ (1992) A subtype of nicotinic cholinergic receptor in rat brain is composed of α4 and β2 subunits and is upregulated by chronic nicotine treatment. *Molecular Pharmacology* **41**: 31–37

30. Giros B and Caron MG (1993) Molecular characterisation of the dopamine transporter. *Trends in Pharmacological Sciences* **14**: 43–49

31. Göthert M (1979) Modification of catecholamine release by anaesthetics and alcohols. In: Paton DM (ed), *The Release of Catecholamines from Adrenergic Neurons*, pp 241–261, Pergamon Press, Oxford

32. Göthert M and Fink K (1989) Inhibition of N-methyl-D-aspartate (NMDA) and L-glutamate induced noradrenaline and acetylcholine

release in the rat brain by ethanol. *Naunyn-Schmiedeberg's Archives of Pharmacology* **340:** 516–521

33. Gonzales RA and Hoffmann PL (1991) Receptor-gated ion channels may be selective CNS targets for ethanol. *Trends in Pharmacological Sciences* **12:** 1–3

34. Grady S, Marks M, Wonnacott S and Collins AC (1992) Characterization of nicotinic receptor mediated [³H]dopamine release from synaptosomes prepared from mouse striatum. *Journal of Neurochemistry* **59:** 848–856

35. Gross RA and Macdonald RL (1988) Differential actions of pentobarbitone on calcium current components of mouse sensory neurones in culture. *Journal of Physiology* **405:** 187–203

36. Grudt TJ and Williams JT (1993) Kappa-opioid receptors also increase potassium conductance. *Proceedings of the National Academy of Sciences USA* **90:** 11429–11432

37. Heikkila RE, Orlansky H and Cohen G (1975) Studies on the distinction between uptake inhibition and release of (³H)dopamine in rat brain tissue slices. *Biochemical Pharmacology* **24:** 847–852

38. Herz A and Shippenberg TS (1989) Neurochemical aspects of addiction: opioids and other drugs of abuse. In: Goldstein A (ed), *Molecular and Cellular Aspects of the Drug Addictions*, pp 111–141, Springer-Verlag, New York

39. Hughes JAH, Smith TW, Kosterlitz HW, Fothergill LA, Morgan B and Morris HR (1975) Identification of two related pentapeptides from brain with potent opiate agonist activity. *Nature* **258:** 577–579

40. Imperato A, Mulas A, and Di Chiara G (1986) Nicotine preferentially stimulates dopamine release in the limbic system of freely moving rats. *European Journal of Pharmacology* **132:** 337–338

41. Jaffe JH (1990) Drug addiction and drug abuse. In: Goodman LS, Gilman A, Rall Th W, Nies A S, Taylor P (eds), *Goodman and Gilman's The Pharmacological Basis of Therapeutics*, pp 522–573, Pergamon Press, New York

42. Jaffe JH and Martin WA (1991) Opioid analgesics and antagonists. In: Gilman A, Rall TW, Nies AS and Taylor P (eds), *Goodman and Gilman's The Pharmacological Basis of Therapeutics*, 8th edn, pp 485–521, Pergamon Press, New York

43. Jessell TM and Iversen LL (1977) Opiate analgesics inhibit substance P release from rat trigeminal nucleus. *Nature* **268:** 549–551

44. Johnson RG (1988) Accumulation of biological amines into chromaffin granules: a model for hormone and neurotransmitter transport. *Physiological Reviews* **68:** 232–307

45. Johnson SM and Fleming WW (1989) Mechanisms of cellular adaptive sensitivity changes: applications to opioid tolerance and dependence. *Pharmacological Reviews* **41:** 435–488

46. Krnjevic K (1986) Cellular and synaptic effects of general anesthetics. In: Roth SH and Miller KW (eds), *Molecular and Cellular Mechanisms of Anesthetics*, pp 3–16, Plenum Press, New York

47. Lapchak PA, Araujo DM, Quirion R and Collier B (1989) Effect of chronic nicotine treatment on nicotinic autoreceptor function and N-[³H]methylcarbamylcholine binding sites in the rat brain. *Journal of Neurochemistry* **52:** 483–491

48. Lena C, Changeux J-P and Mulle C (1993) Evidence for 'preterminal' nicotinic receptors on GABAergic axons in the rat interpeduncular nucleus. *Journal of Neuroscience* **13:** 2680–2688

49. Leslie SW, Friedman MB, Wilcox RE and Elrod SV (1980) Acute and chronic effects of barbiturates on depolarization-induced calcium influx into rat synaptosomes. *Brain Research* **185:** 409–417

50. Liang NY and Rutledge CO (1982) Comparison of the release of [³H]dopamine from isolated corpus striatum by amphetamine, fenfluramine and unlabeled dopamine. *Biochemical Pharmacology* **31:** 983–992

51. Macdonald RL, Rogers CJ and Twyman RE (1989) Barbiturate regulation of kinetic properties of the GABA$_A$ receptor channel of mouse spinal neurones in culture. *Journal of Physiology* **417:** 483–500

52. Mansour A, Khachaturian H, Lewis ME, Akil H and Watson SJ (1988) Anatomy of CNS opioid receptors. *Trends in Neurosciences* **11:** 308–316

53. Marks MJ, Grady SR and Collins AC (1993) Downregulation of nicotinic receptor function after chronic nicotine infusion *Journal of Pharmacology and Experimental Therapeutics* **266:** 1268–1276

54. Mathers DA and Barker JL (1980)

(−)Pentobarbital opens ion channels of long duration in cultured mouse spinal neurons. *Science* **209:** 507–509

55. Moore KE (1978) Amphetamines: biochemical and behavioural actions in animals. In: Iversen LL, Iversen SD and Snyder SH (eds), *Handbook of Psychopharmacology*, pp 41–98, Plenum Press, New York

56. Mulder AH and Schoffelmeer ANM (1993) Multiple opioid receptors and presynaptic modulation of neurotransmitter release in the brain. In: Akil H and Simon EJ (eds), *Handbook of Experimental Pharmacology*, vol 104, *Opioids I*, pp 125–144, Springer-Verlag, Berlin

57. Nicholson GM, Spence I and Johnston GAR (1988) Differing actions of convulsant and nonconvulsant barbiturates: an electrophysiological study in the isolated spinal cord of the rat. *Neuropharmacology* **27:** 459–465

58. Nicoll RA (1975) Presynaptic action of barbiturates in the frog spinal cord. *Proceedings of the National Academy of Sciences USA* **72:** 1460–1463

59. Nicoll RA (1980) Sedatives-hypnotics: animal pharmacology. *Handbook of Psychopharmacology* **12:** 187–234

60. Nomikos GG, Damsma G, Wenkstern D and Fibiger HC (1990) *In vivo* characterisation of locally applied dopamine uptake inhibitors by striatal microdialysis. *Synapse* **6:** 106–112

61. North RA (1993) Opioid actions on membrane ion channels. In: Akil H and Simon EJ (eds), *Handbook of Experimental Pharmacology*, vol 104, *Opioids II*, pp 773–797, Springer-Verlag, Berlin

62. North RA and Williams JT (1983) How do opiates inhibit transmitter release? *Trends in Neurosciences* **6:** 337–339

63. Oderda GM and Klein-Schwartz W (1982) Central nervous stimulants. In: Skoutakis VA (ed), *Clinical Toxicology of Drugs: Principles and Practice*, pp 183–199, Lea and Febiger, Philadelphia

64. Ollat H, Parvez H and Parvez S (1988) Alcohol and central neurotransmission. *Neurochemistry International* **13:** 275–300

65. Olsen RW, Sapp DM, Bureau MH, Turner DM and Kokka N (1991) Allosteric actions of central nervous system depressants including anesthetics on subtypes of the inhibitory γ-aminobutyric acid$_A$ receptor–chloride

channel complex. *Annals of the New York Academy of Sciences* **625:** 145–154

66. Parker EM and Cubbedu LX (1988) Comparative effects of amphetamine, phenylethylamine and related drugs, on dopamine efflux, dopamine uptake and mazindol binding. *Journal of Pharmacology and Experimental Therapeutics* **245:** 199–210

67. Pincus JH and Insler NF (1981) Barbiturates and transmitter release at the frog neuromuscular junction. *Brain Research* **213:** 127–137

68. Raiteri M, Angelini F and Levi G (1974) A simple apparatus for studying the release of neurotransmitters from synaptosomes. *European Journal of Pharmacology* **25:** 411–414

69. Raiteri M, Cerrito F, Cervoni AM, del Carmine R, Ribera MT and Levi G (1978) Studies on dopamine uptake and release in synaptosomes. In: Roberts PJ, Woodruff GN and Iversen LL (eds), *Advances in Biochemical Psychopharmacology*, pp 35–56, Raven Press, New York

70. Rall Th W (1990) Hypnotics and sedatives; ethanol. In: Goodman LS, Gilman A, Rall Th W, Nies A S, Taylor P (eds), *Goodman and Gilman's The Pharmacological Basis of Therapeutics*, pp 345–382, Pergamon Press, New York

71. Rang HP and Dale MM (1991) Analgesic drugs. In: *Pharmacology*, 2nd edn, pp 706–732, Churchill Livingstone, Edinburgh

72. Reisine T and Bell GI (1993) Molecular biology of opioid receptors. *Trends in Neurosciences* **16:** 506–510

73. Robinson TE and Becker JB (1986) Enduring changes in brain and behaviour produced by chronic amphetamine administration: a review and evaluation of animal models of amphetamine psychosis. *Brain Research* **396:** 157–198

74. Roth SH, Tan K and MacIver B (1986) Selective and differential effects of barbiturates on neuronal activity. In: Roth SH and Miller KW (eds), *Molecular and Cellular Mechanisms of Anesthetics*, pp 43–56, Plenum Press, New York

75. Rowell PP and Wonnacott S (1990) Evidence for functional activity of up-regulated nicotine binding sites in rat striatal synaptosomes. *Journal of Neurochemistry* **55:** 2105–2110

76. Rudnick G and Wall SC (1992) The molecular mechanism of 'ecstasy' [3,4-methylene-

dioxymethamphetamine (MDMA)]: serotonin transporters are targets for MDMA-induced serotonin release. *Proceedings of the National Academy of Sciences USA* **89:** 1817–1821

77. Rudnick G and Wall SC (1992) Chloramphetamine induce serotonin release through serotonin transporters. *Biochemistry* **31:** 6710–6718

78. Sargent PB (1993) The diversity of neuronal nicotinic acetylcholine receptors. *Annual Reviews of Neuroscience* **16:** 403–443

79. Seiden LS, Sabol KE and Ricuarte GA (1993) Amphetamine: effects on catecholamine systems and behavior. *Annual Review of Pharmacology and Toxicology* **32:** 639–677

80. Shen K-F and Crain SM (1989) Dual opioid modulation of the action potential duration of mouse dorsal root ganglion neurons in culture. *Brain Research* **491:** 227–242

81. Shulz DW and Macdonald RL (1981) Barbiturate enhancement of GABA-mediated inhibition and activation of chloride ion conductance: correlation with anticonvulsant and anesthetic actions. *Brain Research* **209:** 177–188

82. Stein C (1993) Peripheral mechanisms of opioid analgesia. In: Akil H and Simon EJ (eds), *Handbook of Experimental Pharmacology*, vol 104, *Opioids II*, pp 91–104, Springer-Verlag, Berlin

83. Suarez-Roca H and Maixner W (1992) Morphine produces a multiphasic effect on the release of substance P from rat trigeminal nucleus slices by activating different opioid receptor subtypes. *Brain Research* **579:** 195–203

84. Sulzer D and Rayport S (1990) Amphetamine and other psychostimulants reduce pH gradients in midbrain dopaminergic neurons and chromaffin granules: a mechanism of action. *Neuron* **5:** 797–808

85. Taylor P, Culver P, Brown RD, Herz J and Johnson DA (1986) An approach to anesthetic action from studies of acetylcholine receptor function. In: Roth SH and Miller KW (eds), *Molecular and Cellular Mechanisms of Anesthetics*, pp 99–110, Plenum Press, New York

86. Teichberg VI, Tal N, Goldberg O and Luini A (1984) Barbiturates alcohols and the CNS excitatory neurotransmission: specific effects on the kainate and quisqualate receptors. *Brain Research* **291:** 285–292

87. Watson SJ, Trujillo KA, Herman JP and Akil H (1989). Neuroanatomical and neurochemical substrates of drug-seeking behavior: overview and future directions. In: Goldstein A (ed), *Molecular and Cellular Aspects of the Drug Addictions*, pp 29–91, Springer-Verlag, New York

88. Weakly JN (1969) Effect of barbiturates on 'quantal' synaptic transmission in spinal motoneurones. *Journal of Physiology* **204:** 63–77

89. Wilkie GI, Stephens MW, Hutson PJ, Whiting P and Wonnacott S (1993) Hippocampal nicotinic autoreceptors modulate acetylcholine release. *Biochemical Society Transactions* **21:** 429–431

90. Willow M and Johnston GAR (1983) Pharmacology of barbiturates: electrophysiological and neurochemical studies. *International Reviews of Neurobiology* **24:** 15–45

91. Winkler H (1988) Occurrence and mechanism of exocytosis in adrenal medulla and sympathetic nerve. In: Trendelenburg U and Weiner N (eds), *Catecholamines I*, pp 43–118, Springer-Verlag, New York

92. Wonnacott S (1990) The paradox of nicotinic acetylcholine receptor upregulation by nicotine. *Trends in Pharmacological Sciences* **11:** 216–219

93. Wonnacott S, Drasdo A, Sanderson E and Rowell P (1990) Presynaptic nicotinic receptors and the modulation of transmitter release. In: Marsh J (ed), *Ciba Foundation Symposium 152: The Biology of Nicotine Dependence*, pp 87–101, John Wiley, Chichester

94. Wooten GF (1993). Functional anatomy of opiate withdrawal. In: Hammer RP (ed), *The Neurobiology of Opiates*, pp 165–174, CRC Press Boca Raton, FL

95. Yu ZJ and Wecker L (1994) Chronic nicotine administration differentially affects neurotransmitter release from rat striatal slices. *Journal of Neurochemistry* **63:** 186–194

# 17 Beneficial therapeutic interventions via manipulation of presynaptic modulatory mechanisms

Thomas C. Westfall

If, as suggested in Chapters 14 and 15, alterations in neurotransmitter release-modulating mechanisms underlie some pathophysiological conditions, then drugs acting at the receptors that trigger the mechanisms offer a potentially important means for therapeutic intervention. In this final chapter, Thomas Westfall considers some of the human conditions that have been treated therapeutically with drugs that are thought to act in major part by pharmacologically manipulating neurotransmitter release at certain types of synapse, by stimulating or blocking presynaptic receptors that modulate release. Important issues are raised that are of relevance to treating other conditions that result from hypo- or hypersecretion of neurotransmitters or neurohormones.

## 1   Introduction

The previous chapters of this volume have discussed the overwhelming evidence for the existence of presynaptic receptors, and their pharmacological characterisation, physiological significance and the mechanisms by which they exert their action. Moreover the clinical relevance of presynaptic receptors has also been addressed. As discussed in the preceding chapters, it is known that these receptors may be located on the soma, dendrites or axons of neurones, where they may respond to neurotransmitters or modulators released from the same neurone or from adjacent neurones or cells. Soma-dendritic receptors are those receptors located on, or near, the cell body and dendrites and, when activated, primarily modify functions of the soma-dendritic region, such as protein synthesis and generation of action potentials. Presynaptic receptors, by convention, are those receptors presumed to be located on, in, or near axon

terminals or varicosities and when activated modify functions of the terminal region, possibly transmitter synthesis and certainly transmitter release. Two main classes of presynaptic receptor have been identified: heteroreceptors are those presynaptic receptors that respond to neurotransmitters or modulators released from adjacent neurones or cells, or distant tissues (see Chapters 6 and 7), while autoreceptors are those receptors located on or close to those axon terminals of a neurone through which the neurone's own transmitter can and, under appropriate conditions may, modify transmitter synthesis or release (see Chapter 5). Fig. 17.1 and Table 17.1 summarise in general terms the possible auto- and heteroceptors, the result of their activation with appropriate agonists and the result of their blockade by antagonists. If a maintained increase or decrease in neurotransmitter release contributes to the pathophysiology or symptoms of a disease, then drugs that act at autoreceptors or hetero-

**Table 17.1.**  *Types of presynaptic receptors*

| Location of receptor | Type of receptor | Effect of activation of receptor | Effect of blockade of receptor |
| --- | --- | --- | --- |
| Soma-dendritic | Inhibitory autoreceptor | Decrease in impulse traffic | Increase in impulse traffic |
| Soma-dendritic | Excitatory autoreceptor | Increase in impulse traffic | Decrease in impulse traffic |
| Soma-dendritic | Inhibitory heteroreceptor | Decrease in impulse traffic | Increase in impulse traffic |
| Soma-dendritic | Excitatory heteroreceptor | Increase in impulse traffic | Decrease in impulse traffic |
| Terminal region | Inhibitory autoreceptor | Decrease in release/synthesis | Increase in release/synthesis |
| Terminal region | Excitatory autoreceptor | Increase in release/synthesis | Decrease in release/synthesis |
| Terminal region | Inhibitory heteroreceptor | Decrease in release/synthesis | Increase in release/synthesis |
| Terminal region | Excitatory heteroreceptor | Increase in release/synthesis | Decrease in release/synthesis |

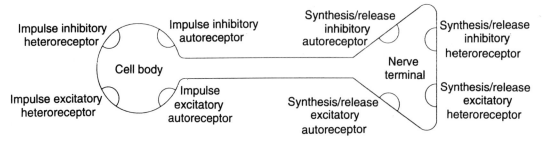

Fig. 17.1. A representation of the cell body and terminal region of a hypothetical neurone. Impulse-modulating inhibitory and excitatory heteroreceptors or impulse-modulating inhibitory or excitatory autoreceptors exist on the soma or dendrites of neurones. Likewise in the terminal region, there may be inhibitory or excitatory heteroreceptors and inhibitory or excitatory autoreceptors that regulate synthesis and/or release of the transmitter.

receptors that modulate the release might alleviate the symptoms and/or improve the outcome of the disease. In this chapter some examples are discussed where such therapeutic interventions or strategies have been tried, or have the potential to be useful therapy. Examples are provided for the treatment of three types of disease and serve as examples of therapeutic manipulation of presynaptic receptors. These are: schizophrenia, non-insulin-dependent diabetes and essential hypertension.

## 2  Dopamine receptors and schizophrenia

### 2.1  Dopamine autoreceptors

The one area that has probably generated the greatest interest in the manipulation of presynaptic receptors for therapeutic benefit has been in the field of dopamine autoreceptors. The term autoreceptor was first coined by Arvid Carlsson in the early 1970s, at which time it was suggested that the released neurotransmitter, in this case dopamine, could activate presynaptic receptors, which then decreased subsequent nerve stimulation-induced release of the transmitter[9]. This concept has been substantiated through the years and is now used to describe this type of feedback modulation for all transmitters in the nervous system.

Currently dopamine autoreceptors are thought to carry out three functions: inhibition of impulse flow (e.g. a decrease in propagated action potentials down the neurone), inhibition of synthesis, and inhibition of release of dopamine. The impulse-regulating autoreceptors are thought to be located on the soma-dendritic region of dopamine neurones, while synthesis- and release-regulating autoreceptors are thought to be present on the terminal region (e.g. presynaptic receptors, see Fig. 17.1 and Table 17.1). Within the brain, there are regional differences in the representation of these three types of dopamine autoreceptor. This is thought to explain the differences in basal dopaminergic activity (e.g. amount of impulse traffic, synthesis and release of dopamine) that exists in dopamine neurones in different brain regions. However, it is unclear whether these three types of functional autoreceptor correspond to distinctly different receptor subtypes (see below).

### 2.2  The dopamine hypothesis of schizophrenia

Alterations in dopamine function are thought to underlie various psychiatric illnesses including some subtypes of schizophrenia. Since the 1970s, it has been hypothesised that there is increased dopaminergic neurotransmission in schizophrenia, the so called dopamine hypothesis of schizophrenia[34].

Although some of the evidence does not fit, this hypothesis has held up well through the years. Since the 1960s, it has been suggested that the mechanism for the therapeutic usefulness of antischizophrenic drugs (often referred to as neuroleptics) is that they block soma-dendritic $D_2$ receptors located on neurones receiving dopaminergic innervation (postsynaptic $D_2$ receptors)[11,35]. Long-term use of these drugs appears to produce also depolarisation–inactivation of the dopamine neurones themselves. This is thought to be the result of a reduction in activity of the neurones that feedback (long-loop feedback) onto dopamine cell bodies and normally inhibit their firing rate. Inhibition of this pathway would result initially in activation of the dopamine neurones; long-term activation results in the depolarising block and inactivation via mechanisms not clearly understood[11,35]. More recently it has been hypothesised that it is the positive symptoms of schizophrenia (e.g. hallucinations, paranoia, etc.) that are associated with increased dopaminergic neuronal activity with consequent increased release of dopamine (the original Dopamine Hypothesis) and it is these symptoms that are alleviated by neuroleptics. In contrast, the negative symptoms of the disease (flat affect, withdrawal, lack of motivation, etc.) are associated with decreased dopaminergic neuronal activity with consequent decreased dopamine release. These are not benefitted by neuroleptic drugs[34]. Newer neuroleptic agents such as clozapine have been found more useful in treating negative as well as positive symptoms and have less severe side effects (extrapyramidal effects and tardive dyskinesia, see below)[34]. The mechanism of action of drugs such as clozapine and how they may benefit both positive and regulative symptoms are discussed below.

## 2.3  The role of dopamine autoreceptors in schizophrenia

Since the early days of the autoreceptor concept, evidence has accumulated that presynaptic autoreceptors might be more sensitive to dopamine agonists, including dopamine, than are the postsynaptic dopamine receptors[10]. For instance, it was observed that some dopamine agonists showed biphasic dose–response curves with regard to locomotor activity, with low doses causing inhibition and higher doses causing stimulation. This suggested that the agonists were acting on more than one type of receptor. One type, located presynaptically, led to inhibition of locomotor activity, via inhibition of dopamine release and subsequent reduction in postsynaptic stimulation. Another type, located postsynaptically, led to stimulation of locomotor activity. Subsequently, dopamine receptors were subclassified into $D_1$ and $D_2$ based on pharmacological, biochemical, electrophysiological and behavioural evidence[25]. Dopamine receptors have now been further classified into at least five subtypes ($D_1$, $D_2$, $D_3$, $D_4$ and $D_5$) based on molecular cloning strategies[12].

Although the dopamine autoreceptor is thought to be of the $D_2$ receptor subtype, its precise character is still not completely established. If the autoreceptor is a $D_2$ type, then the receptor either has both a presynaptic and postsynaptic representation or there are further subtypes, with the presynaptic $D_2$ receptor different from the postsynaptic $D_2$ receptor. There has been a concerted effort to develop selective dopamine autoreceptor agonists and a number of such agents are now available. Several drugs have been developed that show autoreceptor selectivity, although many are, at best, only partial agonists and behave as weak $D_2$ antagonists at postsynaptic receptors[10,13,45]. Many of these drugs are now undergoing clinical trials in the treatment of schizophrenia and there is evidence suggesting that they are effective. According to Carlsson[10], the autoreceptor partial agonists may be useful clinically because of the combination of postsynaptic antagonism and presynaptic agonist properties. At the autoreceptor, they may behave as agonists because of the low endogenous dopamine present in the vicinity of these receptors. Their action here would be to decrease dopamine release. At the same time, at postsynaptic receptors where they behave as antagonists, they would prevent the action of dopamine present in the synapse. This may allow these drugs to have antipsychotic activity but with the production of minimal extrapyramidal symptoms and perhaps less production of the severe side effect of tardive dyskinesia.

## 2.4   The development and potential of dopamine autoreceptor agonists for the treatment of schizophrenia

There is increasing interest in developing selective dopamine autoreceptor full agonists free of postsynaptic antagonism properties. Such drugs have the potential to be important new therapeutic agents for the treatment of the positive symptoms of schizophrenia (where increased dopaminergic activity is suspected) and possibly other neuropsychiatric illnesses.

Herbert Y. Meltzer has recently summarised the effects on dopamine autoreceptors that would be desirable for dopamine autoreceptor agonists[34]. These include: selective effects on different types of autoreceptor (release, synthesis and impulse-inhibiting autoreceptors); selective effects in various brain regions; down-regulation of only some types of dopamine autoreceptor; ability to produce differences in the postsynaptic feedback mechanisms that overcome the presynaptic effects of the agonists; ability to induce changes in postsynaptic dopamine receptor sensitivity; and, finally, possessing differences in the extent of the ability to produce degeneration of dopamine neurones in different neuropsychiatric illnesses.

Although it is not possible to predict how useful selective dopamine autoreceptor agonists will be and for which subtypes of schizophrenia or other psychiatric disease they will be useful, this is nevertheless a very exciting time and more information should soon be forthcoming on the utility of these agents since several drugs are now in clinical trial. It is hoped that this will result in improved treatment strategies for controlling the positive symptoms of schizophrenia alongside less side effects. These agents may also be useful as antimanic drugs, as well as for controlling the symptoms of Huntington's chorea, Tourette's syndrome and spasmodic torticollis.

## 2.5   Clozapine: a prototypic atypical antipsychotic that acts on multiple dopamine receptors

Within the last few years, the drug clozapine has appeared on the scene and has been found to be more effective in treating both positive and negative symptoms of schizophrenia than the commonly used neuroleptic drugs. Clozapine has also been shown to produce fewer extrapyramidal symptoms such as tremor, bradykinesia and rigidity (similar to that seen in Parkinson's patients). Furthermore, clozapine has not been found to produce tardive dyskinesia and does not increase serum prolactin levels in man[34]. This has been hailed as a major breakthrough and numerous studies have been conducted in order to discover its mechanism of action. Although there are still a large number of conflicting results, it is obvious that clozapine has complex actions and the mechanisms underlying its clinical usefulness are still uncertain.

It is clear that the acute and chronic effects of clozapine are different and that the chronic effects are more relevant to the mechanism(s) of its antipsychotic action. There are a large number of studies suggesting that clozapine is an effective dopamine receptor antagonist, having the capacity to modulate impulse-regulating soma-dendritic and release-inhibiting presynaptic dopamine autoreceptors on dopaminergic neurones. It is also thought that clozapine acts as an antagonist on dopamine heteroreceptors located on cholinergic, serotonergic and noradrenergic neurones, which alter acetylcholine, 5-HT and noradrenaline release. Clozapine also has the ability to antagonise postsynaptic $D_2$ and 5-HT$_2$ receptors. Other studies suggest that clozapine acts on the $D_4$ subtype of dopamine receptor although the location, presynaptic or postsynaptic, of this receptor is unclear. Clozapine also exerts considerable regional selectivity, exerting different effects on dopamine neurones in the prefrontal cortex, mesolimbic regions and striatal neurones. For example, the ability of clozapine to increase dopamine release in the striatum and frontal cortex without diminishing dopamine release in the nucleus accumbens has been suggested to explain the reduced tendency of the drug to produce extrapyramidal side effects and contributes to its better action on positive schizophrenic symptoms[34]. In addition, clozapine's ability to increase the turnover and release of dopamine in the prefrontal cortex may be beneficial in treating negative symptoms of schizophrenia[34]. Although these last points are largely speculative, it would appear that a fruitful area of research is to develop other drugs that (i) have regional selectivity, and (ii) have differential effects on presynaptic receptors (autoreceptors and heteroreceptors) and on postsynaptic receptors, as proposed by Meltzer[34]. This would enable a drug to block certain of the actions of key neurotransmitters but at the same time maintain some level of neurotransmission by that neurotransmitter.

## 3   Treatment of non-insulin-dependent diabetes mellitus and $\alpha_2$-adrenoceptors

### 3.1   Regulation of insulin secretion

Non-insulin-dependent diabetes (NIDDM) is considered to be a heterogeneous group of disorders characterised by impaired insulin secretion, peripheral insulin resistance and increased basal hepatic glucose production[20,26]. The underlying pathogenic mechanisms in NIDDM remains unknown. It is a common disease affecting millions of people worldwide and it appears that the majority of patients with diabetes have NIDDM. Therapeutic strategies for the treatment of NIDDM have included diet control and loss of weight as drugs to promote the release of insulin.

The regulation of insulin release is complex and involves a variety of hormonal and neuronal influences, including those exerted by the autonomic nervous system[1,15]. Insulin is produced by and stored in the $\beta$ cells of the pancreatic islets of Langerhans and its release results in a decrease in blood glucose and hypoglycaemia. The $\beta$ cells of the pancreas, like other cell types present in this organ, receive dual innervation by parasympathetic and sympathetic nerves of the autonomic nervous system and contain a variety of receptors that can be activated by mediators (transmitters and co-transmitters) released from parasympathetic or sympathetic nerves. Stimulation of parasympathetic nerves leads to an increase in insulin release, which is mediated by activation of muscarinic receptors by acetylcholine or via peptides co-stored and co-released with acetylcholine, such as VIP, gastrin and/or cholecystokinin[1,15]. Stimulation of sympathetic nerves, however, can result in either an increase or a decrease in insulin release depending on the receptor activated[1,30]. Stimulation of $\alpha_2$-adrenoceptors by released noradrenaline results in a decrease in insulin release while activation of $\beta$-adrenoceptors results in an increase in insulin release[2,3,4,30,42,43]. Physiologically, it is considered that activation of $\alpha_2$-adrenoceptors predominates following stimulation of sympathetic nerves. In addition to the classical neurotransmitter noradrenaline, it is now known that co-transmitters in sympathetic nerves, such as neuropeptide Y or galanin, may also be released, and that these also modulate insulin release[15,30]. As is the case with sympathetic neurones elsewhere, there are presynaptic $\alpha_2$-autoreceptors on nerves innervating the pancreas. Activation of these autoreceptors results in a decreased noradrenaline release, while blockade of these receptors results in an increase in the evoked release of noradrenaline.

### 3.2 The role of $\alpha_2$-adrenoceptors in mediating insulin secretion

As mentioned above, it has now been demonstrated by numerous groups that post-synaptic $\alpha_2$-adrenoceptors are involved in the inhibition of insulin release by sympathetic nerve stimulation[2,3,4,30,42,43]. This has been demonstrated in several species, including humans, and in isolated islets where insulin release was stimulated by glucose. A variety of $\alpha_2$-adrenoceptor agonists have been shown to exert these inhibitory effects, while $\alpha_1$- or $\beta$-adrenoceptor agonists failed to do so. Likewise, the inhibition of insulin release and the parallel hyperglycaemic response was antagonised by $\alpha_2$-adrenoceptor antagonists but not by $\alpha_1$- or $\beta$-adrenoceptor antagonists. Recently, molecular cloning strategies and biochemical–pharmacological studies have suggested the existence of multiple subtypes of $\alpha$- and $\beta$-adrenoceptors[8,36]. These receptor subtypes arise from different gene products and exhibit differences in the rank order of potency to agonists and antagonists. There is evidence that the inhibition of insulin release is mediated by the $\alpha_{2A}$-adrenoceptor subtype but not by the $\alpha_{2B}$ subtype[42]. This conclusion is supported by the fact that the $\alpha_{2A}$-adreno-ceptor preferential agonist, oxymetazoline but not $\alpha_{2B}$-subtype-selective agonists inhibit-ed the release of insulin from isolated rat pancreatic islets and the hyperglycaemic response *in vivo*. Similarly, neither $\alpha_1$-adreno-ceptor-selective agonists, nor $\beta$-adrenoceptor agonists altered either glucose-evoked insulin release or sympathetic nerve stimulation-induced hyperglycaemia. The effects of both non-specific $\alpha_2$-adrenoceptor agonists and selective $\alpha_{2A}$-adrenoceptor agonists were attenuated by $\alpha_{2A}$-adrenoceptor-selective antagonists such as WB 410, while $\alpha_{2B}$-, $\alpha_1$- or $\beta$-adrenoceptor-selective antagonists failed to block the $\alpha_{2A}$-adrenoceptor-mediated inhi-bition of insulin release or hyperglycaemia.

### 3.3 The development and potential of $\alpha_2$-adrenoceptor antagonists for the treatment of NIDDM

As a result of these studies, the development of drugs to block postsynaptic $\alpha_2$-adrenocep-tors on pancreatic $\beta$ cells as well as to block presynaptic $\alpha_2$-autoreceptors on sympathetic nerves to cause an increase in noradrenaline and co-transmitter release have been under-taken as a strategy for increasing insulin release and to achieve possible therapeutic benefit in NIDDM. The agent SL 84-0418 has been reported to enhance the efflux of nora-drenaline induced by stimulation of the sym-pathetic nerves to the pancreas, presumably as a result of blocking presynaptic receptors on the sympathetic nerve terminals[29]. At the same time, SL 84-0418 antagonised the inhi-bition of insulin secretion that would have resulted from activation of $\alpha_{2A}$-adrenoceptors on the pancreatic $\beta$ cells. The net result of this drug was, as predicted, an increase in insulin release produced by noradrenaline's activation of $\beta$-adrenoceptors, or by recep-tors on the pancreatic islets responding to co-transmitters released along with noradrena-line[29]. The mechanism of the increase in insulin release following sympathetic nerve stimulation in the presence of SL 84-0418 is shown in Fig. 17.2. There are nevertheless some complications in this treatment strate-gy. As noted above, it is now known that both noradrenaline and acetylcholine are co-localised with other mediators (co-transmit-ters) in sympathetic and parasympathetic nerves. It has been suggested that noradrena-line is co-localised with galanin in the pan-creas and that galanin also has the ability to inhibit insulin release even in the absence of noradrenaline. Therefore, the ability of sym-pathetic nerve stimulation to alter the secre-tion of insulin will depend not only upon the degree of $\alpha_{2A}$-adrenoceptor blockade but also upon the balance between the action of nor-adrenaline to increase insulin release via $\beta$-adrenoceptors and galanin's action to inhibit insulin release.

Another potential problem is that patients

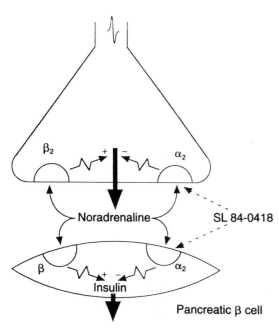

Fig. 17.2. The sympathetic innervation of a β cell of the islets of Langerhans in which insulin is produced. This figure depicts how a selective $\alpha_2$-adrenoceptor antagonist (SL 84-0418) can lead to an increase in the release of noradrenaline and co-transmitter during nerve stimulation by blocking presynaptic release-modulating $\alpha_2$-adrenoceptors[29]. In addition, by blocking postsynaptic $\alpha_2$- adrenoceptors, the activation of which normally inhibits insulin release, there will be an increase in insulin release caused by activation of β-adrenoceptors[29].

with NIDDM are often obese and have elevated blood pressure[19]. If $\alpha_{2A}$-adrenoceptor antagonists were to increase the release of noradrenaline and/or co-transmitters from sympathetic nerves in blood vessels, this could potentially increase blood pressure and cause further complications in these patients. Of course, such a complication could be overcome by developing antagonists that act only on pancreatic β cell $\alpha_{2A}$-adrenoceptors and not on $\alpha_2$-receptors in blood vessels.

# 4 Presynaptic receptors and the aetiology and treatment of essential hypertension

In Chapter 14, the idea was introduced that alterations in presynaptic receptor function may contribute to the pathophysiology of essential hypertension. It was also suggested that drugs which influence presynaptic receptors could be useful therapeutic agents in the treatment of this disease. In this chapter, the role of the sympathetic nervous system in the aetiology of essential hypertension is expanded. Besides presynaptic α- and β-adrenoceptors, other presynaptic receptors, including those for purines, dopamine and peptides, that could potentially be important components in both the development/maintenance or in the treatment of hypertension are discussed.

## 4.1  Role of the sympathetic nervous system in essential hypertension

The mechanism(s) contributing to essential hypertension are still unclear, but it is obvious that it is a multifactorial disease probably involving alterations in the nervous and endocrine systems as well as alterations in vascular smooth muscle function. Although other mechanisms are clearly involved, there is a great deal of evidence from several experimental models, as well as human essential hypertension, which suggests that an increase in sympathetic nerve activity plays a role in the development and maintenance of hypertension. There is experimental evidence for an increase in sympathetic nerve activity and for an increased release of noradrenaline and adrenaline (see ref. 54 for review and references) in the developmental phase and perhaps also in the maintenance phase of elevated blood pressure (see also Chapter 14).

The mechanisms for increased sympathetic nerve activity leading to increased release of noradrenaline (or other co-transmitters) and subsequent increased contraction of vascular smooth muscle has still not been resolved. Throughout this volume there has

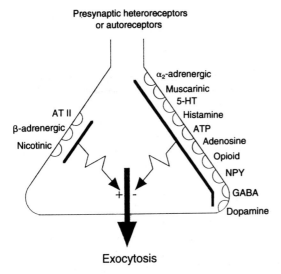

Presynaptic heteroreceptors
or autoreceptors

α₂-adrenergic
Muscarinic
5-HT
Histamine
ATP
Adenosine
Opioid
NPY
GABA
Dopamine

AT II
β-adrenergic
Nicotinic

+  −

Exocytosis

Fig. 17.3. Excitatory and inhibitory autoreceptors and heteroreceptors in a sympathetic nerve terminal at the vascular neuro-effector junction. Three types of excitatory receptors are known to exist, namely β-adrenoceptors, angiotensin II and cholinergic, nicotinic receptors. Activation of each of these receptors leads to increased release of sympathetic neurotransmitter during nerve stimulation. The figure also shows a large number of receptors that, when activated, lead to inhibition of transmitter release during nerve stimulation.

been discussion of autoreceptor and heteroreceptor regulation of noradrenaline release. Figure 17.3 summarises the many presynaptic receptors that have been experimentally demonstrated to increase or decrease the release of sympathetic neurotransmitters.

As discussed earlier in this chapter, a decrease in the activity of inhibitory modulators or an increase in the activity of facilitatory modulators could theoretically result in an increase in the nerve-induced release of noradrenaline or its co-transmitters and a subsequent increase in the contraction or tone of blood vessels. Although examination of all of these possibilities has not been carried out, there is evidence for changes in the activity of some presynaptic modulators in various experimental hypertension models.

## 4.2 Presynaptic facilitatory receptors in hypertension

### 4.2.1 Presynaptic β-adrenoceptors

The evidence that β-adrenoceptor-mediated augmentation of noradrenergic neurotransmission occurs in blood vessels has been summarised in Chapter 14. Such an action results in an increase in the release of noradrenaline and/or co-transmitters (neuropeptide Y; ATP – see below) and, consequently, an increased contraction of vascular smooth muscle, vasoconstriction and elevated blood pressure. There is a great deal of support for this concept, which has been summarised in recent reviews[7,31,38,54]. It has been demonstrated that increases in circulating adrenaline result in the amine being taken up by sympathetic nerve endings on blood vessels, where it is stored as a co-transmitter and subsequently released upon nerve stimulation. This scenario has been shown to occur in normotensive rats and to cause hypertension. There is an increase in circulating adrenaline and noradrenaline in young SHR, a genetic model in which hypertension develops spontaneously in animals at 6–8 weeks of age. A similar increase in circulating adrenaline and noradrenaline has been observed in young, borderline hypertensive humans. Bilateral adrenal medullectomy of SHR reduced the circulating adrenaline and attenuated the development of hypertension. However, hypertension can be restored by implantation of sustained release forms of adrenaline in these rats. Moreover, the facilitatory effect of β-adrenoceptor agonists on noradrenergic transmission from blood vessels is enhanced in young or developing SHR and β-adrenoceptor antagonists attenuate the development of hypertension in these animal models. Increases in the facilitatory effect of β-adrenoceptor agonists would result in an increase in the nerve stimulation-induced release of noradrenaline and presumably produce vasoconstriction and hypertension. The fact that β-adrenoceptor antagonists prevent the increased release of noradrenaline as well as attenuating the development of hypertension suggests that such a mechanism may play a role in the development of hypertension in these animals. In fact β-adrenoceptor antagonists produced a greater inhibition of the evoked release of noradrenaline from the vascular neuro-effector junction of SHR compared both with WKY rats (a normotensive genetic strain developed at the same time as SHR) and with other normotensive rats.

A role for adrenaline has been suggested by other rat hypertension models. For example, there was an increase in the cardiac adrenaline content in a model of hypertension produced by immobilising rats and placing them in an isolated environment. The increase in cardiac adrenaline was prevented by adrenal medullectomy or by the amine-uptake inhibitor desipramine. The hypertension in this model was also prevented by β-adrenoceptor antagonists or by the destruction of peripheral noradrenergic nerves with 6-hydroxydopamine.

Adrenaline has also been implicated in essential hypertension in humans. For instance, it was mentioned above that there is an increase in circulating adrenaline and noradrenaline in young borderline hypertensive and hypertensive patients (under the ages of 40). Moreover, the β-adrenoceptor agonist isoprenaline produced an increase in plasma noradrenaline. This effect was antagonised by propranolol. The infusion of adrenaline during the cold pressor test or during isometric exercise resulted in elevated levels of noradrenaline and a greater increase in blood pressure than the cold pressor test or isometric test alone. These studies in humans gave results that were consistent with those obtained in the animal models described above.

The role of increased release of noradrenaline caused by activation of presynaptic β-adrenoceptors in adult SHR (animals that have been hypertensive for sometime) is less clear and there are conflicting data. For example, it has been reported that there is an enhancement of the isoprenaline-induced increase in [³H]-noradrenaline release and

pressor response to periarterial nerve stimulation in the perfused mesenteric artery of young SHR compared with WKY rats[23]. In contrast, such enhancement was not observed in the perfused kidney, portal vein, superfused spleen, or renal or mesenteric arteries from adult SHR compared with WKY rats[18,27,55]. Moreover, β-adrenoceptor antagonists failed to inhibit the increment in the evoked release of [³H]-noradrenaline release from the renal artery of adult SHR as compared with WKY rats[37].

Therefore, the data suggest that there is increase in circulating adrenaline as well as an enhancement of β-adrenoceptor-mediated release of noradrenaline in young hypertensive rats and in borderline and young essential hypertensive humans and that such mechanisms may contribute to the development but not the maintenance of hypertension. The effectiveness of β-adrenoceptor antagonists in the treatment of early essential hypertension may be the result of blockade of presynaptic β-adrenoceptors, leading to interruption of the facilitatory loop. It is important to determine whether or not a specific subtype of presynaptic β-adrenoceptor mediates the enhancement of noradrenaline release during nerve stimulation. This characterisation could result in the development of drugs with greater specificity for these presynaptic β-adrenoceptors and would constitute an exciting potential therapeutic intervention for the prevention or treatment of essential hypertension.

### 4.2.2 Angiotensin II receptors

It is well established that angiotensin II acts at pre- and postsynaptic sites to enhance tissue responses to both sympathetic nerve stimulation and exogenous agonists[44,46] (see also Chapter 7). In addition to being a potent vasoconstrictor, angiotensin II is known to have a facilitatory effect on sympathetic neurotransmission by acting on presynaptic receptors in sympathetic neurones[44,46,59]. Data exist which demonstrate that there is an increase in the facilitatory effect of

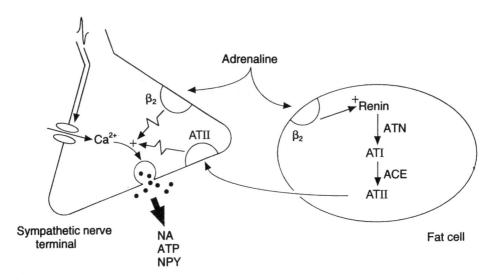

Fig. 17.4. Facilitation of sympathetic neurotransmitter release by β-adrenoceptor or angiotensin II receptor activation. Angiotensin II receptors and β-adrenoceptors may be located on sympathetic nerve terminals. In addition, β-adrenoceptors may be present on other cell types, such as fat cells, in which, following activation, there is an increase in the synthesis and release of angiotensin II. This can stimulate receptors on the sympathetic terminal thus leading to increased release of neurotransmitter during nerve stimulation.

angiotensin II on the nerve stimulation-induced release of noradrenaline from blood vessels of the SHR[22,55,57]. Recently, it has been demonstrated that each of the components necessary for the synthesis of angiotensin II (e.g. angiotensinogen; angiotensin converting enzyme, etc.) are present locally in many cell types found in and around blood vessels[16,39,41]. Moreover, the release of angiotensin II from blood vessels has been demonstrated[39,41] and there is evidence for a β-adrenoceptor-mediated enhancement of angiotensin II synthesis and release from blood vessels[24,54]. This mechanism could contribute to the β-adreno-ceptor-mediated enhancement of noradrenaline release seen in control rats, which is increased in the SHR.

The interaction between β-adrenoceptors and the angiotensin II pathway has led to the hypothesis that activation of β-adrenoceptors in blood vessels leads to the formation and/or release of angiotensin II. This released angiotensin II activates receptors on sympathetic neurones leading to enhanced noradrenaline release. Fig. 17.4 depicts this pos-sibility schematically. In this scheme, β-adrenoceptors are located on fat cells within blood vessels, where both angiotensinogen mRNA and angiotensin converting enzyme have been found. In the presence of renin, taken up from the circulation, activation of β-adrenoceptors stimulates the synthesis cascade, resulting in the formation of angiotensin II, which leaves the fat cells and activates receptors on sympathetic neurones. Interruptions of this local angiotensin II synthesis by inhibitors of angiotensin converting enzyme (such as enalapril) would prevent the angiotensin II-mediated enhancement of noradrenaline release. This could explain the therapeutic usefulness of these drugs as anti-hypertensives.

Another potential site for therapeutic intervention within this pathway would be the development of specific antagonists for the presynaptic angiotensin II receptor, but, as is the case for other autocoids, hormones and neurotransmitters, subtypes of angiotensin II receptor are known to exist. If presynaptic angiotensin II receptors are a distinct subtype, then development of selective antagonists would form the basis for a viable therapeutic strategy.

## 4.3 Presynaptic inhibitory receptors in hypertension

### 4.3.1 Presynaptic α-adrenoceptors

As has been mentioned in other chapters, $\alpha_2$-adrenoceptor-mediated inhibition of the evoked release of noradrenaline is thought to be the major physiologically relevant negative feedback mechanism that modulates sympathetic neurotransmission. Several groups have investigated the possibility that alterations in the operation of $\alpha_2$-adrenoceptor-mediated inhibition of noradrenaline may occur in hypertensive animals, but there is little evidence that this is the case in humans. In contrast to the situation that appears to occur with β-adrenoceptors and angiotensin II receptors in young or prehypertensive animals, there is little evidence that indicates an altered responsiveness of $\alpha_2$-adrenoceptors in young SHR. For example, the enhancement of noradrenaline release by the $\alpha_2$-adrenoceptor antagonist yohimbine in the portal vein or caudal artery was similar in young SHR and in the normotensive WKY rat[47,54,55]. On the other hand, yohimbine produced less enhancement of evoked noradrenaline release from blood vessels of adult SHR compared with WKY rats, suggesting a decrease in the functional activity of presynaptic $\alpha_2$-adrenoceptors in the hypertensive animal[47,54,55]. In contrast, yohimbine was found to produce the same degree of enhancement of evoked release of noradrenaline in two other animal models of hypertension (the 'one clip–one kidney' renal hypertensive rat and the 'DOCA-salt' hypertensive rat) as in their respective sham controls[49]. The 'one clip–one kidney' renal hypertensive model is produced by removing one kidney and placing a clip that reduces blood flow to the other kidney. It produces hypertension in 1 to 3 weeks caused by activation of the renin–angiotensin II system and

expansion of extracellular volume. The 'DOCA-salt' model involves removing one kidney and feeding the rats desoxycorticosterone plus sodium chloride. Hypertension is produced in 1 to 3 weeks as the result of salt retention and volume expansion. The results obtained from the experiments using these model systems suggest that alterations in presynaptic $\alpha_2$-adrenoceptors do not contribute to the development of hypertension but may participate in the maintenance of hypertension in older animals. The data further suggest that a decrease in presynaptic $\alpha_2$-adrenoceptor function and a reduction in inhibition of neurotransmitter release may play a role in the maintenance of hypertension in the SHR but not in the other animal models. It is unclear whether a specific subtype of $\alpha_2$-adrenoceptor is involved.

There is now considerable evidence for subclassification of α-adrenoceptors based on the results of molecular cloning experiments as well as from biochemical and pharmacological studies[8,36]. For example, it is now known that there are $\alpha_{1A}$- and $\alpha_{1B}$-adrenoceptors as well as $\alpha_{2A}$- and $\alpha_{2B}$-adrenoceptors. Subtypes provide the possibility that more selective drugs can be developed (as for the treatment of NIDDM above). As more understanding of the type of $\alpha_2$-adrenoceptor that modulates neurotransmitter release is gained, selective drugs will no doubt be developed and a re-examination of the role of $\alpha_2$-adrenoceptors in hypertension will be undertaken.

### 4.3.2 Purine receptors

Sympathetic neurotransmission is decreased by purine compounds, such as adenosine and ATP, which act on receptors located on sympathetic nerve terminals (Chapter 6). ATP has been shown to be a co-transmitter with noradrenaline and neuropeptide Y in sympathetic nerves innervating blood vessels (Chapter 2) and, together with adenosine, can also be released from vascular smooth muscle and endothelial cells (Chapter 7). It is possible, therefore, that both ATP and adenosine are normal modulators of substances released from sympathetic nerves[40,54]. It has been observed that both ATP and adenosine inhibit the neurogenic vasoconstriction of the perfused mesenteric vascular bed resulting from perivascular nerve stimulation in a dose-dependent manner in WKY rat. In a similar preparation, isolated from 17–21-week-old SHR, the inhibitory effects of both adenosine and ATP were significantly smaller than in the WKY rat[21]. In other experiments, with the same experimental preparation, adenosine was found to decrease the efflux of $[^3H]$-noradrenaline caused by sympathetic nerve stimulation[28]. The inhibition was smaller in both pre-hypertensive (5-weeks-old) and hypertensive (15–18-weeks-old) SHR compared with age-matched WKY rats. A decrease in the adenosine effect was not seen in Wistar rats made hypertensive by left renal artery occlusion. Studies carried out with the perfused kidney or portal vein are at variance with observations made with the mesenteric vascular bed[17,56]. In these studies, it was observed that adenosine was equally effective in the SHR and WKY rats in causing inhibition of the stimulation-induced release of noradrenaline.

As with other receptors, there are subtypes of both ATP and adenosine receptor. Regardless of whether or not there are alterations in the function of presynaptic ATP or adenosine receptors in hypertension, drugs selective for these presynaptic receptors may have some usefulness in the treatment of hypertensive disease. However, there is little information currently available concerning the investigation of such agents in human hypertension trials.

### 4.3.3 Neuropeptide Y receptors

Neuropeptide Y is a peptide of 36 amino acid residues (see ref. 14 for review and references) known to be co-localised with noradrenaline in some sympathetic nerves. Perivascular nerves innervating blood vessels are particularly rich in NPY. NPY is now accepted to be a co-transmitter/co-modulator since it is released together with noradrenaline following nerve stimulation and produces both pre- and postsynaptic effects. Currently, there are three NPY receptor subtypes described ($Y_1$, $Y_2$ and $Y_3$), based on differences in ligand binding and pharmacological activity of a variety of agonists. NPY inhibits the evoked release of noradrenaline by acting presynaptically on the $Y_2$ subtype[33,48,50,53]. There is evidence that NPY can inhibit its own release. Postsynaptically, NPY causes direct contraction of some blood vessels and potentiates the contractile effect of a wide variety of vasoactive agents, such as α-adrenoceptor agonists, angiotensin II, vasopressin, histamine, $K^+$ and ATP[33,50,53]. It is thought that the principal, although not exclusive, postjunctional receptor is the $Y_1$ subtype.

The pre- and postsynaptic effects of NPY in the perfused mesenteric arterial bed of 8-week-old SHR and normotensive controls has been studied. The presynaptic neurotransmitter release-inhibiting effect of NPY was attenuated in SHR compared with WKY rats (Fig. 17.5). In contrast, the ability of NPY to potentiate nerve-induced or agonist-induced increases in perfusion pressure (i.e. postsynaptic effects) was enhanced (Fig. 17.6)[51,52]. These results implicate NPY in the pathophysiology of hypertension development and/or maintenance in SHR. The net effect of the reduction in the inhibitory effect of NPY on noradrenaline release and the enhanced contractile effects on vascular smooth muscle would be a greater increase in blood pressure.

NPY is also able to alter blood pressure by acting at other sites in the neural axis to regulate vascular tone. In the spinal cord, NPY has been shown to decrease blood pressure by decreasing sympathetic outflow; in the posterior hypothalamic nucleus, NPY increases blood pressure by stimulating centrally mediated sympathetic outflow. It is unclear if these effects of NPY are at pre- or postsynaptic sites, or both. It is of great interest that the depressor effect following the intrathecal injection of NPY was attenuated

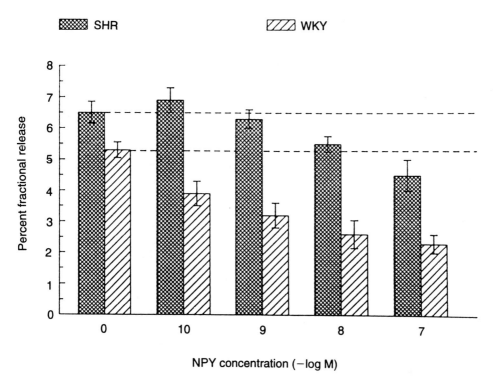

Fig. 17.5. The effect of NPY on periarterial nerve stimulation-induced release of endogenous noradrenaline from the perfused mesenteric arterial bed of 8–10-week-old SHR and WKY rats. Data are plotted as the percentage fractional release of noradrenaline versus NPY concentration. Each bar shows the mean ± SEM of 5–7 preparations. NPY produced significantly less inhibition of evoked release of noradrenaline in SHR. (From ref. 52, with permission.)

in SHR but not in WKY rats, while the pres sor response to microinjections of NPY into the posterior hypothalamic nucleus was enhanced[32,52]. These results strengthen the proposed role for NPY in the development/maintenance of hypertension.

It is clear that NPY agonists and antagonists when developed would be potential therapeutic agents in the treatment of essential hypertension. The development of nonpeptide agonists or antagonists is in its infancy and such a discussion would be speculative; it is certainly beyond the scope of the present chapter. However, because of the wide variety of actions produced by NPY there are numerous potential therapeutic targets for such drugs.

### 4.3.4  Dopamine receptors

It is known that, in addition to acting on presynaptic $\alpha_2$-adrenoceptors (at which it is less effective than noradrenaline), dopamine acts on specific receptors on sympathetic nerve endings that, upon activation, inhibit the release of noradrenaline[58]. Some experimental data suggest that the dopamine receptors do not generally participate in negative feedback control of noradrenaline release, although such modulation may occur in specific tissues[58]. The dopamine receptor that inhibits noradrenaline release is different from that mediating vascular relaxation, and the two types of receptor have been classified as $DA_1$ (vascular relaxation) and $DA_2$

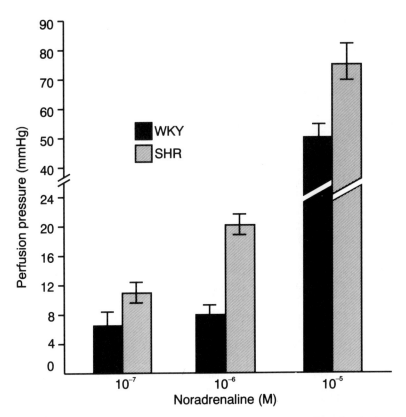

Fig. 17.6. The effect of NPY (100 nM) in potentiating the response to noradrenaline in the perfused mesenteric arterial bed of 8–10-week-old SHR and WKY rats. Data are plotted as the mean increase in perfusion pressure ± SEM caused by increasing concentrations of noradrenaline (0.1–10 μM). NPY produced significantly greater increases in perfusion pressure in the mesenteric arterial bed of the SHR versus WKY rats with all three concentrations of noradrenaline. (From ref. 52, with permission.)

(inhibition of sympathetic neurotransmission)[58]. This terminology is similar but not identical to the original classification of central dopamine receptors $D_1$ and $D_2$. The presence of the $DA_2$ receptors on sympathetic nerves seems to be tissue and species dependent, in contrast to the ubiquitousness of the presynaptic $\alpha_2$-adrenoceptor. Note that $DA_2$ receptors have also been found in sympathetic ganglia[58]. Even in those situations where it is thought that peripheral dopamine might play a physiological role, the source of the dopamine is unclear. In autonomic ganglia, dopamine has been found in small intensely fluorescent (SIF) cells as well as in interneu-

rones. There is some evidence for dopaminergic innervation in the kidney (see below) and dopamine may be synthesised in non-neuronal tissue.

In addition to dopamine receptors located on sympathetic nerves, there are $DA_2$ receptors that inhibit neurotransmission in peripheral dopamine neurones, such as those in the kidney[5,6]. Although the physiological role of peripheral dopaminergic neurones in general is still unclear, in the kidney there is convincing evidence that dopamine stimulates natriuresis. Notwithstanding the above comments, $DA_2$ receptor agonists have been demonstrated to lower blood pressure in conscious and anaesthetised animals, but the site of action of the agonists is uncertain. There are data suggesting that these effects may arise from activation of presynaptic $DA_2$ receptors on noradrenergic terminals or inhibitory receptors on autonomic ganglia or, alternatively, within the CNS[58]. Unfortunately, most of the agents that act on $DA_2$ receptors also activate dopamine receptors present in the chemoreceptor trigger zone located in the area postrema in the lower brain stem. Activation of these receptors leads to emesis (vomiting). Despite this problem, the development of tissue-specific dopamine agonists with specificity for $DA_2$ receptors on sympathetic nerves in blood vessels is at least a theoretically feasible approach for the development of drugs for the treatment of essential hypertension. However, given that there are many other ways to lower blood pressure, and taking into account the potential side effects of peripherally acting dopamine agonists, it is perhaps unlikely that this would be a very productive approach to the treatment of hypertension.

### 4.3.5 Other presynaptic receptors

Although stimulation of a variety of other receptors can decrease noradrenergic neurotransmission (Fig. 17.3), such as 5-HT, muscarinic–cholinergic, prostaglandin $E_2$, prostacyclin, etc., there is little evidence that they play a role physiologically. Furthermore, there is little convincing evidence that there are alterations in the function of any of these receptors in hypertensive disease and, therefore, little to suggest that they contribute to the development or maintenance of hypertension in experimental hypertensive animal models or human essential hypertension[56]. Nevertheless, activation of these receptors clearly leads to a decrease in noradrenergic transmission. Therefore, development of drugs selective for these presynaptic receptors and free of side effects still remains as a possible therapeutic target for the treatment of hypertension.

## 5   Summary

In this chapter, only a few for the many possibilities for the manipulation of presynaptic receptors as a beneficial therapeutic intervention in disease states have been discussed. Content was limited to the treatment of schizophrenia, non-insulin-dependent diabetes mellitus and essential hypertension, for which conditions considerable experimental data have been accumulated. However, it is now known that practically every central and peripheral neurone contains presynaptic autoreceptors and heteroreceptors that can modulate, in an excitatory or inhibitory way, the release of the transmitter. It is clear that increases or decreases in neurotransmitter release may contribute to the pathophysiology of various diseases. Therefore, development of selective agents that can activate or antagonise these presynaptic receptors would appear to be a beneficial therapeutic strategy. Successful application of this strategy has been discussed in this chapter, but there are numerous additional possibilities, and these would indicate a useful direction for future research.

Another useful direction would be to consider further the role of co-transmitters, since it is now quite clear that most, if not all, neurones contain more than one mediator. Research to date has concentrated on the classical or primary neurotransmitters, yet functional neurotransmission may be maintained by the co-transmitter in the absence of the primary or classical transmitter. The development of drugs that act as agonists or antagonists at receptors targeted by these co-transmitters offers an additional way to influence neurotransmission in normal and pathophysiological situations.

Another area for future research is to gain a better understanding of putative neurotransmitters, such as nitric oxide and carbon monoxide, which do not behave like classical transmitters in that they are not synthesised, stored in vesicles or released by exocytosis. In contrast, they are synthesised on demand and diffuse out of neurones by non-exocytocic processes. Nitric oxide has been suggested to be a neurotransmitter in the enteric nervous system, the vasculature and CNS. Carbon monoxide is also thought to be a neurotransmitter in the CNS. In addition to being thought of as neurotransmitters, they are known to produce neurotoxicity and cell death. The discovery of these two mediators has changed our thinking of neurotransmitters. It is not known if the production and release of either mediator is regulated by presynaptic receptors, although both the synthesis and postsynaptic actions can be altered by various agents. A better understanding of the physiological and pathophysiological role of mediators such as these and their pharmacological manipulation is an additional important area for future research.

# References

1. Ahren B, Taborsky GJ Jr and Porte D Jr (1986) Neuropeptidergic versus cholinergic and adrenergic regulation of islet hormone secretion. *Diabetologia* **29:** 827–836
2. Angel I, Bidet S and Langer SZ (1988) Pharmacological characterization of the hyperglycemia induced by alpha$_2$ adrenoceptor agonists. *Journal of Pharmacology and Experimental Therapeutics* **246:** 1098–1103
3. Angel I and Langer SZ (1988) Adrenergic induced hyperglycemia in anesthetized rats: involvement of peripheral alpha2 adrenoceptors. *European Journal of Pharmacology* **154:** 191–196
4. Angel I, Niddam R and Langer SZ (1990) Involvement of alpha2 adrenergic receptor subtypes in hyperglycemia. *Journal of Pharmacology and Experimental Theraputics* **254:** 877–882
5. Bell C (1988) Dopaminergic vasomotor nerves. In: Burnstock G and Griffith SG (eds), *Nonadrenergic Innervation of Blood Vessels*, vol 1: *Putative Neurotransmitters*, pp 41–64, CRC Press, Boca Raton, FL
6. Bell C (1991) Peripheral dopaminergic nerves. In: Bell C (ed), *Novel Peripheral Neurotransmitters. International Encyclopedia of Pharmacology and Therapeutics,* pp 135–160, Pergamon Press, Oxford
7. Borkowski KR (1990) Presynaptic receptors in hypertension. *Annals of the New York Academy of Sciences* **604:** 389–397
8. Bylund DB (1988) Subtypes of α$_2$ adrenoceptors: pharmacological and molecular biological evidence converge. *Trends in Pharmacological Sciences* **9:** 356–361
9. Carlsson A (1975) Receptor-mediated control of dopamine metabolism. In: Usdin E and Bunney WE (eds), *Pre and Postsynaptic Receptors*, pp 49–65, Marcel Dekker, New York
10. Carlsson A (1977) Presynaptic dopaminergic autoreceptor as targets for drugs. In: Langer SZ, Galzin AM and Custentin J (eds), *Presynaptic Receptors and Neuronal Transporters*, pp 43–46, Pergamon Press, Oxford
11. Chiodo LA and Bunney BS (1983) Typical and atypical neuroleptics: differential effects of chronic administration of the activity of A9 and A10 mid brain dopaminergic neurons. *Journal of Neuroscience* **3:** 1607–1619
12. Civelli O, Bunzow JR and Grandy DK (1993) Molecular diversity of the dopamine receptors. *Annual Reviews of Pharmacology and Toxicology* **32:** 281–307
13. Clark DO, Hjorth S and Carlsson A (1985) Dopamine receptor agonists: mechanisms underlying autoreceptor selectivity, II: theoretical considerations. *Journal of Neural Transmission* **62:** 171–207
14. Colmers WF and Wahlestedt C (eds) (1993) *The Biology of Neuropeptide Y and Related Peptides*, pp 1–564, Humana Press, Totwa, NJ
15. Dunning BE, Ahren B, Veith RC and Taborsky GJ (1988) Noradrenergic sympathetic neural influences on basal pancreatic hormone secretion. *American Journal of Physiology* **255:** E785–E792
16. Dzau VJ (1984) Vascular renin-angiotensin: a possible autocrine or paracrine system in control of vascular function. *Journal of Cardiovascular Pharmacology* **6:** S377–S382
17. Ekas RD, Steenberg ML and Lokhandwala MJ (1983) Increased norepinephrine release during sympathetic nerve stimulation and its inhibition by adenosine in the isolated perfused kidney of spontaneously hypertensive rats. *Clinical and Experimental Hypertension* **A5:** 41–48
18. Ekas RD, Steenberg MC, Woods MS and Lokhandwala MF (1983) Presynaptic α and β adrenoceptor stimulation of norepinephrine

release in the spontaneously hypertensive rat. *Hypertension* **5**: 198–204

19. Epstein M and Sowers JR (1992) Diabetes mellitus and hypertension. *Hypertension* **19**: 403–418

20. Garvey WT (1989) Insulin resistance and non-insulin dependent diabetes mellitus: which horse is pulling the cart? *Diabetes and Metabolism Reviews* **5**: 727–742

21. Kamikawa Y, Cline WH Jr and Su C (1990) Diminished purinergic modulation of the vascular adrenergic neurotransmission in the spontaneously hypertensive rat. *European Journal of Pharmcology* **66**: 342–353

22. Kawasaki H, Cline WH Jr and Su C (1982) Enhanced angiotensin mediated facilitation of adrenergic neurotransmission in spontaneously hypertensive rats. *Journal of Pharmacology and Experimental Therapeutics* **221**: 112–116

23. Kawasaki H, Cline WH Jr and Su C (1982) Enhanced presynaptic beta adrenoceptor mediated modulation of vascular adrenergic neurotransmission in spontaneously hypertensive rats. *Journal of Pharmacology and Experimental Therapeutics* **223**: 721–728

24. Kawasaki H, Cline WH and Su CJ (1984) Involvement of the vascular renin–angiotensin system in beta adrenergic receptor-mediated facilitation of vascular neurotransmission in spontaneously hypertensive rats. *Journal of Pharmacology and Experimental Therapeutics* **231**: 23–32

25. Kebabian JW and Calne DB (1979) Multiple receptors for dopamine. *Nature* **277**: 93–96

26. Kolterman OG, Gray RS, Griffin J et al. (1981) Receptor and postreceptor defects contribute to the insulin resistance in non-insulin dependent diabetes mellitus. *Journal of Clinical Investigation* **68**: 957–699

27. Kubo T, Kuwahara M and Misu Y (1984) Effect of isoproterenol on vascular adrenergic neurotransmission in prehypertensive and hypertensive spontaneously hypertensive rats. *Japanese Journal of Pharmacology* **36**: 419–421

28. Kubo T and Su C (1983) Effects of adenosine on $^3$H-norepinephrine release from perfused mesenteric arteries of SHR and renal hypertensive rats. *European Journal of Pharmacology* **87**: 349–352

29. Langer SZ, Angel I, Schoemaker H et al. (1992) Pharmacological interventions at the level of presynaptic receptors. *Proceedings of the 7th International Catecholamine Symposium*, p 178

30. Lorrain J, Angel I, Duval N, Eon MT, Oblin A and Langer SZ (1992) Adrenergic and nonadrenergic cotransmitters inhibit insulin secretion during sympathetic stimulation in dogs. *American Journal of Physiology* **263**: E72–E78

31. Majewski H and Rand MJ (1986) A possible role of epinephrine in the development of hypertension. *Medical Research Reviews* **6**: 467–486

32. McAuley MA, Chen X and Westfall TC (1993) Central cardiovascular action of neuropeptide Y. In: Colmers WF and Wahlestedt C (eds), *The Biology of Neuropeptide Y and Related Peptides*, pp 399–418, Humana Press. Totowa, NJ

33. McAuley MA and Westfall TC (1992) Possible location and function of neuropeptide Y receptor subtypes in the rat mesenteric arterial bed. *Journal of Pharmacoogy and Experimental Therapy* **261**: 863–868

34. Meltzer HY (1990) Presynaptic receptors: relevance to psychotropic drug action in man. *Annals of the New York Academy of Sciences* **604**: 353–371

35. Meltzer HY and Stahl SM (1976) The dopamine hypothesis of schizophrenia. *Schizophrenia Bulletin* **2**: 19–26

36. Minneman KP (1988) $\alpha_1$-Adrenergic receptor subtypes, inositol phosphates and sources of cell $Ca^{2+}$. *Pharmacological Reviews* **40**: 87–119

37. Misu Y, Kuawahara M and Kubo T (1987) Some relevance of presynaptic β-adrenoceptors to development of hypertension in spontaneously hypertensive rats. *Archives Internationale de Pharmacodynamie* **287**: 299–308

38. Misu Y and Kubo T (1991) Presynaptic β-adrenoceptors in the peripheral sympathetic nervous system and hypertension. In: Feigenbaum J and Hanani M ( eds), *Presynaptic Regulation of Neurotransmitter Release: A Handbook*, vol II, pp 1147–1174, Freund Publishing

39. Mizumo K, Nakamaru M, Higashimohi K and Inagami T (1988) Local generation and release of angiotensin II in peripheral vascular tissue. *Hypertension* **11**: 223–229

40. Moylan RD and Westfall TC (1979) Effect of adenosine on adrenergic neurotransmission in the superfused rat portal vein. *Blood Vessels* **16**: 302–310

41. Nakamaru M, Jackson EK and Inagami T (1986) β-Adrenoceptor-mediated release of

angiotensin II from mesenteric arteries. *American Journal of Physiology* **250:** H144–H148

42. Niddam R, Angel I, Bidet S and Langer SZ (1990) Pharmacological characterization of alpha 2 adrenergic receptor subtype involved in the release of insulin from isolated rat pancreatic islets. *Journal of Pharmacology and Experimental Therapeutics* **254:** 883–887

43. Roy MW, Lee KC, Jones MS and Miller RE (1984) Neural control of pancreatic insulin and somatostatin secretion. *Endocrinology* **115:** 770–775

44. Story DF and Ziogas J (1987) Interaction of angiotensin with noradrenergic neuroeffector transmission. *Trends in Pharmacological Sciences* **8:** 269–271

45. Svensson K, Johansson AM, Magnusson T and Carlsson A (1986) (+)-AJ 76 and (+)-UH232: central stimulants acting as preferential dopamine autoreceptor antagonists. *Naunyn-Schmiedeberg's Archives of Pharmacology* **334:** 234–245

46. Westfall TC (1977) Local regulation of adrenergic neurotransmission. *Physiological Reviews* **57:** 659–728

47. Westfall TC, Badino L, Naes L and Meldrum MJ (1987) Alterations in the field stimulation-induced release of endogenous norepinephrine from the coccygeal artery of spontaneously hypertensive and Wistar-Kyoto rats. *European Journal of Pharmacology* **135:** 433–437

48. Westfall TC, Carpentier S, Chen X, Beinfeld MC, Naes L and Meldrum MJ (1987) Prejunctional and postjunctional effects of neuropeptide Y at the noradrenergic neuroeffector junction of the perfused mesenteric arterial bed of the rat. *Journal of Cardiovascular Pharmacology* **10:** 716–722

49. Westfall TC, Carpentier S, Naes L and Meldrum MJ (1986) Comparison of norepinephrine release in hypertensive rats II caudal artery and portal vein. *Clinical and Experimental Hypertension* **A8:** 221–237

50. Westfall TC, Chen X, Ciarleglio A *et al.* (1990) *In vitro* effects of neuropeptide Y at the vascular neuroeffector junction. *Annals of the New York Academy of Sciences* **611:** 145–155

51. Westfall TC, Han SP, Chen X *et al.* (1990) Presynaptic peptide receptors and hypertension. *Annals of the New York Academy of Sciences* **604:** 372–388

52. Westfall TC, Han SP, Knuepfer M *et al.* (1990) Neuropeptides in hypertension: role of neuropeptide Y and calcitonin gene related peptide. *British Journal of Clinical Pharmacology* **30:** 75S–82S

53. Westfall TC, Martin JM, Chen X *et al.* (1988) Cardiovascular effects and modulation of noradrenergic neurotransmission following central and peripheral administration of neuropeptide Y. *Synapse* **2:** 299–307

54. Westfall TC and Meldrum MJ (1985) Alterations in the release of norepinephrine at the vascular neuroeffector junction in hypertension. *Annual Reviews of Pharmacology* **25:** 621–641

55. Westfall TC, Meldrum MJ, Badino L and Earnhardt JT (1984) Noradrenergic transmission in the isolated portal vein of the spontaneously hypertensive rat. *Hypertension* **6:** 267–274

56. Westfall TC, Qualy JM, Meldrum MJ, Zhang S-Q, Carpentier S and Naes L (1987) Central and peripheral alterations in noradrenergic transmission in experimental hypertension: modulation by prejunctional receptors. *Journal of Cardiovascular Pharmacology* **10:** 562–567

57. Westfall TC, Xue C-S, Meldrum MJ and Badino L (1985) Effect of low sodium diet on the facilitatory effect of angiotensin on $^3$H-norepinephrine release in the rat portal vein. *Blood Vessels* **22:** 13–24

58. Wiffert B and de Jonge A (1991) Inhibitory prejunctional dopamine receptors on sympathetic nerves In: Feigenbaum J and Hanani M (eds), *Presynaptic Regulation of Neurotransmitter Release: A Handbook*, pp 1071–1083, Freund Publishing

59. Zimmerman BG (1978) Actions of angiotensin on adrenergic nerve endings. *Federation Proceedings* **37:** 199–202

# Index

References in **bold** denote illustrations.

347